Cases in
Health Services
Management

Cases in Health Services Management

FOURTH EDITION

edited by

Jonathon S. Rakich, Ph.D.
Indiana University Southeast

Beaufort B. Longest, Jr., Ph.D., FACHE
University of Pittsburgh

Kurt Darr, J.D., Sc.D., FACHE
The George Washington University

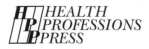

HEALTH PROFESSIONS PRESS

Baltimore • London • Winnipeg • Sydney

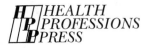
*HEALTH
PROFESSIONS
PRESS*

Health Professions Press, Inc.
Post Office Box 10624
Baltimore, MD 21285-0624

www.healthpropress.com

Typeset by Auburn Associates, Inc., Baltimore, Maryland.
Manufactured in the United States of America by
Victor Graphics, Baltimore, Maryland.

This casebook can be used alone or in conjunction with other texts. To help instructors use the cases most effectively in the classroom, the editors have prepared an instructor's guide, *Instructor's Manual for Cases in Health Services Management*, available on CD-ROM from Health Professions Press (see website and address above or call 1-888-337-8808 or 1-410-337-9585). *Cases in Health Services Management* can also be used in conjunction with the editors' textbook, *Managing Health Services Organizations and Systems*, also published by Health Professions Press.

The cases presented in this volume are based on the case authors' field research in a specific organization or are composite cases based on experiences with several organizations. In most instances, the names of organizations and individuals and identifying details have been changed. Cases are intended to stimulate discussion and analysis and are not meant to reflect positively or negatively on actual persons or organizations.

Library of Congress Cataloging in Publication Data

Cases in health services management / edited by Jonathon S. Rakich, Beaufort B. Longest, Jr., Kurt Darr.—4th ed.
    p. cm.
    Includes bibliographical references.
    ISBN 1-878812-89-0
    1. Health services administration—United States—Case studies. 2. Health facilities—United States—Administration—Case studies. 3. Hospitals—United States—Administration—Case studies. I. Rakich, Jonathon S. II. Longest, Beaufort B. Jr. III. Darr, Kurt.

    [DNLM: 1. Hospital Administration—United States. 2. Organizational Case Studies—United States. 3. Total Quality Management—United States. WX 150 C338 2004]
    RA971.C34 2004
    362.1'0973—dc22
                                                 2003060584

British Library Cataloguing in Publication data are available from the British Library.

To managers willing to share the lessons
of their experience with the next generation

Contents

PART I   STRATEGIC MANAGEMENT

Jonathon S. Rakich and Alan S. Wong

Organization life cycle of a 96-bed hospital is traced from inception by community leaders, facility decline and sale to a for-profit system, and regeneration with the city's acquisition and change to not-for-profit status. CEO reflects on strategies that returned MCSI to profitability and ponders future strategic alternatives.

Anthony R. Kovner

General acute care, not-for-profit 400-bed hospital in economically depressed section of city struggles with rising costs and deteriorating quality of care; two major issues are the need for investment in facilities and technology and continuing support for six off-site clinics partially funded by the city.

William E. Aaronson

Not-for-profit church-affiliated continuing care retirement community seeks help with long-range planning; consultant encounters resistance to change, questionable financial management practices, and lack of business acumen in the board of directors.

Confident that the board would support him in a contract dispute with hospital-based radiologists seeking to build a competing off-site imaging center, he is surprised to have been fired. He underestimated the power of the medical staff and the four physician board members.

Kent V. Rondeau and Jonathon S. Rakich

Vice president of nursing services at a 285-bed for-profit hospital determines what action to take regarding items in her in-basket, including correspondence, phone messages, and interruptions ranging from an angry physician, to a wandering patient, staff shortages, and increasing OR infections.

Kurt Darr

Management of a community hospital is unwilling to recognize and address the major problems in its radiology department, which is being directed by a radiologist whose preoccupation with income, stock market speculation, and disruptive behavior has greatly diminished the quality of radiograph interpretations with tragic results.

Kent V. Rondeau

CEO of Westmount has difficulty overcoming barriers and pitfalls in implementing TQM in a chain of seven nursing homes. The embroilment of the TQM initiative in negotiations with the union representing nurses threatens the initiative's future.

William Q. Judge and Curtis P. McLaughlin

Responsible for building and maintaining a network of providers and overseeing quality in the southeast region of a national insurance and HMO company, the medical director is "constantly putting out unexpected fires" that detract from addressing strategic issues.

patients. Unchecked, the practice will create a large deficit for the community hospital. Turning these patients away will create a double bind of serious public relations problems for the hospital.

About the Editors

Jonathon S. Rakich, Ph.D., Professor of Management, School of Business, Indiana University Southeast, New Albany, Indiana 47150
Dr. Rakich received his master of business administration from the University of Michigan–Ann Arbor and his doctorate from Saint Louis University. His university instructional areas are strategic management and health services administration. During his 36-year teaching career, Dr. Rakich has coauthored 3 books in 12 editions, 40 journal articles (including those in *Health Care Financing Review, Health Care Management Review, Hospital & Health Services Administration, Journal of Health & Society Policy*, and *Hospital Topics*), and more than 35 conference proceedings and professional papers.

Professor Rakich has been awarded a postdoctoral federal faculty fellowship with the U.S. Department of Health and Human Services and has served on the board of trustees of a home health agency and health systems agency. During academic sabbaticals, he served an administrative residency at Summa Health System and conducted on-site research of the Canadian health care system.

Professor Rakich is a member of the Academy of Management, the Association for Health Services Research, and the Decision Sciences Institute. He holds personal membership in the Association of University Programs in Health Administration and is a faculty affiliate of the American College of Healthcare Executives.

Professor Rakich is Distinguished Professor Emeritus of Management and Health Services Administration at the University of Akron, where he taught from 1972 to 1999. During that period he held administrative positions as Director of Graduate Programs in Business, Director of Executive Development Programs, and Coordinator of the MBA-Health Services Administration option program.

Beaufort B. Longest, Jr., Ph.D., FACHE, M. Allen Pond Professor and Director, Health Policy Institute, Graduate School of Public Health, University of Pittsburgh, Pittsburgh, Pennsylvania 15261
Dr. Longest's primary faculty appointment is in the Department of Health Policy and Management in the University of Pittsburgh's Graduate School of Public Health. He holds a secondary appointment as Professor of Business Administration in the Katz Graduate School of Business.

He received an undergraduate education at Davidson College and received a master of health administration and a doctorate from Georgia

State University. Professor Longest is a fellow of the American College of Healthcare Executives and holds memberships in the Academy of Management, AcademyHealth, American Public Health Association, and the Association for Public Policy Analysis and Management. He has the unusual distinction of having been elected to membership in the Beta Gamma Sigma Honor Society in Business as well as in the Delta Omega Honor Society in Public Health.

His research on issues of health policy and management has generated substantial grant support and has led to the publication of numerous peer-reviewed articles. In addition, he has authored or co-authored 9 books and 26 chapters in other books. His book *Health Policymaking in the United States* (Health Administration Press, 2002) is among the most widely used textbooks in graduate health policy programs.

He consults with health care organizations and systems, universities, associations, and government agencies on health policy and management issues.

Kurt Darr, J.D., Sc.D., FACHE, Professor of Hospital Administration, Department of Health Services Management and Leadership, School of Public Health and Health Services, The George Washington University Medical Center, Washington, D.C. 20037
Dr. Darr holds a doctor of science from The Johns Hopkins University and a master of hospital administration and a juris doctor from the University of Minnesota.

Professor Darr completed his administrative residency at Rochester (Minnesota) Methodist Hospital and subsequently worked as an administrative associate at the Mayo Clinic. After being commissioned in the U.S. Navy, he served in administrative and educational assignments at St. Albans Naval Hospital and Bethesda Naval Hospital. He completed his postdoctoral fellowships with the Department of Health and Human Services, the World Health Organization, and the Accrediting Commission on Education for Health Services Administration.

Professor Darr is a fellow of the American College of Healthcare Executives, is a member of the District of Columbia and Minnesota State Bar Associations, serves as an arbitrator and mediator for the American Health Lawyers Association, and is a mediator for the Superior Court of the District of Columbia.

He regularly presents seminars on health services ethics, hospital organization and management, quality improvement, and the application of the Deming method in health services. Professor Darr is the author and editor of books used in graduate health services administration programs and numerous articles on health services topics.

Professors Longest, Rakich, and Darr are co-authors of the textbook, *Managing Health Services Organizations and Systems, Fourth Edition* (2000), published by Health Professions Press. The editors have collaborated in writing this and other texts for more than 25 years.

Contributors

William E. Aaronson, Ph.D.
Associate Professor of Healthcare
  Management
Temple University
409 Ritter Annex (006-00)
1810 North 13th Street
Philadelphia, PA 19122

Mark D. Applebaum
(see co-contributor Elizabeth M.
  A. Grasby)

Bryan Boliard, M.B.A.
Sykes College of Business
University of Tampa
401 West Kennedy Boulevard
Tampa, FL 33606

Carol Anne Brothers
(see co-contributor Murray J.
  Bryant)

Murray J. Bryant, Ph.D.
Associate Professor, Director—
  MBA Programs
Richard Ivey School of Business
The University of Western
  Ontario
1151 Richmond Street North
London, Ontario N6A 3K7
CANADA

Joseph F. Castellano, Ph.D.
Professor of Accounting
School of Business Administration
University of Dayton
300 College Park
Dayton, OH 45469

George S. Cooley, M.B.A.
President
Long Green Associates, Inc.
Post Office Box 15
Long Green, MD 21092

Kathryn H. Dansky, Ph.D.
Associate Professor of Health
  Policy and Administration
Department of Health Policy and
  Administration
The Pennsylvania State
  University
114-H Henderson Building
University Park, PA 16802

Kurt Darr, J.D., Sc.D.
Professor
Department of Health Services
  Management and Leadership
School of Public Health and
  Health Services
The George Washington
  University
2175 K Street, N.W., Suite 700
Washington, D.C. 20037

Bonnie Eng-Suess, M.H.A.
Contract and IPA Specialist
Central Health MSO, Inc.
1051 Parkview Drive, Suite 220
Covina, CA 91723

Bruce D. Evans, M.B.A.
Professor of Management
Graduate School of Management
University of Dallas
Braniff Building, Room 260
1845 East Northgate
Irving, TX 75062

Elizabeth M.A. Grasby, Ph.D.
Richard Ivey School of Business
The University of Western
    Ontario
1151 Richmond Street North
London, Ontario N6A 3K7
CANADA

Raymond L. Hilgert, D.B.A.
Professor Emeritus
John M. Olin School of Business
Washington University
    in St. Louis
St. Louis, MO 63130

Donna Lind Infeld, Ph.D.
Professor of Public
    Administration and of Health
    Services Management and
    Leadership
Department of Public
    Administration
The George Washington
    University
2175 K Street, N.W.
Washington, D.C. 20037

**Mike Jasperson, M.B.A.,
M.S.H.A.**
Sykes College of Business
University of Tampa
401 West Kennedy Boulevard
Tampa, FL 33606

**Richard L. Johnson, FACHE,
FAAHC, M.B.A.**
Executive Vice President
Physician Management
    Resources, Inc.
Post Office Box 188
Clarendon Hills, IL 60514

William Q. Judge, Ph.D.
Professor of Management and
    Director of Senior Executive
    MBA Program
University of Tennessee
411 Stokely Management Center
916 Volunteer Boulevard
Knoxville, TN 37996

Anthony R. Kovner, Ph.D.
Professor of Public and Health
    Management
Robert F. Wagner Graduate
    School of Public Service
New York University
40 West 4th Street
600 Tisch Hall
New York, NY 10003

Edwin C. Leonard, Jr., Ph.D.
Professor of Management
Department of Management and
    Marketing
School of Business and
    Management Sciences
Indiana University–Purdue
    University Fort Wayne
Fort Wayne, IN 46805

Cynthia Levin, M.H.S.A.
Kaiser Permanente

Cyril C. Ling, D.B.A.
Professor Emeritus
Illinois Wesleyan University
1312 Park Street
Bloomington, IL 61701

Curtis P. McLaughlin, D.B.A.
Professor Emeritus of Health
    Policy and Administration
Kenan-Flagler School of Business
University of North
    Carolina–Chapel Hill
Chapel Hill, NC 27599

Dorothy J. Moon

Robert C. Myrtle, D.P.A.
Professor of Health Services
  Administration and
  Gerontology
School of Policy, Planning, and
  Development
University of Southern California
Lewis Hall 312
Los Angeles, CA 90089

Randi Priluck, Ph.D.
Assistant Professor of Marketing
Lubin School of Business
Pace University
One Pace Plaza W482
New York, NY 10038

Jonathon S. Rakich, Ph.D.
Professor of Management
School of Business
Indiana University Southeast
4201 Grant Line Road
New Albany, IN 47150

Harper A. Roehm, Ph.D.,
  C.P.A.
Professor Emeritus of Managerial
  Accounting
School of Business Administration
University of Dayton
300 College Park
Dayton, OH 45469

Michael F. Rolph, M.B.A.,
  C.P.A.
Senior Vice President and Chief
  Financial Officer
First Health of the Carolinas
Post Office Box 3000
Pinehurst, NC 28374

Kent V. Rondeau, Ph.D.
Assistant Professor
Department of Public Health
  Sciences
Faculty of Medicine and
  Dentistry
University of Alberta
13-103 Clinical Sciences Building
Edmonton, Alberta T6G 2G3
CANADA

Kimberly A. Rucker, M.H.S.A.
Health Care Consultant
Washington, D.C.

Earl Simendinger, Ph.D.
Professor of Management
Sykes College of Business
University of Tampa
Campus Box 148F
401 West Kennedy Boulevard
Tampa, FL 33606

William E. Stratton, Ph.D.
Professor of Management
College of Business
Idaho State University
Campus Box 8020
Pocatello, ID 83209

Cara Thomason, M.H.A.,
  M.S.G.
Dementia Care Coordinator
Park Terrace Senior Living
21952 Buena Suerte
Rancho Santa Margarita, CA
  92688

Rosalie Wachsmuth, M.H.A.,
  M.S.G.
Program Manager
Aging and Disability Services
  Administration
9315 58th Avenue Court S.W.
  #R-204
Lakewood, WA 98499

Mary Anne Watson, Ph.D.
Associate Professor of
  Management
Sykes College of Business
University of Tampa
Campus Box 122F
401 West Kennedy Boulevard
Tampa, FL 33606

Gary R. Wells, Ph.D.
Professor of Finance
College of Business
Idaho State University
Campus Box 8020
Pocatello, ID 83209

Michael Wiltfong

Alan S. Wong, Ph.D.
Professor of Finance
School of Business
Indiana University Southeast
4201 Grant Line Road
New Albany, IN 47150

Preface

Like its predecessors, the fourth edition of *Cases in Health Services Management* describes management issues and problems in a variety of settings. The cases included were selected and grouped into four parts in order to provide a comprehensive set of health services management cases in one volume. The primary criterion was that each case be rich in applied lessons. Selection was tempered by the editors' 90 years of combined experience in teaching with the case method.

This edition reflects the dramatic shifts that have occurred in how and where health services are delivered. Of the 28 cases, more than half (16) are new. Classic cases that have stood the test of time have been retained in this edition. Almost half of the cases feature nonhospital settings, including long-term care facilities, an HMO, several health networks, a continuing care retirement community, an emergency department, relocation of a hospital burn unit, a pharmaceutical company's distribution of a new AIDS drug, a city health department, and a home health agency. Two of the new cases are set within the Canadian health care system.

The range of acute care hospitals includes a variety of sizes; types; ownerships; and geographic locations, including rural and inner-city hospitals. There is also a case set in a multi-institutional system. The principles and applications of continuous quality improvement are reflected in another case. An in-basket exercise simulates the time pressures and the importance of prioritizing that may confront managers. Vignettes in administrative and clinical ethics sensitize and educate readers about ethical issues that managers face.

Depending on depth of analysis and the amount of time available for out-of-class preparation, most cases can be addressed adequately in 1 or 2 class hours. A few of the cases are short and present single issues. Most, however, are integrative and complex, and involve multiple problems and issues. Analyses will require applying several discrete disciplines and knowledge areas. Users must synthesize and apply knowledge, skills, and experience gleaned from social-behavioral sciences; administrative and clinical ethics; individual, social, and environmental determinants of health; management and administration (e.g., strategic planning and policy formulation, marketing, organizational and administrative relationships, problem solving, resource allocation and utilization, control, financial management, human resources management); and health services organization, financing, and delivery.

The primary audience for this book is students in programs educating health services managers. Cases are especially effective in integrating the curriculum, and many students will use this book in a capstone course. Case analysis bridges theory and practice. In this regard, new and experienced managers will find the cases informative as they hone analytical and problem-solving skills. These cases are also useful in continuing professional development seminars for practicing managers. (A broad definition of *managers* is appropriate here because department heads and mid- and senior-level managers perform similar generic activities).

By their nature, cases present events, situations, problems, and issues. It is the dynamics of the analysis, especially group discussion, that make the case method such a powerful and rich learning tool. Therefore, users are urged to review the introductory material that describes the case method and case analysis.

The cases included in this volume are intended to stimulate class discussion and analysis. In most instances, the names of organizations and individuals are disguised. The authors of these cases have prepared well-written factual situations based on field research in a specific organization or a composite case based on experience with several organizations. None of these cases is meant to reflect positively or negatively on actual persons or organizations or to depict either effective or ineffective handling of administrative situations.

The 28 cases are grouped into four parts:

Part I: Strategic Management (six cases)
Part II: Administration, Medical Staff, and Governing Body (eight cases)
Part III: Resource Utilization and Control (seven cases)
Part IV: Human Resource Management and Organizational Dynamics (seven cases)

The table of contents includes a synopsis of each case, which identifies the organizational setting and predominant themes and issues.

As experiential learning in health services management education has given way to more discipline-based didactic education and as younger, less experienced students have entered graduate programs, cases that apply didactic work have become more important. No case study can replace experience, but this collection, combined with a solid academic grounding in health services and management disciplines, will greatly aid in preparing students for situations they are certain to encounter as health services managers.

The core task in teaching others to manage effectively in the health services field is to provide them with the insight to identify and define problems and the judgment to apply the skills and methods needed to solve them. With instructor or seminar leader guidance, cases such as the ones in this volume are an important means to that end.

To assist in the task of teaching by the case method, students and teachers may find the editors' textbook *Managing Health Service Organizations and Systems*, published by Health Professions Press, a useful supplement. It can provide a solid grounding in the health care system and many of the managerial topics applicable to issues presented in the cases.

To assist instructors, the editors have compiled an Instructor's Manual, available on CD-ROM from Health Professions Press, to accompany *Cases in Health Services Management*. It contains teaching notes for each case that have been prepared by the case authors. It is available to instructors who adopt the casebook.

Acknowledgments

The editors wish to acknowledge the generous contribution of the authors whose cases are included in this book. They are listed alphabetically beginning on page xix. We thank them for granting permission to use their cases. Thanks also to the book and journal publishers who allowed us to reprint the cases to which they hold the copyright. We are indebted to the staff of Health Professions Press for their help in producing the book; specifically Mary Magnus, director of publications; Tim Dunn, book production editor; and Lisa Rapisarda, production manager. Special appreciation is given to those at our respective universities who assisted us: Susanna Bauder, Linda Kalcevic and Denise Warfield, and Sarah Palmer. Finally, we thank our respective deans and chairpersons for providing the organizational environment that made this work possible.

Introduction

The case method has played an important role in the study of law, medicine, and business for many years. It now is well established as a useful educational technique in health administration programs as well. The cases in this book have been selected specifically for use in such programs because they describe problems and situations that have been faced by managers in the past and provide useful learning opportunities for tomorrow's managers. The cases were selected because their use will permit the following:

- Assistance to students to develop assessment, analytical, and conceptual skills necessary for effective problem solving and decision making

- Support of students in their efforts to synthesize and integrate theory and application

- Encouragement of dynamic and interactive discussion among students that challenges their experience and values

- Acquisition of knowledge and insights by students in a short period of time that would otherwise be gained much more slowly

Traditional didactic education provides background and foundation in disciplines and methodologies relevant to health services management. For many students, management fellowships, residencies, and other field experiences supplement didactic learning with experience. Case study blends both didactic and experience-based learning, enhancing both in the process.

This introduction 1) briefly describes the various types of case, 2) lists some of the benefits of the case method, 3) discusses the roles of instructors and students in properly using cases, and 4) suggests a case analysis procedure.

TYPES OF CASES

Cases are situation-specific descriptions of issues and problems that students can identify and evaluate from a managerial perspective. Because they are based on events that have already occurred, cases are descriptions of the past. Although set in the past, the cases in this book deal with contemporary situations, issues, and problems that managers will confront again in the future. Thus, cases have the capacity to impart valuable lessons and insights relatively unfettered by temporal change. Individuals can apply lessons learned in the study of cases throughout their professional careers. Skills in using evaluative and analytical processes are of enduring usefulness to managers.

Some of the cases are comprehensive and integrative, involving a variety of areas and a range of issues and problems affecting entire organizations. Others are more narrowly focused. All of the cases, however, permit students to do the following:

- Operationally define the issue(s) or problem(s) involved

- Separate important from unimportant considerations

- Winnow through quantities of information to determine which facts are pertinent and make reasonable assumptions when information is absent

- Apply appropriate disciplines and methodologies

- Identify with managers in the cases (or, in some instances, adopt the role of outside consultants) when considering alternatives, offering recommendations, and designing implementation plans for solving problems

BENEFITS OF THE CASE METHOD

Use of the case method provides a number of benefits for students. Perhaps none is more important than students having the opportunity to develop and sharpen their analytical and thought processes. The essence of case analysis is assessment and problem solving. Thus, cases enable students to hone their skills in situation assessment, problem diagnosis and definition, alternative solution evaluation and selection, and development of workable plans to implement solutions. Other supportive skills and insights are developed as well. Because students must articulate and defend their recommendations, logic and communication skills are enhanced.

The case method also permits students to synthesize and integrate knowledge. Compartmentalized subject areas and underlying disciplines such as organizational behavior, accounting, economics, marketing, finance, and law must be linked, blended, and applied in a holistic way in case analysis. Cases also permit students to apply theory to realistic situations. Case study provides an opportunity to practice being a manager. It puts the students at the scene of the events depicted in the case and provides the opportunity to apply theory. Case study exposes students to many different organizational settings and managerial problems and often provides a vehicle for the introduction and discussion of corollary subject matter pertinent to the case but not included in it.

Finally, cases provide a good opportunity for students to practice their interactions in groups. The case method is applied in group forums. In either a structured or unstructured fashion, all participants discuss the case, offer their views, and critique those of others. The free flow of facts, opinions, perceptions, and values results in productive student learning, including learning how to be a more effective participant in groups.

ROLES OF INSTRUCTORS AND STUDENTS

In using the case method, instructors depart from their familiar role of lecturer, becoming discussion leaders and facilitators. The instructor's task in the case method is to encourage students to think independently and to formulate and defend their decisions. The burden of learning is on the students. Learning will take place in the case method only if the students use the opportunity provided by analysis and discussion to sharpen their skills.

This does not mean that instructors are unimportant. They contribute in a number of ways: selecting cases and the order in which they are assigned; providing a classroom environment that permits students to gain maximum benefit from the case analysis and interactive discussions; and giving directions to class discussion—expanding or contracting it, or changing the direction and focus when appropriate. To do this effectively, a thorough familiarity with the case is essential. Instructors may also define and address collateral issues and focus the discussion by posing key questions about the cases. Following the discussion, the instructor may provide comments about the class discussion, the analytical process, elements ignored or over- or underemphasized, and the quality of recommendations. Such critiques improve the ability of students to use the case analysis method properly.

Although instructors differ in the evaluation of student performance in the case method, most use a combination of the following criteria:

- Mastery of background information provided in the case (and, in some instances, not provided but acquired by the student from other sources) and the use of that information

- Application of discipline and analytical methodologies

- Soundness of assumptions and logic

- Thoroughness in identifying problems and issues and the clarity and precision with which they are articulated

- Consistency and compatibility of analysis and recommendations

- Quality of alternative solutions to the problems identified and the comprehensiveness of decision criteria by which alternative solutions are judged

- Plans for implementing and evaluating results

- Degree to which recommendations and implementation plans are reasonable and relevant to the issue(s) involved; whether they consider pertinent forces, internal and external to the organization; and whether they are feasible

Pedagogically, instructors may choose a structured or unstructured approach to case study. In the latter approach, the instructor assigns a case. Students read and prepare to discuss the case in class. The instructor initiates discussion by asking open-ended questions to the class in general, or of specific students: What issues are involved? What variables should be considered? What information is important, unimportant? If you were a manager what would you do? Why? How would you implement your recommendation(s)?

More structured approaches to case study might require each student to prepare a written report using a specific format or outline. To initiate discussion of a case, the instructor chooses one person to present his or her case analysis. Alternatively, the instructor assigns the case to groups of three or four students. Together, the students in each group prepare a written case analysis. Then a group can be asked to present its analysis to the class as a means of initiating the discussion. In either approach, general discussion follows.

The pedagogical technique chosen by the instructor will be influenced by several factors, including the instructor's preference; class size and length of the class period; academic mix and previous experience of students, their familiarity with the case method, and their grounding in underlying disciplines. Over time, the approach may vary from structured to unstructured depending on learning objectives, the degree to which the instructor introduces corollary subject matter by lecturing or through controlled and directed discussion, and the progress students make in adapting to the case analysis method.

Whichever approach is used, two attributes of case study surprise some students. First, case writers cannot possibly describe all of the relevant information and circumstances of a particular situation in a case. In this sense, cases are always incomplete. Thus, students must make reasonable and justifiable assumptions, reaching decisions based on available information. This is the usual situation that confronts managers.

Second, by design, cases generally do not have right or wrong answers. It is this attribute that makes case study so dynamic, interesting, integrating, and powerful. Initially, students may feel frustrated because there are no correct answers to the problems or issues in a case. Increased experience with case study will show them that small differences in situation assessment, assumptions, or problem definition can lead to very different conclusions and recommendations, all of which may be argued.

The role of students in case study is demanding. They bear the responsibility of learning. For many, the most challenging and sometimes anxiety-laden aspect is presenting their views in the classroom, where peers and the instructor question their analyses and recommendations. If class discussion is to be productive, students must prepare extensively before class, and they must be active participants in discussions. Effective participation means contributing substance, not merely talking or rehashing points already made.

CASE ANALYSIS APPROACH

There are several suitable case analysis models, and instructors typically have developed their own. Most, however, require students to identify with the organization or setting described in the case, assume the perspective of the manager(s) involved, and apply a systematic analytical approach.

Typically, students begin their analysis by assessing the information in the case and organizing it by category. Appropriate categories may include organizational objectives, expectations about organizational performance held by internal and external stakeholders, past and present results of operations, internal organizational strengths and weaknesses, external influences such as regulations or the actions of competitors, and other relevant factors. For some cases, each category may be important in the assessment. For others, only selected categories are important. Regardless, the initial task is to gather and group information into a meaningful form. Once done, attention can be turned to identifying the problems and issues in the case.

The case may have one issue or problem or many, which can be explicit or implicit. Properly identifying the issue or problem is crucial to the case analysis. It can be a difficult task, but the skill is developed and facilitated through experience with case analysis. Success in the task depends on a thorough and effective assessment of the information base. Care must be taken to distinguish symptoms and root causes of problems or issues. Some cases have exhibits that contain pertinent data and information, and these should be thoroughly assessed—to the point of performing calculations—so that they may be fully used in understanding the case situation and the problems and issues embedded in it.

The next step in the case analysis is the formulation of alternatives that might solve the problem(s) or suitably address the issue(s). As in problem/issue identification, information base assessment continues to be important. Particularly useful is information that delimits or distinguishes obvious infeasible alternatives from those that can be considered further. Facility expansion, for example, may be infeasible if assessment of the current financial situation indicates capital funds are unavailable or the organization's market area will not sustain the growth. Quantitative and financial analytical methods should be used to compare alternatives whenever these techniques are appropriate.

Once a set of feasible solutions has been developed, the analyst can turn to evaluating alternatives and recommending a course of action. Evaluating alternative solutions requires applied decision criteria that judge relative merit and suitability in solving a problem or addressing an issue. Appropriate questions to guide the choice include

- Which alternative provides the greatest benefits?

- What are the relative costs of alternatives?

- How consistent are the alternatives with organizational philosophy, culture, and objectives?

- Are internal capabilities to implement alternatives equal?

- Will external influences constrain or support implementation of the alternatives differentially?

Using the answers to these and other questions, solutions to the problem(s) or issue(s) in the case are selected.

Once the alternatives have been chosen, implementation plans are designed. These should include evaluation of the results of implementation. How will we know if the problems are solved or the issues addressed? In some cases, the primary focus may be on implementation, and much greater detail about implementation plans is required. In others, evaluating alternative solutions and choosing one is primary focus. In these cases, implementation may be addressed more generally. Regardless of the case emphasis, attention must be given to implementation and to the evaluation of the implemented solutions. This makes the case analysis experience more realistic, which is, after all, the central reason for using the case analysis method.

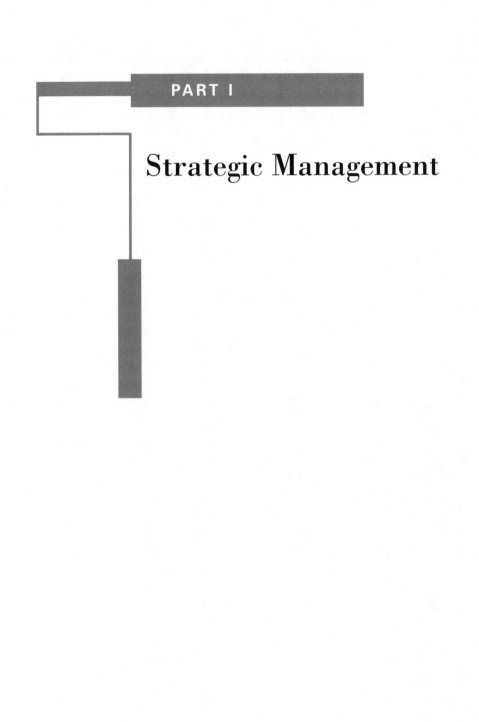

PART I

Strategic Management

Medical Center of Southern Indiana

Community Commitment and Organization Revival

Jonathon S. Rakich

Alan S. Wong

Indiana University Southeast, New Albany, Indiana

At the signing of the Declaration of Independence, it is reported that Benjamin Franklin told John Hancock, "We must indeed all hang together, or, most assuredly we shall hang separately." The words of our Founding Fathers were indeed noble. They were, however, more than mere words; they reflected a deep and abiding commitment to creating something unprecedented. It was their collective spirit, their devotion to a common good, that made a revolutionary notion viable.

In an interview with the case writers, Kevin Miller, the current President and CEO of the Medical Center of Southern Indiana (MCSI) (www.mcsin.org), reflected on the results of the hospital's performance for the

Used by permission of the authors. Copyright © 2004 by Jonathon S. Rakich and Alan S. Wong.

Note to the reader: Historical portions of this case are largely based on local newspaper accounts and internal hospital documents. These sources are cited throughout. To enhance readability, there is liberal use of accounts' wording absent quotation notation. Observations and statements attributed to persons identified in the case carry quotation notation.

year ending 1998. He stated, "We feel very much the same about our hospital that the nation's Founding Fathers did. Of course, our revolutionary notion—to build, and preserve a hospital dedicated to enhancing the quality of life of the community—pales before that of creating a new nation. However, our local founding fathers, that is, our tight-knit community has fought over the years to plan, build, and sustain our hospital, and, more critically, has fought to keep it open when all odds pointed to its closure just a few years ago. Through the commitment of business leaders, local government, physicians, hospital employees, and citizens, our hospital forged a new beginning when the community purchased it in 1991, weathered the 'critical care' years through 1997, and accomplished the turnaround with a 1998 operating profit of $480,545, our largest ever."[1]

Miller further observed, "It was that irrepressible will that carried our hospital and community through the toughest of times. This unconquerable spirit forms the foundation of the partnership—between the hospital and its constituents, between its physicians and management—that has brought our hospital back from the brink of extinction to a position of unparalleled growth and unmatched station in a growing, forward-looking community."[2]

When asked, "What's new?" at the MCSI, the answer is "plenty." As reported in the June 25, 1993, issue of the *Evening News*, "There's a new owner, new management, a renewed commitment to the community, new services, a new look and, of course a new name! The facility was formerly known as North Clark Community Hospital."[3] Miller observed, "It is evident that the strategy of investing over $3.0 million between 1992 and 1998 in new equipment, new services, and expanded operations finally paid off. The MCSI was built, suffered setbacks, recovered, and made an impressive comeback, and now has a promising future."

In 1998, MCSI had a bed complement of 96 beds, 270 full-time equivalent (FTE) employees, and $22.6 million in net patient revenues, with an operating profit of $480,545. It had achieved its highest ever number of patient days (15,915), outpatient surgeries (883), and primary care clinic visits (11,314). Its occupancy rate was 45.4%.[4]

HISTORY

The Dream

The building of a hospital in the City of Charlestown, Indiana, was the dream of many community members, especially Eli Goodman, a local physician, and John K. Bowen, the city's mayor then. From its inception in 1973, the hospital was known as North Clark Community Hospital

(NCCH). Its name was changed in late 1991 to the Medical Center of Southern Indiana when the facility was purchased by the City of Charlestown. Initial plans for a 120-bed acute-care hospital plus a 118-bed extended care facility were announced by Mayor Bowen in July of 1973.[5] Events that precipitated this ambitious project were the desire by community members and local physicians to have their own hospital; the donation of a 21-acre site by a local citizen, Mrs. Sylvester Greissel; and a decision by Clark Memorial Hospital, the county's only other acute-care hospital, not to oppose the building of the facility. On September 17, 1973, the board of Clark Memorial Hospital, a 232-bed, county-owned, acute-care hospital indicated that it would not seek to expand satellite services to the northern portion of the county, nor would it lodge an objection with the area's comprehensive planning agency—the Southeast Indiana Comprehensive Planning Council—to the building of a new facility in the northern part of the county, in which the City of Charlestown is located.[6]

In September 1973, the non-profit Charlestown North Clark Community Corporation (CNCCC) was formed to operate the planned hospital. William L. Voskuhl, M.D., was elected chair and Mayor John K. Bowen as vice chair of the board of trustees. Initial consideration was given to having the hospital built by the Denver Corporation, with financing by a City of Charlestown revenue bond issue. Ownership would revert to the city after the retirement of the bonds in 20–25 years. In the interim, the hospital would be leased by the non-profit CNCCC.[7]

The next 9 months of planning resulted in substantive changes, including scaling back the size of the facility. The CNCCC was reincorporated as the North Clark County Hospital Board (NCCHB) and in July of 1974, a contract was signed with The Planned Systems Technology Company (PlanTech) of Indiana to build the hospital.[8] The agreement with PlanTech included a 2.5% development fee and a 1-year management contract. In January, the North Clark Community Hospital Board entered into an agreement with the John Nuveen Company of Chicago to sell $8.1 million in tax-free revenue bonds for the building of a 96-bed, acute-care hospital. Finally, the dream of so many community members had become a reality. Ground breaking occurred in July of 1975. North Clark Community Hospital opened its doors in September 1976. Among the 200 individuals attending the ceremony were Dr. William L. Voskuhl, Mayor John K. Bowen, and Col. Harlan Sanders, the founder of Kentucky Fried Chicken.[9]

The Struggle

As reported in the November 29, 1977, issue of the *Indiana Times*, North Clark Community Hospital ran into troubled times. It had lost money since its opening 14 months before. On an average day, only 40–50 of its 96 beds were filled—62 filled beds were required to meet expenses—and only 5 of the county's 50 physicians used the hospital exclusively. Furthermore, the other large hospital located in the southern part of the county, Clark Memorial Hospital, announced a planned expansion of an additional 26 beds to its existing complement of 232 beds.

The combination of losses, low census, and potential increased competition did not bode well for NCCH. The board considered several alternatives, including selling the facility or retaining a professional hospital management company to manage the hospital.[10] The board chose the latter by signing a 3-year contract with the Hospital Corporation of America (HCA) to manage NCCH. At the time, HCA owned or managed 95 hospitals that operated in 25 states. Thomas F. Frist, President of HCA, stated, "This [North Clark Community Hospital] is an excellent hospital with an outstanding medical staff, a fine group of employees and a superior reputation for high quality care. We do not anticipate any major changes in the hospital operating philosophy . . . except to incorporate the systems and procedures which we have developed and used effectively throughout our own [HCA] hospital network."[11]

The Sale

North Clark Community Hospital's struggle for survival continued during the next 6 years until its sale to HCA for $15 million in March 1985. Benefits of being part of HCA were access to purchasing systems, physician recruitment, capital, and other resources of HCA. At the time, HCA owned 4 hospitals in Southern Indiana and it owned or managed more than 400 hospitals nationwide.[12] At the time of purchase, HCA was pursuing a strategy of horizontal and vertical integration.

The Spin-Off

Restructuring by HCA in mid-1987 through an Employee Stock Ownership Plan (ESOP) resulted in the creation of HealthTrust. This company, owned principally by employees with minority interest by HCA, was formed by the spin-off of 100 HCA hospitals, including North Clark Community Hospital.[13] Based in Nashville, HealthTrust hospitals had aggregate revenues of $1.5 billion. With continued poor financial performance, however, HealthTrust indicated in May of 1991 that North Clark Community Hospital would be divested, that is, either sold or closed. The reasons for this action were declining census caused by encroachment of larger Louisville, Kentucky, hospitals into NCCH's service area, outmigration of patients traveling to larger city facilities, the impact of managed care contracting by Indiana businesses with Kentucky insurers, the economic climate, and Medicare cutbacks.[14] The stark reality was that in Fiscal Year 1991 (ending August 31), the 96-bed North Clark Community Hospital had an average occupancy of 15.6 patients per day and a net loss of $1,743,000.[15]

Beginning the Turnaround

As in the past, the community rallied around its hospital. With citizen and hospital employee support, the City of Charlestown purchased NCCH from HealthTrust for $2 million on December 31, 1991. The hospital was renamed the Medical Center of Southern Indiana, was leased to a newly formed non-profit company, Charlestown Hospital Inc., and managed by American MedTrust of Atlanta.[16] A new chapter in the hospital's history had begun.

MEDICAL CENTER OF SOUTHERN INDIANA

The Setting

Clark County, Indiana, is predominately rural. It covers 369 square miles of the southern portion of the state with its southernmost border on the Ohio River, separating it from Kentucky. The city of Louisville is the closest large metropolitan area, with a population of approximately 300,000.[17] Clark County is one of seven counties in the Louisville Standard Metropolitan Statistical Area with a population of 1 million, and, consequently, its proximity to Louisville results in patient outmigration to the large number of medical facilities in the city. In 1998, Clark County's population was 93,805, having increased approximately 9% since 1990.[18] The employed labor force was 50,000 with a low unemployment rate of just 2.7%.[19] Nearly 75% of Clark County's residents live in rural areas. The county's largest cities are Jeffersonville with a population of 27,000; Clarksville with a population just over 20,000; along with Sellersburg and Charlestown with populations of 6,000 each.[20] In 1997, county household income was $36,726, ranking 49th among Indiana's 92 counties.[21] Two institutions of higher education are located in the area. Ivy Tech's Sellersburg campus, which is part of Indiana's 23 regional campus, vocational and associate-degree educational system, enrolled 2,000 students in 1997. Indiana University Southeast, part of the eight-campus Indiana University system, enrolled approximately 6,000 students. Even with these institutions of higher education, only 11% of the county's population has earned a bachelor's degree or higher.[22] Thus, the county is predominately rural, has a Medicare population percentage equal to that in the state as a whole, has a low household income, and has relatively few numbers of individuals who have earned higher education degrees.

In 1998, medical facilities in Clark County included Clark Memorial Hospital, located in Clarksville in the southern portion of the county. It is a full-service, acute-care facility with 285 beds including 52 skilled nursing beds, a 47-bed inpatient psychiatric unit, and an active medical staff of 132 physicians.[23] The second full-service hospital located in the northern part of the county is the Medical Center of Southern Indiana with 96 beds, including 18 skilled nursing beds, and an active medical staff of 75 physicians. Employment at MCSI was 270 full-time equivalents making it the largest employer in the City of Charlestown. Other facilities include Jefferson Hospital—a 100-bed psychiatric and substance abuse facility—and Lifespring Mental Health Services, an outpatient mental health facility located in Jeffersonville.[24] Even though MCSI's primary competitor is Clark Memorial Hospital, substantial numbers of residents seek treatment in Louisville, which is 15 miles from Charlestown.

The 1992–1998 Years

A 1992 article in the *Community Showcase Evening News* (6/23/92) headlined the Medical Center of Southern Indiana as the "Pride of Charlestown." Rebounding from the 1991 fiscal year loss of $1,743,000 and purchase of the hospital by the City of Charlestown from HealthTrust to prevent its closure, Donna Mullins, Director of Human Resources and the hospital's first employee, stated, "We felt small; we were a tax write-off for HealthTrust, and that attitude extended to staff, doctors and patients. It was devastating. Despite the divestiture by HealthTrust, the community that had fought to build the hospital fought even harder to keep it open. The community spirit was overwhelming."[25] The purchase of the hospital by the city, its leasing to a non-profit organization, and the retaining of a for-profit firm, American MedTrust, to manage the hospital was, as indicated by Mullins, "an act of courage on the part of Mayor Bob Braswell and the city. The mayor—a long time supporter of the hospital and a hospital board member—had no hesitation in making the partnership with American MedTrust work."[26]

American MedTrust

American MedTrust (AMT), which took over the management of the Medical Center of Southern Indiana in 1992, is an Atlanta-based for-profit management corporation that specializes in revitalizing community hospitals. It is composed of experienced executives who have a track record of successfully turning around troubled hospitals. The firm's operating philosophy is to ". . . enhance customer satisfaction by integrating the hospital management team, the community, and the medical staff. AMT's core concept is to establish a strong value-based relationship with key constituencies (i.e., physicians, patients and their families, employees, and the community) that are both personal and effective." The revitalization initiatives AMT pursues are as follows:[27]

- Providing a rapid assessment plan based on operating priorities, including initiating new financial and operating systems to control costs immediately

- Increasing revenues by increasing the number of managed care contracts

- Investing in new equipment and renovations to support growth in programs and services

- Developing simple, accurate cost and statistical systems to track patient outcomes and the success of new programs

- Assisting affiliated physicians and group practices manage their practices more effectively

- Forming affiliations with large, integrated delivery systems to expand market reach, provide better access to care, and solidify links with hospital medical staff

Kevin J. Miller, a principal with AMT, became President and CEO of the Medical Center of Southern Indiana in 1994. Prior to accepting that position, he held senior corporate development positions for two major health care systems and had occasionally served as an interim director of hospitals in transition. He holds a master's degree in health services administration and is a Fellow in the American College of Healthcare Executives.[28]

In an interview with the case researchers, Miller indicated that "1992 was a do or die year for the Medical Center of Southern Indiana. The time immediately after the buyout was critical. By laying important groundwork right away, AMT was able to turn an operating profit of $197,499 on net patient revenues of $7,822,046 the first year without any layoffs." He stated further, "Under ownership of HealthTrust, the previous administration backed off on marketing. There were no public relations, no meetings with groups in the community, and no meetings with businesses. Furthermore, with the anticipated closing of the hospital, managed care contracts were not renewed. In this business, managed care contracts are critical for survival."

Health Care Expenditures and Managed Care

Aggregate health care expenditures in the United States were $1,146 billion dollars in 1998, representing 13.0% of Gross Domestic Product (GDP) and $4,093 on a per capita basis. Of aggregate health care expenditures, 54.4% were private and 45.6% were publicly paid by federal, state, and local governments. Medicare, the health insurance program for the elderly and certain individuals with disabilities, accounted for $213.6 billion. Medicaid, a joint federal–state program for indigent individuals, had expenditures of $186.9 billion.

Broken down by sector, the 1998 aggregate health care expenditures for hospital care were $377.1 billion; physician and clinical services were $254.2 billion; nursing home care was $88.0 billion; and home health care was $33.5 billion. Projections for 2003 are aggregate health care expenditures of $1.591 billion, representing 15.2% of GDP and $5,456 per capita.[29]

In 1997, there were 6,097 hospitals of all types in the United States. Of that number, 5,057 were classified as community general hospitals, which are nonfederal and short-term, with an average length of stay of less than 30 days. Twenty-two percent of the community general hospitals had a bed size between 50 and 99 beds. Seventeen percent were sized 25–49 beds and 5.5% had fewer than 25 beds. Correspondingly, there were only 807 (16%) that had more than 300 beds.[30]

During the period from 1980 to 1997, there were a large number of hospital closures. In aggregate, the 1980 base of 5,830 community general hospitals decreased by 13% by 1997 with the largest number of closures occurring in the 50 to 99 bed size. This category, the one in which the Medical Center of Southern Indiana falls, decreased by 24%. The implication is that the health care environment was not sympathetic to smaller hospitals, especially those less than 100 beds. The health care delivery landscape turned more onerous for these institutions. In the mid-1980s, the federal government instituted a fixed-price reimbursement program for paying provider organizations that treated Medicare beneficiaries. The implementation of the prospective pricing system based on diagnosis-related groups replaced the cost-based reimbursement system previously used by the federal government. The implication was that hospitals had to decrease costs. Furthermore, the 1990s witnessed the rise of managed care. The fact that the MCSI survived during this turbulent period is a testament to its strengths and the commitment of the community to the hospital.

Managed care is an insurer's arrangement with physicians, hospitals, and other health care providers to provide a defined set of health care services to plan members for a fixed annual amount or prospectively agreed fees and charges. Managed care plans can take on many forms ranging from health maintenance organizations (HMOs), in which providers receive a fixed capitated amount and enrolled beneficiaries must use plan specified providers, to preferred provider organizations (PPOs), in which beneficiaries' copayments and deductibles are generally less if the plan's approved providers are used; they are higher if providers outside the network are used by patients. In an HMO or PPO managed care plan, a hospital, for example, will negotiate a set fee for its services with the plan. The net effect of managed care plans was to direct its subscribers (i.e., those covered individuals) to hospitals and physicians that had prenegotiated fees, which are quite frequently substantially lower than traditional charges. As Miller previously indicated, a hospital without managed care contracts with insurers is at a distinct disadvantage since potential patients would be directed (as in the case of an HMO) or have a large financial incentive (as in the case of a PPO) to seek services at a participating hospital.[31]

Most of the nation's 269 million people had employer-provided or government-provided health insurance in 1998. Sixteen percent, or 42 million, had no insurance. Of those insured, Medicare covered 30.9 million people and Medicaid covered 24.5 million.[32] Of the estimated 214 million people insured through private insurance programs, mostly through employment, an astounding number were members of managed care programs. HMO enrollment, for example, was 105.3 million people in 1998, having increased from 12.5 million in 1983. PPO enrollment was 98.3 million people, having increased from 28.5 million in 1987.[33]

Rebuilding the MCSI Managed Care Business

"My primary priority when assuming the position of CEO in January 1994 was to increase the number of managed care contracts," said Miller when being interviewed by the case writers. Since HealthTrust planned to close the hospital, it canceled existing contracts. In 1994, the hospital had only two. In 1998 it had 25. Miller indicated that it has taken a great deal of effort to restore relationships with managed care companies. "I pulled out all the stops," he said, "by being sensitive to insurers, earning their respect, and proving to them why it was to their benefit to contract with MCSI. Initially, a lot of plans wouldn't even return my phone calls. Because of our past track record under HealthTrust, many of them wouldn't give me the time of day." Enlisting the support of the local state senator, a bill titled *Any Willing Provider,* was passed by the Indiana legislature in 1995 that required managed care companies to negotiate with providers such as MCSI. With the assistance of that legislation and persuasion from the state insurance commissioner, Miller worked with the legislature to require insurers to present the conditions under which they contract with hospitals, and to give written notice explaining why they declined to sign up with hospitals. This initiative not only helped MCSI but also dozens of other hospitals around the state. "As a policy," Miller indicated, "MCSI will continue to do what is appropriate to keep the trust of managed care insurers." Today, relations with insurers are much improved and the hospital's affiliation with the Norton Health System, a major regional hospital system located in Louisville, is an added boost to MCSI's managed care business. "The alliance provides the acceptance of more insurers, treatment in new areas (including chemotherapy and teleradiology), access to more physicians and, most importantly," Miller said, "it has driven up the hospital's status up with the community, physicians, and managed care plans."[34]

The Mission

The published mission of the Medical Center of Southern Indiana follows: "We at the Medical Center dedicate our lives, our hearts, and resources to enhancing the quality of life in Southern Indiana. The Medical Center's physicians and employees commit to providing excellent medical care, community education and advanced diagnostic and emergency services to the communities of southern Indiana. We will bring together medical technology and compassion to treat each of our patients competently and with dignity."[35]

As outlined in its 1998 strategic plan document, the objectives of the MCSI are to 1) improve the quality of services provided, 2) improve market share in its service area; and 3) improve the hospital's image. Specific initiatives to accomplish these objectives follow:[36]

1. *Increase physician recruitment, retention, and collaboration:* Among the action plans are developing a primary care physician office site and specialty clinic in nearby Scottsburg; expanding and aggressively marketing a physician referral and health information program; aggressively marketing primary care physicians, family practice centers, and specialty clinics through direct mail and print ads; and exploring options for development of two new primary care clinics in the western part of the service area.

2. *Continue managed care contracting:* The action plans include developing North Clark Physicians, Inc. (NCP), by adding new physicians, marketing the medical staff organization services, and matching the hospital's managed care list with the NCP managed care list; pursuing a managed care contract with Humana, a major health insurance company, to facilitate servicing Medicare patients who are members of Humana's Medicare Select program; obtaining managed care contracts for specialty services (i.e., skilled nursing, home health, and behavioral health services); increasing occupational medicine contracts; improving financial and clinical information systems; and investigating and developing a community-based insurance product and/or direct contracting with employers.

3. *Improve existing services and pursue new product/service development and marketing:* Planning activities include increasing utilization of the

emergency department through aggressive marketing; increasing outpatient visits and ancillary services volumes; growing the occupational medicine program by providing on-site services and marketing of hand surgery availability; developing a wound care center; implementing a quality improvement team to examine and improve dietary services, environmental services, antibiotic usage review, and clinical information reports; developing a senior care program and investigating a geriatric assessment center; and continuing to expand the hospital's "quality of caring" program and enhance patient/customer relations.

Other potential service area expansion programs to undergo preliminary feasibility studies are an assisted living center, adult day care, child care (for-profit), migraine headache center, counseling, and a retail pharmacy. In addition, the 1998 strategic plan dealing with improving and expanding services calls for investigating: the possibility of affiliating key products with branded services (i.e., oncology with Sloan-Kettering Cancer Center); the development of disease specific outreach programs such as cancer and diabetes; the development of Women's and Men's services (i.e., gynocology, an alternative birthing center, a urological center); and developing affiliation with the community hospice program and local long-term care facilities. Finally, a major initiative to be considered is a feasibility study of AMT acquiring Charter-Jefferson Hospital and referral of adult psychiatric and geropsychiatric patients to MCSI.

The Organization and Medical Staff

In 1998, the Medical Center of Southern Indiana had 329 employees representing 270 full-time equivalents. Due to community "ownership," both literally and figuratively, turnover among its employees was a low 11%. The hospital's structure is characterized by a lean organization. This is in keeping with AMT's operating policy of controlling costs. Exhibit 1 presents the MCSI organization chart and identifies the hospital's various functions.

The medical staff is composed of 140 individuals, 75 of whom are active. One AMT initiative upon assuming management of the hospital was to rebuild physician-administration relationships. Under HealthTrust, these relationships had deteriorated. As a result, a partnership—independent practice association (IPA)—was formed with 10 primary care physicians. The main objective was to enable these physicians to keep their own practices, yet compete through the IPA for managed care contracts. Furthermore, the IPA offers practice management services to these physicians.[37]

Miller observed, "Over the years we have helped our medical staff expand access to patients. There are three primary care and two specialty clinics located throughout the county and owned by MCSI. Our biggest

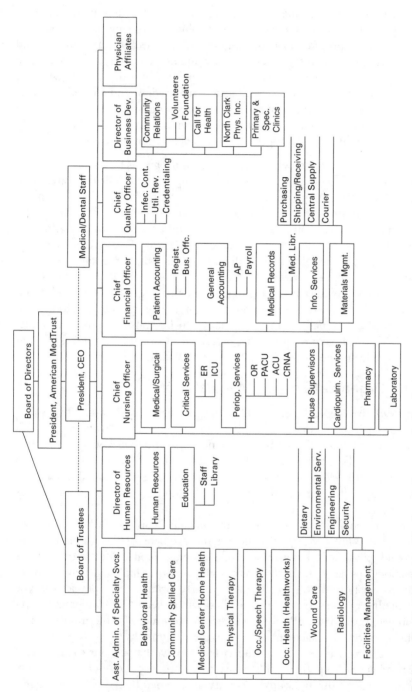

Exhibit 1. The Medical Center of Southern Indiana organization chart.

14

improvement, however, has been involving physicians in issues central to quality and their day-to-day practices. Our attitude is one of cooperation and involvement in major organizational decisions that affect the medical staff." He went on to say, "Just as managed care contracts are critical to the survival of any hospital, so too is medical staff relations. Nothing happens in a hospital until a patient is admitted and a physician orders treatment. Doctors are absolutely critical to our hospital's success. Consequently, we are continuously seeking to have more physicians join our medical staff." To make the point, he referred to the data in Exhibit 2. It shows the hospital's 1998 revenue generated by physicians.

Service Enhancement and Investment

As a full-service hospital, MCSI offers inpatient medical/surgical care, outpatient diagnostic testing and care, 24-hour emergency services, radiology, skilled nursing care, psychiatric care, home health care, laboratory services, occupational medicine, pain management therapy, social services/discharge planning, and specialty clinics. Exhibit 3 presents the full range of services.[38] It is not surprising that the service lines were expanded under the management of American MedTrust. In fact, it is consistent with its operating philosophy to invest in new programs and services and is essential to the hospital fulfilling its mission. CEO Miller indicated that "beyond expanding traditional inpatient and outpatient medical/surgical services, it was critical to respond to the needs of our Medicare patient base through the creation of 3 cost-based programs: a home health agency (1993), a skilled nursing facility (1993) with 24 beds, and a geriatric psychiatry inpatient/outpatient hospitalization program in 1994. These programs have made a significant impact on patient care, meeting community needs, and our bottom line."[39]

Home Health Agency

MCSI's accredited home health agency filled a chronic community need for care outside the hospital. In 1998, more than 15,000 visits were made to patients in a five-county region. Even though visits dropped from 21,000 in 1997 due to government funding cutbacks, the agency enhances continuity of care by providing basic care, psychiatric care, respite care, physical therapy, and homemaker services. In the past 4 years, its gross revenue has grown from about $422,000 to $1.75 million in 1998. Home health and homemaker respite visits totaled 28,700 in 1998.

Skilled Nursing Facility

MCSI's skilled nursing facility also serves a critical need in the larger community, receiving referrals in the region and throughout the metropolitan

Physician	Discharges	Patient Days	O/P Registration	Revenue (in dollars)
1	243	2,313	1,355	$4,667,850
2	199	3,570	207	4,634,015
3	376	2,312	1,786	4,464,752
4	45	260	3,310	3,477,125
5	128	1,028	1,205	2,236,740
6	131	1,770	6	2,084,305
7	220	942	109	1,974,429
8	142	910	594	1.806,472
9	96	596	1,500	1,615,923
10	75	340	2,877	1,369,355
11	33	159	2,645	1,123,274
12	74	527	121	964,095
13	–	–	470	868,175
14	64	441	184	776,929
15	38	153	3,861	760,447
16	4	54	65	443,268
17	18	40	189	342,562
18	17	40	80	336,688
19	5	24	608	324,944
20	21	96	306	303,228
21	5	26	125	298,867
22	–	–	174	242,421
23	10	30	613	235,524
24	3	11	114	210,477
25	19	56	381	189,882
26	1	2	165	148,272
27	–	–	52	134,660
28	4	2	259	133,885
29	–	–	120	132,508
30	1	1	333	128,175
31	4	14	77	120,848
32	1	1	47	108,640
33	3	24	31	101,881
All others	36	172	5,785	2,918,740
Total	2,016	15,914	29,754	$39,679,356

Exhibit 2.   MCSI 1998 physician utilization and gross hospital revenue generated by physician.

Behavioral Health Services (inpatient geropsychiatric unit, outpatient counseling)

Call for Health (physician referral service)

Cardiopulmonary

Community Education

Community Skilled Care (skilled nursing and subacute care unit)

Diabetic Education

Echocardiography/TEE

Electrocardiography (EKG, stress test)

Electroencephalography (EEG)

24-hour Emergency Services

Endoscopy

Home Health Care (nursing, physical therapy, respite/homemaker, mental health, pediatric nursing)

Inpatient/Outpatient Surgical Services (cardiology-pacemaker, ENT, gastroenterology, general surgery, GYN, neurosurgery, orthopedic, plastic/reconstructive, pediatric, thoracic, vascular)

Intensive Care Unit

Laboratory Services

Leatherman Spine Center

Medical-Surgical Unit (pediatric, adult, geriatric)

Nutritional/Dietary Counseling

Occupational Medicine

Occupational Therapy

Orthopedic Options (joint replacement program, sports medicine)

Outpatient Chemotherapy

Outpatient Diagnosis and Treatment Services

Pain Management

Physical Therapy

Podiatry

Pulmonary Function Lab

Radiology (bone densitometry, CT scanning, magnetic resonance imaging, mammography, nuclear medicine, ultrasound)

Respiratory Therapy

Social Services/Disharge Planning

Speakers' Bureau

Specialty Clinic (Charlestown)

Speech Therapy

Urology

Volunteer Services

Wound Care

Exhibit 3. Services offered by MCSI.

area. The 18-bed unit is fully Medicare certified, having received two deficiency-free survey ratings since its opening in March 1994. The program provides extensive care for stroke and postsurgical patients, and has proven an excellent complement to both hospital and community nursing home programs. Its gross revenues increased from $1.07 million in 1994 to $4.7 million, with 262 admissions in 1998 and an average length of stay of 16.8 days.

Geropsychiatric Services

In 1994, an inpatient geropsychiatry partial hospitalization program was implemented. The 17-bed facility is equipped to treat adults over the age of 54 who require 24-hour monitoring. The partial hospitalization program provides intensive, adult day-care services and helps reduce inpatient hospitalization. Gross revenue for behavioral health programs totaled $4.56 million in 1998, based on 337 admissions and an average length of stay of 19.1 days.

Outpatient Mall

In response to the need to provide the most cost-efficient, accessible care possible to the community, an outpatient mall was created in the hospital. Nearly $300,000 was spent to remodel and equip 4,000 square feet of storage space and to open the mall in the fall of 1995. The multi-departmental facility provides the one-stop outpatient shop that patients need, and enhances radiology, physical therapy, cardiopulmonary and laboratory services. One room in the center doubles as a daytime room for partial psychiatric therapy and as a nighttime public education facility.

Capital Expenditures and Improvements

It takes money to make money. When Mr. Miller became CEO in 1994, he found that very little had been spent to make improvements in the hospital. During the period of 1995–1998, management spent about $2.25 million on equipment and renovations to support newly implemented programs and services. Included in those purchases was $450,000 to lease an advanced computerized tomography system (CT scanner) to support the radiology department's ability to care for patients on site, without having to refer them to hospitals 20 minutes or more away. A new mammography system, a new SPECT nuclear medicine camera, a new remote primary and specialty care clinic, and numerous other ventures were funded.

Key Indicators and Finances

1998 was the first year in many in which MCSI had an operating profit. It was $480,545, based on net patient revenues of $22.5 million and gross patient revenues of $39.6 million. The difference between gross and net patient revenue is known in the trade as contractual allowances and discounts (the difference between charges for services and the amount received). Peter Feimer, Assistant Administrator of Specialty Services, likened it to the difference between list price and negotiated price. Essentially a phenomenon of managed care contracting, it is not uncommon for hospitals to have such a large disparity between charges and contracted prices. Consequently, for analysis purposes, net patient revenue is a better indicator of a hospital's fiscal status.

Exhibit 4 presents selected operating statistics for the MCSI for the years from 1994 to 1998. Inspection reveals increasing trends in net patient revenue, FTE employees, patient admissions, patient days, outpatient surgeries, and occupancy rate.

Financial information for the seven year period of 1992–1998 is presented in the following exhibits. Exhibit 5 contains the MCSI's balance sheet. Exhibit 6 presents each balance sheet item as a percentage of the total assets. Exhibit 7 contains the income statement and Exhibit 8 presents the income statement items as a percentage of net revenue. Exhibit

STATISTIC	1994	1995	1996	1997	1998
Net patient revenue (in millions)	$13.0	$14.3	$15.8	$18.9	$22.4
Total patient revenue (in millions)	$19.5	$23.7	$27.7	$34.3	$39.6
Accounts receivable (days)	64	66	80	66	66
Total employee hours	380,668	444,497	478,400	548,958	581,906
Total number (full, part, and PRN)	264	294	380	351	329
Full time equivalent employees	183	214	230	258	270
Total patient admissions	1,471	1,871	1,936	2,086	2,016
Total patient days	11,335	14,194	15,402	15,680	15,915
Outpatient surgeries	529	600	573	709	883
Primary care clinic visits	2,085	3,197	6,831	8,694	11,314
Home health visits	8,067	12,928	16,967	21,104	15,197
Medical staff	–	104	121	129	119
Occupancy rate (based on 96 beds)	32.4	40.5	44	44.7	45.4
Occupancy rate (based on 77 beds)	40.3	50.5	54.8	55.8	56.6
Outpatient visits	8,883	11,793	10,447	10,501	10,851
Wages and benefits (in millions)	$6.3	$7.3	$8.5	$9.9	$11.2

Exhibit 4. MCSI operating statistics, 1994–1998.

Balance Sheet—MCSI

	1992	1993	1994	1995	1996	1997	1998
Assets:							
Cash & Cash Equivalents	$ 357,266	$ 312,769	$1,032,531	$ 631,844	$ 905,077	$ 639,558	$ 447,297
Receivables	1,748,403	1,966,056	2,276,182	2,034,829	3,410,861	3,379,851	2,479,264
Inventories	289,995	291,333	349,260	378,020	342,441	333,041	395,347
Other Current Assets	27,688	39,062	48,439	54,864	53,757	43,633	60,697
Total Current Assets	$2,423,352	$2,609,220	$3,706,412	$3,099,557	$4,712,136	$4,396,083	$3,382,605
Prop., Plant & Equip (net)	$ 252,185	$ 572,818	$1,059,143	$1,791,723	$2,300,939	$2,444,674	$2,791,278
Net Acquisition & Start Up Costs (net)	268,268	394,236	385,472	291,768	198,552	127,681	56,950
Other Assets	100	2,000	0	0	0	0	0
Total Assets	$2,943,905	$3,578,274	$5,151,027	$5,183,048	$7,211,627	$6,968,438	$6,230,833
Liabilities and Fund Balance:							
Current Maturies of LT Debt	$ 103,983	$ 158,814	$ 196,748	$1,222,637	$1,192,278	$ 702,032	$ 665,314
Account Payable	305,134	893,943	969,486	812,054	986,736	694,982	1,289,160
Accrued Salaries & Wages	216,136	265,092	363,575	143,203	320,134	167,982	375,647
Accrued compensated absences					163,521	202,398	201,786
Due to Affiliate	329,341	422,515	1,174,463	1,044,947	1,344,625	1,394,119	1,767,346
Estimated 3rd Party Settlements, Net		(69,650)	746,389	1,011,684	1,944,301	2,667,118	433,320
Other Current Liabilities	185,724	198,022	236,755	293,075	478,488	516,336	410,333
Total Current Liab.	$1,140,318	$1,868,736	$3,687,416	$4,527,600	$6,430,083	$6,344,967	$5,142,906
LT Debt, Less Curr. Mat.	$1,165,128	$1,175,052	$1,331,454	$ 565,504	$ 776,541	$ 937,662	$ 976,689
Total Liabilities	2,305,446	3,043,788	5,018,870	5,093,104	7,206,624	7,282,629	6,119,595
Deferred Revenue	$ 440,960	$ 385,839	$ 330,723	$ 275,604	$ 220,307	$ 165,372	$ 110,256
Fund Balance	197,499	148,647	(198,566)	(185,660)	(215,304)	(479,563)	982
Total Liabilities & Fund Balance	$2,943,905	$3,578,274	$5,151,027	$5,183,048	$7,211,627	$6,968,438	$6,230,833

Exhibit 5. MCSI balance sheet for the years 1992–1998.

Common Size Balance Sheet—MCSI

	1992	1993	1994	1995	1996	1997	1998
Assets:							
Cash & Cash Equivalents	12.1%	8.7%	20.0%	12.2%	12.6%	9.2%	7.2%
Receivables	59.4%	54.9%	44.2%	39.3%	47.3%	48.5%	39.8%
Inventories	9.9%	8.1%	6.8%	7.3%	4.7%	4.8%	6.3%
Other Current Assets	0.9%	1.1%	0.9%	1.1%	0.7%	0.6%	1.0%
Total Current Assets	82.3%	72.9%	72.0%	59.8%	65.3%	63.1%	54.3%
Prop., Plant & Equip (net)	8.6%	16.0%	20.6%	34.6%	31.9%	35.1%	44.8%
Net Acquisition & Start Up Costs (net)	9.1%	11.0%	7.5%	5.6%	2.8%	1.8%	0.9%
Other Assets	0.0%	0.1%	0.0%	0.0%	0.0%	0.0%	0.0%
Total Assets	100.0%	100.0%	100.0%	100.0%	100.0%	100.0%	100.0%
Liabilities and Fund Balance:							
Current Maturies of LT Debt	3.5%	4.4%	3.8%	23.6%	16.5%	10.1%	10.7%
Account Payable	10.4%	25.0%	18.8%	15.7%	13.7%	10.0%	20.7%
Accrued Salaries & Wages	7.3%	7.4%	7.1%	2.8%	4.4%	2.4%	6.0%
Accrued compensated absences	0.0%	0.0%	0.0%	0.0%	2.3%	2.9%	3.2%
Due to Affiliate	11.2%	11.8%	22.8%	20.2%	18.6%	20.0%	28.4%
Estimated 3rd Party Settlements, Net	0.0%	-1.9%	14.5%	19.5%	27.0%	38.3%	7.0%
Other Current Liabilities	6.3%	5.5%	4.6%	5.7%	6.6%	7.4%	6.6%
Total Current Liab.	38.7%	52.2%	71.6%	87.4%	89.2%	91.1%	82.5%
LT Debt, Less Curr. Mat.	39.6%	32.8%	25.8%	10.9%	10.8%	13.5%	15.7%
Total Liabilities	78.3%	85.1%	97.4%	98.3%	99.9%	104.5%	98.2%
Deferred Revenue	15.0%	10.8%	6.4%	5.3%	3.1%	2.4%	1.8%
Fund Balance	6.7%	4.2%	-3.9%	-3.6%	-3.0%	-6.9%	0.0%
Total Liab. & Fund Bal.	100.0%	100.0%	100.0%	100.0%	100.0%	100.0%	100.0%

Exhibit 6. Balance sheet items as a percentage of the total assets for the years 1992–1998.

Income Statement—MCSI

	1992	1993	1994	1995	1996	1997	1998
Unrestricted Rev., Gains, & Others:							
Net patient service revenue	$7,822,046	$8,395,734	$13,014,714	$14,377,223	$15,874,463	$18,941,727	$22,458,259
Income on investments	14,446	9,682	2,746	23,818	33,403	42,475	34,735
Rental income	63,202	56,827	28,452	53,028	50,910	60,946	71,965
Gains on sale of assets	55,120	55,121	55,116	55,116	65,511	68,366	55,116
Other revenue	108,795	100,200	112,154	106,451	63,261	107,410	106,604
Unrestricted gifts & bequests	10,000						
Total Unrestricted rev., gains & others	$8,073,609	$8,617,564	$13,213,182	$14,615,636	$16,087,548	$19,220,924	$22,726,679
Expenses:							
Salaries & wages	$3,331,447	$3,954,002	$5,622,103	$6,660,827	$7,644,074	$8,731,566	$9,882,526
Employee benefits	420,665	540,080	718,876	857,072	883,645	1,129,760	1,345,784
Professional fees	920,021	1,061,889	2,071,691	1,721,574	2,397,032	2,720,071	3,121,787
Supplies and other	1,959,520	2,048,803	3,022,647	3,522,281	3,230,159	4,167,609	4,610,041
Maintenance and utilities	302,438	293,644	401,017	244,250	481,402	452,080	241,587
Lease expense	200,000	200,000	200,000	200,000	200,000	250,000	250,000
Depreciation & amortization	71,089	88,275	226,695	328,103	438,628	577,776	663,130
Interest	147,511	151,481	214,670	228,943	255,828	281,878	293,225
Provision of bad debt	523,419	328,242	1,082,696	839,680	586,424	1,174,443	1,838,054
Total expenses	$7,876,110	$8,666,416	$13,560,395	$14,602,730	$16,117,192	$19,485,183	$22,246,134
Excess (Defic.) of Rev. Over Exp.	$197,499	($48,852)	($347,213)	$12,906	($29,644)	($264,259)	$480,545
Unrestricted net assets (deficit), begin.	$0	$197,499	$148,647	($198,566)	($185,660)	($215,304)	($479,563)
Unrestricted net assets (deficit), year end	$197,499	$148,647	($198,566)	($185,660)	($215,304)	($479,563)	$982

Exhibit 7. MCSI income statement for the years 1992–1998.

22

Common Size Income Statement—MCSI

	1992	1993	1994	1995	1996	1997	1998
Unrestricted Rev., Gains, & Others:							
Net patient service revenue	96.9%	97.4%	98.5%	98.4%	98.7%	98.5%	98.8%
Income on investments	0.2%	0.1%	0.0%	0.2%	0.2%	0.2%	0.2%
Rental income	0.8%	0.7%	0.2%	0.4%	0.3%	0.3%	0.3%
Gains on sale of assets	0.7%	0.6%	0.4%	0.4%	0.4%	0.4%	0.2%
Other revenue	1.3%	1.2%	0.8%	0.7%	0.4%	0.6%	0.5%
Unrestricted gifts & bequests	0.1%	0.0%	0.0%	0.0%	0.0%	0.0%	0.0%
Total Unrestricted rev., gains & others	100.0%	100.0%	100.0%	100.0%	100.0%	100.0%	100.0%
Expenses:							
Salaries & wages	41.3%	45.9%	42.5%	45.6%	47.5%	45.4%	43.5%
Employee benefits	5.2%	6.3%	5.4%	5.9%	5.5%	5.9%	5.9%
Professional fees	11.4%	12.3%	15.7%	11.8%	14.9%	14.2%	13.7%
Supplies and other	24.3%	23.8%	22.9%	24.1%	20.1%	21.7%	20.3%
Maintenance and utilities	3.7%	3.4%	3.0%	1.7%	3.0%	2.4%	1.1%
Lease expense	2.5%	2.3%	1.5%	1.4%	1.2%	1.3%	1.1%
Depreciation & amortization	0.9%	1.0%	1.7%	2.2%	2.7%	3.0%	2.9%
Interest	1.8%	1.8%	1.6%	1.6%	1.6%	1.5%	1.3%
Provision of bad debt	6.5%	3.8%	8.2%	5.7%	3.6%	6.1%	8.1%
Total expenses	97.6%	100.6%	102.6%	99.9%	100.2%	101.4%	97.9%
Excess (Defic.) of Rev. Over Exp.	2.4%	-0.6%	-2.6%	0.1%	-0.2%	-1.4%	2.1%

Exhibit 8. MCSI Income statement items as a percentage of net revenue for the years 1992–1998.

23

Statement of Cash Flow—MCSI

	1992	1993	1994	1995	1996	1997	1998
CF from Operating Activities							
Excess (deficiency) of Rev. Over Expense	$197,499	($48,852)	($347,213)	$12,906	($29,644)	($264,259)	$480,545
Adjust. to Reconcile above to Net Cash:							
Depreciation & Amortization	$71,089	$88,275	$226,695	$328,103	$438,628	$577,776	$663,130
Disposal of fixed assets							
Provision for bad debt	$523,419	$328,242	$1,082,696	$839,680	$586,424	$1,174,443	$1,838,054
Changes in:							
Receivables					($1,962,456)	($1,143,433)	($937,467)
Inventories					$35,579	$9,400	($62,306)
Other current assets					$1,107	$10,124	($17,062)
Accounts Payable					$174,682	($291,754)	$594,178
Estimated 3rd Party settlements					$932,617	$722,817	($2,233,798)
Accrued salaries & wages					$825,543	($25,933)	$474,277
Deferred Revenue					($55,296)	($54,935)	($55,116)
Total Changes	($228,218)	$113,080	$322,620	($819,037)	($48,224)	($773,714)	($2,237,294)
Amortization of Gains	($55,120)	($55,121)	($55,116)	($55,116)			
Net Cash Provided by Operating Activities	$508,669	$425,624	$1,229,682	$306,536	$947,184	$714,246	$744,435
CF from Investing Activities							
Purchase of property & equipment	($243,143)	($211,182)	($283,995)	($532,945)	($298,743)	($478,855)	($939,005)
Acquisition & Start-up Costs	($19,528)	($169,503)	($73,398)	($76)			
Net Cash Provided by Investing Activities	($262,671)	($380,685)	($357,393)	($533,021)	($298,743)	($478,855)	($939,005)
CF from Financing Activities							
Proceeds from issuance of long term debt	$302,170					$914,125	$832,543
Principal payments on long term debt	($340,902)	($89,436)	($152,527)	($174,202)	($375,208)	($1,415,035)	($830,234)
Net Cash Provided by Financing Activities	($38,732)	($89,436)	($152,527)	($174,202)	($375,208)	($500,910)	$2,309
Net Increase (Decrease) in Cash	$207,266	($44,497)	$719,762	($400,687)	$273,233	($265,519)	($192,261)
Cash & Cash Equivalents, beg. Of year	$150,000	$357,266	$312,769	$1,032,531	$631,844	$905,077	$639,558
Cash & Cash Equivalents, end Of year	$357,266	$312,769	$1,032,531	$631,844	$905,077	$639,558	$447,297
Supplemental Disclosures of CF Informat.							
Cash Paid for Interest	$62,742	$120,654	$245,497	$207,083	$257,552	$303,085	$293,225
Suppl. Discl. Of Non-Cash Inv. & Fin. Activit							
Capital lease obligat. incurred for Equip	$36,696	$154,191	$346,863	$434,140	$555,886	$171,785	
Debt obligation incurred for building							

Exhibit 9. MCSI statement of cash flow for the years 1992–1998.

9 contains the statement of cash flows. Finally, Exhibit 10 presents selected financial ratios for MCSI and industry averages.[40]

When asked why the hospital had operating losses in five of the last seven years, Miller provided the following reasons:

1. During the past 7 years, the MCSI made substantial expenditures to expand services, not only by type, but also in satellite locations, and to improve technology. Obviously, the startups have taken time to break even. Absent such initiatives, the hospital's financial performance would have been worse. In fact, the hospital would not have survived. The initiatives were included in the MCSI's 1998 strategic plan to provide evidence of just how aggressively MCSI has pursued expansion. A critical mass and mix of services are necessary in order to provide the level of patient care consistent with its mission.

    Referring to the financial exhibits, Miller noted, in 1992, the percentage of net property, plant, and equipment over total assets was just 8.6% (see Exhibits 5 and 6). It jumped to 34.6%, however, in 1995 and the percentage continued to rise until it reached 44.8% in 1998. As a result of the investments over time, the MCSI was able to offer more services and the net patient service revenue increased from $7.8 million in 1992 to $22.5 million in 1998. The 1998 revenue was almost three times the 1992 revenue.

    With the increase in revenue, expenses also increased (see Exhibits 7 and 8). Salaries and wages increased from $3,331,447 in 1992 to $9,882,526 in 1998, almost three times that of 1992. Employee benefits, professional fees, and provision for bad debts also increased by the same magnitude. As expected, depreciation and amortization expenses increased about 9 times, from $71,089 in 1992 to $663,130 in 1998. Interest expenses led to several years of negative income.

    Net cash obtained from operating activities primarily funded the increase in investments. Although MCSI experienced negative income in 4 out of 7 years of operations from 1992 to 1998, the annual net cash provided by operating activities has been positive (see Exhibit 9). The free-operating-cash-flow-over-revenue and the free-operating-cash-flow-over-assets ratios indicate a brighter picture than the income statement (statement of operations and changes in net assets). The increasing burden of servicing debt and leases, and investing in equipment and property, however, has largely absorbed the net cash provided by operating activities.

    MCSI has done an efficient job of managing its assets. All asset efficiency ratios show that MCSI has outperformed the industry average in this area. It also holds true for the fixed assets and current assets (see Exhibit 10).

Selected Financial Ratios—MCSI

	1992	1993	1994	1995	1996	1997	1998
Profitability Ratios:							
Total Margin	2.45%	-0.57%	-2.63%	0.09%	-0.18%	-1.37%	2.11%
Industry		*3.80%*	*3.90%*	*4.40%*	*5.00%*	*5.80%*	*3.80%*
ROI	6.71%	-1.37%	-6.74%	0.25%	-0.41%	-3.79%	7.71%
Free Oper CF Over Revenue		3.87%	1.92%	8.01%	1.25%	1.64%	2.07%
Industry				*4.70%*	*2.90%*	*2.40%*	*0.70%*
Free Oper CF Over Assets		5.17%	3.03%	21.10%	2.69%	3.43%	6.52%
Industry				*4.60%*	*3.60%*	*2.60%*	*0.60%*
Liquidity Ratios:							
Current Ratio	2.13	1.40	1.01	0.68	0.73	0.69	0.66
Industry		*2.23*	*2.20*	*2.19*	*2.19*	*2.19*	*2.21*
Days in Patient Accounts Receivable	81.59	85.47	63.84	51.66	78.43	65.13	40.29
Industry		*65.70*	*67.90*	*64.20*	*62.10*	*63.20*	*65.00*
Days Cash On Hand	17.91	13.84	30.76	17.17	21.89	13.16	8.27
Industry		*24.00*	*22.50*	*25.30*	*27.70*	*34.70*	*27.90*
Capital Structure Ratios:							
Fixed Asset Financing Ratio	223.87%	121.51%	92.17%	27.14%	31.07%	36.45%	34.29%
Industry		*42.60%*	*44.10%*	*42.50%*	*40.80%*	*37.70%*	*38.10%*
Cash Flow to Total Debt	11.65%	1.30%	-2.40%	6.70%	5.68%	4.30%	18.69%
Industry		*26.50%*	*26.50%*	*29.80%*	*29.50%*	*33.90%*	*25.20%*
Times Interest Earned	2.34	0.68	-0.62	1.06	0.88	0.06	2.64
Industry		*4.24*	*4.43*	*5.08*	*5.25*	*4.69*	*3.14*
Debt Service Coverage	0.85	0.79	0.26	1.41	1.05	0.35	1.28
Industry		*3.16*	*3.36*	*3.39*	*3.56*	*4.24*	*4.07*
Asset Efficiency Ratios:							
Total Asset Turnover	2.74	2.41	2.57	2.82	2.23	2.76	3.65
Industry				*1.13*	*1.12*	*1.04*	*1.03*
Fixed Asset Turnover	15.49	8.91	9.15	7.01	6.44	7.47	7.98
Industry				*2.44*	*2.52*	*2.29*	*2.33*
Current Asset Turnover	3.33	3.30	3.56	4.72	3.41	4.37	6.72
Industry		*3.52*	*3.47*	*3.51*	*3.52*	*3.40*	*3.36*
Inventory Turnover	27.81	29.58	37.83	38.66	46.98	57.71	57.49
Industry		*44.18*	*43.84*	*44.49*	*45.69*	*46.47*	*46.35*
Other Financial Ratio:							
Capital Expense Growth Rate Ratio		130.61%	97.79%	75.79%	38.10%	20.97%	25.06%
Industry		*6.20%*	*6.50%*	*5.80%*	*6.40%*	*6.90%*	*7.40%*
Gross Property & Equipment	279740.00	64513.00	1275971.00	2243056.00	3097684.00	3747184.00	4686189.00

Exhibit 10. Selected financial ratios for MCSI and industry averages for the years 1992–1998.

2. MCSI needed to offer managed care contract allowances (difference between charges such as list price and contractual amounts) in order to reobtain managed care contracts. Because so much of its patient base is covered by these types of plans, it was essential to aggressively pursue managed care contracts in order to survive.

3. Because 65% of MCSI's patient base is Medicare, the federal government's cutbacks on fixed reimbursement has hurt MCSI's revenue stream as well as that of all other hospitals. In the industry, few hospitals were reporting positive net income.

THE FUTURE

On a hot summer day as Miller met with the case writers in his office, he looked out the window and commented, "The Medical Center of Southern Indiana is like the mythical Phoenix—it was near death and arose again. This hospital, the pride of Charlestown, has gone through very difficult times and multiple phases in its organizational life cycle: conception in 1973; birth in 1976 when it opened; adoption by HCA and HealthTrust through acquisitions, abandonment when it was divested by them; and finally, revival, growth, and maturity since being purchased by the City of Charlestown in 1991. As evidenced by our 1998 strategic plan and positive financial results, we aggressively expanded services to meet the needs of our patients, medical staff, employees, and the community of Charlestown. I believe that we have made the investment in our core services that will allow MCSI to thrive in the future." In thinking about the future, Miller wondered:

1. Should MCSI slow down its aggressive expansion strategy of adding new services and consolidate the gains from those presently in place, or continue the aggressive expansion strategy of adding and investing in even more services?

2. Should MCSI reassess present services and retrench those that are not yet breaking even?

3. Should MCSI change its fiscal orientation and focus on cost reduction versus revenue enhancement?

4. Should MCSI pursue a joint venture with physicians in limited partnerships?

ENDNOTES

1. Quotes attributed to Kevin Miller are from interviews with the case writers or from published sources in which case the source are cited.

2. "The Comeback," an internal hospital document, p. 1.
3. "Medical Center of Southern Indiana is Pride of Charlestown," Evening News, June 25, 1992.
4. Internal hospital records.
5. "Progress Report: City to Own Hospital," The Leader, 17:34, September 20, 1973, pp. 1, 3.
6. "Progress Report: City to Own Hospital," The Leader, 17:34, September 20, 1973, pp. 1, 3 and "Experts Take Part in Medical Complex Hearing," The Leader, 17:35, September 27, 1973, pp. 1–2.
7. "Progress Report: City to Own Hospital," The Leader, 17:34, September 20, 1973, pp. 1, 3.
8. "Low Bid Accepted for Hospital Plan," The Leader, 18:23, July 11, 1974, pp. 1, 3.
9. "Agreement Signed for Bond Sale to Finance New Hospital in C-Town," The Leader, July 23, 1975, pp. 1+.
10. "North Clark Hospital May Go on the Block," Indiana Times, November 29, 1977, p. 1.
11. "HCA Takes Over: New Management Contract Signed for North Clark Community Hospital," The Charlestown Courier, January 19, 1979, p. 1.
12. "Hospital Sale is Closed," The Evening News, March 6, 1985.
13. "North Clark Hospital Becomes Part of New ESOP Company," The Leader, 31:11, June 10, 1987, p. 1.
14. "HealthTrust Negotiating to Sell North Clark Hospital," The Leader, 35:10, May 22, 1991, p. 1.
15. "North Clark Hospital Has New Owner," The Leader, 35:43, January 8, 1992, p. 1.
16. "HealthTrust Negotiating to Sell North Clark Hospital," The Leader, 35:10, May 22, 1991, p. 1.
17. "Stats Indiana," Southern Indiana Development Corporation Fact Sheet.
18. www.stats.Indiana.edu/profiles.pr1809.html, p. 1.
19. "1987–2000 Labor Force Estimates Clark and Floyd Counties," Indiana, Southern Indiana Development Council.
20. "1987–2000 Labor Force Estimates Clark and Floyd Counties," Indiana, Southern Indiana Development Council.
21. www.stats.indiana.edu/profiles.pr1809.html, p. 2.
22. www.stats.indiana.edu/profiles.pr1809.html, p. 2.
23. "Health Care Facilities Clark and Floyd Counties, Indiana," Southern Indiana Development Council.
24. "Health Care Facilities Clark and Floyd Counties, Indiana," Southern Indiana Development Council.
25. "The Comeback," an internal hospital document.
26. *Ibid.*
27. American MedTrust Corporate Document, 2000, p. 3 and Web www.medtrust.com.
28. American MedTrust Corporate Document, 2000, p. 3.
29. Health Care Financing Administration, Office of the Actuary, National Health Statistics Group. Tables 1, 2, and 10. www.hcfa.gov/stats/nhc-oatc/.
30. American Hospital Association, *Hospital Statistics*, various years: Chicago, AHA—tables appearing in Longest, B., Rakich, J., and Darr, K., *Managing Health Services Organizations and Systems*, 4th edition, 2000: Baltimore, Health Professions Press, p. 171.

31. Longest, Rakich, and Darr, pp. 189–191.
32. Longest, Rakich, and Darr, p. 91.
33. Managed Care Digest Series, 2000, Aventis, pp. 3, 13; see also web site www.managedcaredigest.com. *Note:* Segments of the Medicare/Medicaid population were enrolled in HMO and PPO managed care programs.
34. "The Comeback," an internal hospital document.
35. www.mcsin.org.
36. MCSI Internal 1998 Strategic Plan, pp. 1–4.
37. "The Comeback," an internal hospital document.
38. MCSI web site: www.mcsin.org.
39. "The Comeback," an internal hospital document.
40. *Note and source:* Industry averages in the Exhibit 10 are from *2001 Almanac of Hospital Financial & Operating Ratios*, Ingenix Publishing Group/Center for Healthcare Industry Performance Studies (CHIPS). Benchmark ratios used are rural hospitals with fewer than 100 beds.

2

The Case of the Unhealthy Hospital

Anthony R. Kovner
New York University, New York, New York

Bruce Reid, Blake Memorial Hospital's new CEO, rubbed his eyes and looked again at the budget worksheet. The more he played with the figures, the more pessimistic he became. Blake Memorial's financial health was not good; it suffered from rising costs, static revenue, and declining quality of care. When the board hired Reid 6 months ago, the mandate had been clear: improve the quality of care and set the financial house in order.

Reid had less than a week to finalize his $70 million budget for approval by the hospital's board. As he considered his choices, one issue, the future of six off-site clinics, commanded special attention. Reid's predecessor had set up the clinics 5 years earlier to provide primary health care to residents of Marksville's poorer neighborhoods; they were generally considered a model of community-based care. However, although they provided a valuable service for the city's poor, the clinics also diverted funds away from Blake Memorial's in-house services, many of which were underfunded.

As he worked on the budget, Reid's thoughts drifted back to his first visit to the Lorris housing project in early March, just 2 weeks into his tenure as CEO.

Reprinted by permission of *Harvard Business Review*. An excerpt from "The Case of the Unhealthy Hospital" by A.R. Kovner, 69(5) (September–October, 1991). Copyright © 1991 by the Harvard Business School Publishing Corporation; all rights reserved.

The clinic was not much to look at. A small graffiti-covered sign in the courtyard pointed the way to the basement entrance of an aging six-story apartment building. Reid pulled open the heavy metal door and entered the small waiting room. Two of the seven chairs were occupied. In one, a pregnant teenage girl listened to a Walkman and tapped her foot. In the other, a man in his mid-thirties sat with his eyes closed, resting his head against the wall.

Reid had come alone and unannounced. He wanted to see the clinic without the fanfare of an official visit and to meet Dr. Renee Dawson, who had been the clinic's family practitioner for 6 years.

The meeting had to be brief, Dawson apologized, because the nurse had not yet arrived and she had patients to see. As they marched down to her office, she filled Reid in on the waiting patients: the girl was 14 years old, in for a routine prenatal checkup, and the man, a crack addict recently diagnosed as HIV positive, was in for a follow-up visit and blood tests.

On his hurried tour, Reid noted the dilapidated condition of the cramped facility. The paint was peeling everywhere, and, in one examining room, he had to step around a bucket strategically placed to catch a drip from a leaking overhead pipe. After 15 years as a university hospital administrator, Reid felt unprepared for this kind of medicine.

The conditions were appalling, he told Dawson, and were contrary to the image of the high-quality medical care he wanted Blake Memorial to project. When he asked her how she put up with it, Dawson just stared at him. "What are my options?" she finally asked.

Reid looked again at the clinic figures from last year: collectively they cost $1.1 million to operate, at a loss of $256,000. What Blake needed, Reid told himself, were fewer services that sapped resources and more revenue-generating services or at least services that would make the hospital more competitive. The clinics were most definitely a drain.

Of course, there was a surfeit of "competitive" projects in search of funding. Blake needed to expand its neonatal ward; the chief of surgery wanted another operating theater; the chief of radiology was demanding a magnetic resonance imaging (MRI) unit; the business office wanted to upgrade its computer system; and the emergency department desperately needed another full-time physician, and that was just scratching the surface.

Without some of these investments, Blake's ability to attract paying patients and top-grade doctors would deteriorate. As it was, the hospital's location on the poorer, east side of Marksville was a strike against it. Blake had a high percentage of Medicaid patients, but the payments were never sufficient to cover costs. The result was an ever-rising annual operating loss.

Reid was constantly reminded of the hospital's uncompetitive position by his chief of surgery, Dr. Winston Lee. "If Blake wants more paying patients—and, for that matter, good department chiefs—it at least has to keep up with St. Barnabas," Lee had warned Reid a few days ago.

Lee complained that St. Barnabas, the only other acute care hospital in Marksville, had both superior facilities and better technology. Its financial condition was better than Blake's, in part because it was located on the west side of the city, in a more affluent neighborhood. St. Barnabas had also been more savvy in its business ventures: it owned a 50% share in an MRI unit operated by a private medical practice. The unit was reportedly generating revenue, and St. Barnabas had plans for other such investments, Lee had said.

Although Reid agreed that Blake needed more high-technology services, he was also concerned about duplication of service; the population of the greater Marksville area, including suburban and rural residents, was about 700,000. When he questioned Richard Tuttle, St. Barnabas's CEO, about the possibility of joint ventures, however, he received a very cold response. "Competition is the only way to survive," Tuttle had said.

Tuttle's actions were consistent with his words. Two months ago, St. Barnabas allegedly had offered financial incentives to some of Marksville's physicians in exchange for patient referrals. Although the rumor had never been substantiated, it had left a bad taste in Reid's mouth.

Reid knew he could either borrow or cut costs, but the hospital's ability to borrow was limited as a result of an already high debt burden. His only real alternative, therefore, was to cut costs.

Reid dug out the list of possible cuts from the pile of papers on his desk. At the top of the page was the heading "internal cuts," and halfway down was the heading "11 external cuts." Each item had a dollar value next to it representing the estimated annual savings (see Table 1).

Reid reasoned that the internal cuts would help Blake become a leaner organization. With 1,400 full-time equivalent (FTE) employees and 350 beds, there was room for some cost cutting. Reid's previous hospital had 400 beds and only 1,300 FTE employees. Reid recognized, however, that cutting personnel could affect Blake's quality of care. As it was, patient perception of Blake's quality had been slipping during the last few years, according to the monthly public relations office survey, and quality was an issue that the board was particularly sensitive to these days. Eliminating the clinics, conversely, would not compromise Blake's internal operations.

Everyone knew the clinics would never generate a profit. In fact, the annual loss was expected to continue to climb. Part of the reason was rising costs, but another factor was the city of Marksville's ballooning budget deficit. The city contributed $100,000 to the program and provided the space in the housing projects free of charge. Reid had heard from two city councilmen, however, that funding would likely be cut in the coming year.

Table 1.   Reid's list of possible cuts and savings

Internal cuts	Savings
Cut 2% from nursing staff	$340,000
Cut 2% from support and ancillary staff	$290,000
Cut maximum of 3% from business office staff	$50,000
Freeze all wages and salaries at current level	$1.5 million
Eliminate weekly in-house clinics	$100,000
External cuts	**Savings**
Eliminate all off-site clinics	$256,000

Less city money and a higher net loss for the clinic program would only add to the strain on Blake's internal services.

Reid had to weigh this strain against the political consequences of closing the clinics. He was well aware of the possible ramifications from his regular dealings with Clara Bryant, the recently appointed commissioner of Marksville's health services. Bryant repeatedly argued that the clinics were an essential service for Marksville's low-income residents.

"You know how the mayor feels about the clinics," Bryant had said at a recent breakfast meeting. "He was a strong supporter when they first opened. He fought hard in City Hall to get Blake Memorial the funding. Closing the clinics would be a personal blow to him."

Reid understood the significance of Bryant's veiled threat. If he closed the clinics, he would lose an ally in the mayor's office, which could jeopardize Blake's access to city funds in the future or have even worse consequences. Reid had heard through the City Hall rumor mill that Bryant had privately threatened to refer Blake to Marksville's chief counsel for a tax status review if he closed the clinics. He took this seriously; he knew of a handful of hospitals facing similar actions from their local governments.

When Reid tried to explain to Bryant that closing the clinics would improve Blake's financial condition, which, in turn, would lead to better quality of care for all patients, her response had been unsympathetic: "You don't measure the community's health on an income statement."

Bryant was not the only clinic supporter with whom Reid had to reckon. Dr. Susan Russell, Blake's director of clinics, was equally vocal about the responsibility of the hospital to the community. In a recent senior staff meeting, Reid sat stunned while Dr. Winston Lee, Blake's high-tech champion, exchanged barbs with Russell.

Lee had argued that the off-site clinics competed against the weekly in-house clinics that Blake offered under- and uninsured patients. He proposed closing the off-site clinics.

The four in-house clinics—surgery, pediatrics, gynecology, and internal medicine—cost Blake $200,000 a year in physician fees alone, Lee said. And because Medicaid was not adequately covering the costs of these services, the hospital lost about $100,000 a year from the in-house clinics. Furthermore, in-house clinic visits were down 10% so far this year. A choice had to be made, Lee concluded, and the reasonable choice was to eliminate the off-site clinics and bolster services within the hospital's four walls. "Instead of clinics, we should have a shuttle bus from the projects to the hospital," he proposed.

Russell's reaction had been almost violent. "Most of the clinics' patients wouldn't come to the hospital even if there was a bus running every 5 minutes," she snapped back. "I'm talking about pregnant teenage girls who need someone in their community they recognize and trust, not some nameless doctor in a big, unfamiliar hospital."

Russell's ideas about what a hospital should be were radical, Reid thought, but he had to admit they did have a certain logic. She espoused an entirely new way of delivering health care that involved the mobilization of many of Blake's services. "A hospital is not a building, it's a service. And wherever the service is most needed, that is where the hospital should be," she had said.

In Blake's case, that meant funding more neighborhood clinics, not cutting back on them. Russell spoke of creating a network of neighborhood-based preventive health care centers for all of East Marksville's communities, including both the low-income housing projects and the pockets of middle-income neighborhoods. Besides improving health care, the network would act as an inpatient referral system for hospital services.

Lee had rolled his eyes at the suggestion, but Reid had not been so quick to dismiss Russell's ideas. If a clinic network could tap the paying public and generate more inpatient business, it might be worth looking into, he thought. Besides, St. Barnabas was not doing anything like this.

At the end of the staff meeting, Reid asked Russell to give him some data on the performance of the clinics. He requested numbers of inpatient referrals, birth weight data, and the number of patients seen per month by type of visit—routine, substance abuse, prenatal, pediatric, violence-related injury, and HIV.

Russell's report had arrived the previous day, and Reid was flipping through the results. He had hoped it would provide some answers; instead, it only raised more questions.

The number of prenatal visits had been declining for 16 months. This was significant because prenatal care accounted for more than 60% of the clinics' business. Other types of visits, however, were holding steady. In fact, substance abusers had been coming in record numbers since the clinics began participating in the mayor's needle exchange program 3 months ago.

Russell placed the blame for the prenatal decline squarely on the city. "Two years ago, Marksville cut funding for prenatal outreach and advocacy programs to low income communities. Without supplementary outreach, pregnant women are less inclined to visit the clinics," she wrote.

The birth weight data were inconclusive. There was no difference between birth weights for clinic patients and birth weights for nonclinic patients from similar backgrounds. In fact, average birth weights were actually lower among clinic patients. Russell had concluded that the clinic program was too new to produce meaningful improvements.

On the positive side, inpatient referrals from the clinics had risen in the last few years, but Russell's comments about the reasons for the rise were speculative at best. HIV-related illnesses and violence-related injuries were a large part of the increase, but so were early detection of ailments such as cataracts and cancer. Reid made a note to ask for a follow-up study on this.

He put the report down and stared out his window. Blake had a responsibility to serve the uninsured, but it also had a responsibility to remain viable and self-sustaining. Which was the stronger force? It came down to finding the best way to provide high-quality care to the community and save the hospital from financial difficulties. The consequences of his decision ranged from another year of status quo management to totally redefining the role of the hospital in the community. He had less than a week to decide. What should Reid cut, and what should he keep?

Mueller-O'Keefe Memorial Home and Retirement Village

Strategic Planning in a Continuing Care Retirement Community

William E. Aaronson
Temple University, Philadelphia, Pennsylvania

CASE OVERVIEW

Steve Cantwell was preparing for the next meeting of the long range planning committee of the board of directors of the Mueller-O'Keefe Memorial Home and Retirement Village. Cantwell was a consultant with a major independent long-term care consulting firm who had been given the task of directing this project. It had been a difficult task from the beginning. Although he had dealt with similar situations in the past, this project presented some unique challenges.

The consulting firm for which Cantwell worked dealt almost exclusively with not-for-profit long-term care providers. The majority of clients were church sponsored or affiliated. Although well intentioned, governing

This case and related notes are taken from the long-term care management case study collection found in *Cases in Long-Term Care Management: Building the Continuum*, by Donna Lind Infeld and John Kress, published in 1989 by AUPHA Press and used by permission.

board members of these types of providers were not always well informed about the current challenges and opportunities within the long-term care environment.

The Mueller-O'Keefe Home was one such church-related client. The home was affiliated with the Evangelical Free Church. All members of the board of directors except one were church members. The church district executive was an ex officio board member. Although the board consisted of church members, the home was not sponsored by the church. The board was self-perpetuating and independent but chose to maintain close ties with the church.

During a retreat, the board of directors had determined that they would require outside consulting services. They recognized their personal limitations when it came to the development, selection, and implementation of alternative courses of action. Through a subcommittee, the long-range planning committee, the consulting firm for which Cantwell worked was retained. The consulting firm was to assist the home in developing a long-range plan that included identification of new services and a capital development plan.

Cantwell felt comfortable working with this board. All members whom he had met were dedicated to and concerned about the home. A few of the members were actually looking forward to entering the retirement village when the time would come for their own postretirement moves.

Cantwell was approaching this latest meeting with a great deal of concern. The meeting was to serve as a working session in which his report would be discussed and the feasibility of the action recommendations would be considered. He had spent considerable time researching the market, analyzing the organization, and developing alternatives that he believed fit both the home's mission and the organization's abilities. His report was well prepared and appeared to be congruent with the board's perception of the home's mission. However, despite endless interviews with board members, staff, residents, competitors, and community representatives, and after extensive research on the alternatives, he wondered whether the board would approve and respond to his recommendations. He knew that *he* had every reason to be confident in his counsel, or did he?

HISTORY AND DEVELOPMENT OF THE HOME

The Mueller-O'Keefe Memorial Home was founded in 1905, when Dr. Robert Mueller bequeathed a large brick farmhouse and 90 acres of ground to a benevolent organization of members of the Evangelical Free Church. The purpose of the bequest was to establish a home for aged church members. The Evangelical Free Church "Old Folks Home," as it was called, became well established in the local community. The home is located in a rural setting in a small city in Ohio. Two wings were added to the original farmhouse in the 1930s as a result of an increasing number of requests for admission.

The home continued to care exclusively for members of the Evangelical Free Church until 1951. Because of the fine reputation of the home, and in response to some financial difficulties, Mr. Patrick O'Keefe, a prominent local industrialist, established a 25-year endowment. O'Keefe was Roman Catholic. The purpose of the endowment was to ensure financial stability, to allow expansion of facilities, and to encourage the home to open admissions to non–Free Church members. The endowment principal became fully available to the home last year.

The 1950s brought additional changes. The board began to recognize that residents of the home were requiring more nursing care. The home never had an empty bed. When a resident died, the bed was quickly filled. When residents moved into the home, however, they were generally in poorer health than entering residents had been in the past. Plans were initiated to build a nursing care wing onto the Old Folks Home. A 100-bed addition was built in the early 1960s, which brought the total complement to 140 beds.

Another major innovation for the Mueller-O'Keefe Home occurred in the 1960s. The first retirement cottage was built in 1962, initially as a house for the administrator, whose presence at the home was increasingly required. He retired soon after the house was built, and he was allowed to remain there. When it became known that the grounds could be used for retirement living, retired couples began to apply for lots where they could build houses to their liking. The retirement "cottages" (single-family, ranch-style houses) would become the property of the home on completion. The original residents were offered life care contracts in return for the donation of the constructed cottage to the home. This experiment with life care contracts was short-lived as a result of early recognition of the future potential for financial liability.

One current resident of the nursing home is the last such person to hold a life care contract. She is 96, and the cost of her care long ago exceeded the value of her property. The home continues to honor her contract, however, by providing free care. In the mid-1960s the first "continuing care" contract was written. Contingent liability for care was to be limited to the construction cost or resale value of the cottages. Residents would be given preference for admission to nursing care.

A row of eight apartments was added in the early 1970s. These apartments are similar in appearance to single-story townhouses. In the late 1970s, the first attempt to plan within the retirement village took place. An architect was hired to design a state-of-the-art quadriplex, similar to cottage construction taking place at other retirement communities. However, when the building was completed, it did not fit with the predominant design of the community—it resembled an Aspen ski lodge. The home had difficulty selling the cottages. This reinforced the board's belief that 16 "seat of the pants" decisions generally resulted in better outcomes, a belief that many of the board members continued to hold. Haphazard land development had created its own problems, however, primarily involving efficient land use and sewage disposal.

In the 1970s the ratio of nursing care to residential care in the Old Folks Home changed rapidly. In 1970, only 53 beds were certified for nursing care. By 1977, all of the beds (100) in the nursing care building were certified. In 1985, two additional beds were added, bringing the total nursing care beds to 102. These new beds were to be held in reserve for the use of the retirement village residents. Personal care beds remained fixed at 40. They have continued to be located in the Mueller farmhouse. The buildings were modest, especially when compared to competing long-term care facilities.

By the 1980s the home's staff began to recognize that many of the home's residents had developed Alzheimer's disease or related dementias. Individuals in early and middle stages of the disease were particularly difficult to manage in a congregate living arrangement because of behavioral manifestations that the staff observed to be annoying to other residents. Therefore, a separate unit for confused, ambulatory residents was initiated. The Alzheimer's unit quickly developed a reputation for providing exceptional care. The administrator, Mr. Tom Clark, reported that the board was particularly interested in expanding this unit. However, he personally was uncertain about this option. Although it would certainly bring publicity and possibly additional sources of funding, it might also result in the home developing an image as a mental health facility, which might have negative consequences on future admissions.

According to Clark, the home had maintained a reputation for excellent basic care throughout its history. The Evangelical Free Church is a service-oriented denomination that draws its social philosophy from New Testament teachings. Church members are traditionally conscientious objectors and, like the Quakers and the Amish, are excused from military service when a national draft is in effect. Outward expressions of Christian values among administration, staff, and residents were very evident to Cantwell. According to Clark, this atmosphere, rather than the physical environment and other amenities, had been the key factor attracting residents to the home.

According to the board chairman, Mr. Polk, two important consequences had resulted. Many current residents of the retirement village and nursing care facilities had parents, grandparents, aunts, uncles, and siblings who were or had been residents of the home. Every resident of the home had heard of it by word of mouth and usually was intimately aware of it when making postretirement decisions. Second, the home had been frequently remembered in the wills of residents or relatives of residents who were pleased with the care received.

By the end of last May, the home's investment assets, held in the form of securities, were valued at approximately $3.5 million. Another $230,000 was held in a low interest savings account. Net fixed assets were valued at $1.7 million, for a fund balance of $5.6 million. The home did not have any long-term or short-term debt. This very positive financial picture, combined with an ever-growing demand for the services of the home, convinced the board of directors that some future-oriented growth strategies were required. The Long-Range Planning Committee was charged with the responsibility of developing alternative uses of the available funds.

Mr. O'Donnell, Long-Range Planning Committee chairman, stated that the committee immediately ran into problems. First, the board was not solidly behind any planning efforts. The home's growth in the past had been essentially unplanned. "Seat of the pants" decision making appeared to have worked well. Few free-standing nursing homes or retirement centers were as financially healthy as the home. Also, the debacle of the "ski lodge" cottage was seen as the result of the only planning endeavor ever undertaken.

Second, many board members were opposed to incurring long-term debt for any reason. Polk, who in the 1930s had seen what overextension of credit could do to a business, was especially opposed. It soon became apparent that, without debt, the home's options were severely limited.

Third, the home did not have a formally adopted mission statement. There was disagreement within the board as to whether one was necessary, because they had managed for 90 years without one. However, it did not seem likely that the board would agree on any plans because they were divided on issues related to the basic mission (who was to be served and how) and church relations. Because Mueller-O'Keefe is a church-affiliated home, a common mission was recognized as important by the board chairman and by some members of the committee who were trying to focus on acceptable growth options.

THE CONSULTANT'S ANALYSES

In the midst of these impending changes and conflicting opinions, a consulting firm was hired. The first meeting that Cantwell had with the Long-Range Planning Committee revealed several things. The initial proposal he submitted would have to be modified in response to some committee members' concerns. The chairman of the board, Mr. Polk, had objected to some of the terminology in particular. They would prefer to be called a home, not a facility. The committee requested that statistics and charts be kept to a minimum. They preferred to be given recommendations in common language. Finally, Cantwell had noted with some concern that the administrator, Tom Clark, was exceptionally quiet throughout the meeting. Despite the key role he would play in the planning process and in the implementation of any plans, his interactions and responses were subdued.

Cantwell was given a free hand by the committee to develop the long-range plan. The consulting contract stated that this plan would be developed through a process that ended with the presentation to the committee of several alternative strategies. Useful decision criteria were also to be developed. It was made clear to the board and the committee, however, that they were to make the final strategic choice. The consultants were to provide the professional expertise in areas of market analysis and internal organizational review. That knowledge, in conjunction with an in-depth analysis of the organization, was to result in the proposal of strategic alternatives that would be feasible and consistent with the organization's abilities.

Cantwell observed that the Long-Range Planning Committee was determined to take a passive role in the process. Polk, although not a member of the committee, took the most active role. Clark confided to Cantwell that, although Polk appeared to dominate the board and the committee, he was actually very democratic. He believed that if other members would exert themselves, Polk would yield to the will of the majority. Clark stated that he could see no reason why Polk's philosophy would be any different under these circumstances.

Polk had some very definite ideas about what should or should not be done. He viewed the rather substantial endowment and the excellent financial position of the home to be the result of his prudent financial management. Polk also served as the treasurer, which can be equated with the position of chief financial officer, for the home. In addition, he was the vice president for finance of a family-owned furniture business. His financial acumen was developed through a 45-year career with the furniture company. Experience taught him to be wary of debt of any kind.

In reviewing 4 years' worth of balance sheets (see Table 1), Cantwell noted that the accounts payable balance was identical ($10,360) at the close of each period. When questioned, Polk said that it was a fictitious amount. All bills had been paid on receipt. Consequently, the actual balance on the books in accounts payable at the end of the accounting period was zero. The state Medicaid program auditors, however, would not accept a zero balance.

Cantwell had initiated the planning process knowing that implementation of any plan would be problematic. Any program development, no

Table 1. Comparative balance sheets (in dollars)

	This year	Last year	2 years ago	3 years ago
Assets				
Current				
Cash	231,149	192,013	127,747	77,899
Accounts receivable	159,223	157,975	145,189	190,092
Inventory	400	400	400	400
Prepaid insurance	29,015	10,921	13,632	5,511
Total	419,787	361,309	286,968	273,902
Noncurrent				
Agent account	1,557,386	1,307,386	748,473	642,707
Trust account	1,901,122	1,651,122	1,388,735	1,193,165
Total	3,458,508	2,958,508	2,137,208	1,835,872
Fixed assets				
Land	10,284	10,284	10,284	10,284
Buildings	1,702,214	1,699,214	1,671,621	1,666,787
Water/sewer	204,747	204,747	204,747	178,885
Vehicles	105,532	104,846	54,356	54,356
Equipment	437,171	422,663	386,970	363,487
Cottages	303,452	254,050	230,224	150,494
Total	2,763,400	2,695,804	2,558,202	2,424,293
Depreciation	(1,073,784)	(1,052,207)	(998,329)	(953,807)
Net fixed assets	1,689,616	1,643,597	1,559,873	1,470,486
Total assets	5,567,911	4,963,414	3,984,049	3,580,260
Liabilities				
Accounts payable	10,360	10,360	10,360	10,360
Payroll	39,410	47,037	33,384	29,513
Taxes payable	5,368	5,171	4,912	4,441
Total	55,138	62,568	48,656	44,314
Reserves				
Resident care	(57,505)	(54,137)	(47,388)	(41,451)
Memorials	30,239	30,105	27,920	26,819
Resident expenses	(6,679)	1,372	(703)	0
Total	(33,945)	(22,660)	(20,171)	(14,632)
Fund balance	5,546,718	4,923,506	3,955,564	3,550,578
Total liabilities and fund balance	5,567,911	4,963,414	3,984,049	3,580,260

matter how modest, would result in debt being incurred. Furthermore, because of lack of depth in administration, organizational and management development would be required regardless of which direction was taken. The process was initiated with an organizational review, an analysis of current residents, a demographic analysis, and a financial review. A competitor analysis was also conducted, which included tours of and interviews at competing retirement communities and nursing homes. Staff from the Area Agency on Aging and the health systems agency were interviewed as well. Finally, residents, staff, and board members were selected for more extensive interviews.

Based on the findings from the first part of the study, sessions were to be conducted with the Long-Range Planning Committee in which the working papers would be discussed. These sessions would serve as the basis for preparation of the final document. The results of the working documents are summarized in the following sections.

Organizational Review

The board of directors had final responsibility for the operations of the home. The daily operational responsibilities for all facilities and programs were delegated to the administrator, Mr. Clark. Responsibility for the financial management of the home remained with the board chairman, Mr. Polk. The financial analyst and the bookkeeper, although reporting to Clark on paper, actually reported directly to Polk. Clark did have mid-level managers who were responsible for operations within the nursing unit, but he took full responsibility for the retirement village.

According to Polk, the board allowed Clark considerable latitude in running the home. The previous board chairman (Polk's predecessor) had allowed the previous administrator (Clark's predecessor) very little room for decision making. The home experienced some financial difficulties under the former chairman and administrator. Consequently, about 10 years ago, that board chairman was asked to resign. Later that year, the administrator was asked to resign as well. Polk was then selected as the new chairman and hired Clark as the administrator. Polk and Clark have been in their current positions approximately 10 years. They were both members of the same Evangelical Free Church congregation and had known each other for a considerably longer period of time. Substantial trust between the two men was apparent.

Cantwell observed that Clark exhibited little imagination in dealing with the home's operations. He also observed that Clark did an excellent job with the day-to-day management of the home. Employees were productive and contented with their work. Residents were generally well satisfied with their care. The home enjoyed an excellent reputation for the provision of high-quality basic care. Clark fostered the kind of work environment that made this possible. He did not, however, appear to have a thorough understanding of the current long-term care environment, in particular, the concept of a continuum of care. Clark did not seem to recognize the need to bridge the gap between total independence and total dependence of retirement village residents. He stated that he could not understand why the retirement village residents were becoming more vociferous in their demands for services.

Cantwell observed that financially the home was generally well managed. Polk appeared to be a prudent and well-intentioned individual who had managed to reverse previous financial problems without the benefit of a high-powered financial management staff. However, Polk also appeared to lack an understanding of the distinctions between financial management of a not-for-profit health care facility and that of a small, for-profit business. This was particularly apparent to Cantwell in the way that accounts were defined and segregated. The home actually had two equity accounts—capital contributions and retained earnings—which Cantwell combined into one account, the fund balance, for purposes of the financial review. Fund accounting techniques were not evident. All accounts were integrated despite restrictions placed on certain funds. The distinct financial management needs of the continuing care facility were also not recognized by the home's financial manager. Planning for future financial stability was difficult as a consequence.

Resident Profile

The home provided services at three levels of care. Each level of care had a distinct resident profile.

The retirement village housed residents living in 36 units. Twenty-four of the units were single-family homes. The residents tended to be atypical of those residing in other continuing care retirement communities. The average resident age on admission was 70.6 years, compared with a national average of 76 years. The average current age was 75.7 years, compared with mature communities, where the average age approximates 82 years (see Table 2). Thus, the retirement village had a relatively young resident population. Close to one half of the residents were members of the Evangelical Free Church (see Table 3). Residents also tended to originate from distances further from the home than is typical (see Table 4).

The nursing and personal care units were more typical of other church-related nursing homes. The average age on admission (81 years) and the average current age (86 years) were comparable to national averages. Approximately 30% of nursing care and 25% of residential care residents were members of the Evangelical Free Church. This was similar to

Table 2. Average age of in-house residents as of December of last year versus national data (in years)

Level of care	Age at admission	National age at admission	Current age	National average age
Nursing care[a]	81.0	N/A	86.0	N/A
Personal care	82.0	N/A	86.0	N/A
Retirement village[b]	70.0	76	75.7	82

Source: American Association of Homes for the Aging. [1987]. *Continuing care retirement communities: An industry in action.* Washington, DC: Author.

[a]The age distribution of nursing home residents is skewed as a result of the NF/MR program (facilities for persons with mental retardation). According to the American College of Health Care Administrators Ready Reference Service, the current age is similar to the national experience, but the average length of stay at the Mueller-O'Keefe Home is approximately 3 years longer than the national average.

[b]82 years is the resident average age for those retirement communities that opened between 1963 and 1973.

the experience of other denominational homes. More residents had entered from areas outside of the typical 10-mile radius from the home, however, than would be expected of homes in areas of similar population density.

Despite the home's lack of promotional efforts, the nursing and residential care units and the retirement village remained full. Although 43% of the current residents' care was paid through the Medicaid program (see Table 5), 90% had entered as self-pay residents. According to Clark, the high rate of conversion from self-pay to Medicaid was most likely due to the long lengths of stay in nursing care (4.5 years compared to a national average of just over 2 years). Clark further stated that Medicaid, as a percentage of payer mix, would be higher if the home's private pay rates were equivalent to those of other nursing homes in the area: "Many of our residents are not well off. We want to give them the best care we can at the lowest rates so that we don't use up their assets any faster than necessary."

Table 3. Religious preference by level of care

	Level of care					
	Nursing care		Personal care		Retirement village	
Religious preference	Number	Percent	Number	Percent	Number	Percent
Evangelical Free Church	29	29.0	8	24.2	16	47.2
Methodist	27	27.0	13	39.4	5	14.7
Other Christian	40	40.0	12	36.4	8	23.4
None	4	4.0	0	0.0	5	14.7
Total	100	100.0	33	100.0	34	100.0

Table 4. Resident origin by level of care-in-house residents: December 31, last year

| | Level of care | | | | | |
| | Nursing care | | Personal care | | Retirement village | |
Prior residence	Number	Percent	Number	Percent	Number	Percent
Home county	68	66.7	26	76.5	15	44.1
Contiguous counties	20	19.6	6	17.6	3	8.8
Other	14	13.7	2	5.9	16	47.1
Total	102	100.0	34	100.0	34	100.0

Financial Review

The home appeared to be on firm financial footing. Results of the financial statement analyses are presented in Table 6. Declining net revenues were noted 2 and 3 years ago. According to Polk, this trend resulted from the board's decisions not to raise rates during each of those years. A rate increase was put into effect, however, at the end of last year, which resulted in an increase in net revenue during the opening months of this year.

The home had adopted a rate policy for nursing care that was considered to be unique in the nursing home industry. Private rates were to be set no higher than Medicaid rates for the same patient services classification. This was directly related both to the basic care philosophy and to the social philosophy of the Evangelical Free Church. Clark stated that this policy actually resulted in the home having to refund money to the state's Medicaid program last year when the cost reports were analyzed and the state auditors realized that the rate-setting commission had increased Medicaid rates to the home, but the private rates had not been increased by the board. Federal law does not permit Medicaid rates to exceed self-pay rates.

The retirement village residents, although not guaranteed care according to their contracts, were guaranteed a partial payment source for care based on their entrance fees. Entrance fees were to be depreciated over

Table 5. Nursing care utilization profile by payer classification

| | Self-pay | | Medicaid | |
	Patient days	Percent	Patient days	Percent
Last year	21,731	59.5	14,773	40.5
2 years ago	20,407	57.7	15,383	42.3
3 years ago	22,102	60.6	14,368	39.4

Table 6. Comparative statement of revenues and expenses annualized (in dollars)

	This year	Last year	2 years ago
Operating revenues			
Resident care fees			
Personal care	324,408	312,927	319,186
Self-pay nursing facility	1,094,658	1,020,978	978,382
Medicaid nursing facility	729,772	683,162	698,229
Other operating revenues	50,070	47,131	35,880
Total	2,198,908	2,064,198	2,031,677
Operating expenses			
Employee compensation	1,720,057	1,702,209	1,636,782
Supplies	112,010	107,723	108,080
Maintenance	78,940	69,510	64,694
Utilities	97,295	91,753	91,059
Professional development	4,107	6,204	4,383
Professional services	36,785	35,652	34,757
Insurance	37,099	35,074	17,608
Miscellaneous	4,282	4,625	3,174
Total	2,090,575	2,052,750	1,960,537
Depreciation	73,470	62,704	44,522
Total expenses	2,164,045	2,115,454	2,005,059
Gain (loss) from operations	34,863	(51,256)	26,618
Nonoperating revenue	131,400	72,619	72,705
Net income for period	166,263	21,363	99,323

a 12-year period, with the undepreciated balance available to pay for nursing care if the resident should permanently transfer to the nursing home. Cantwell became quite concerned when he could not track the entrance fees. Consequently, he could not accurately calculate the home's potential liabilities for care. The resident care reserve fund appeared to cover only residents who had actually transferred to nursing care. When questioned, Polk became defensive about this procedure. He stated that fees were deposited directly into one of the trust accounts. Resident care was provided according to the contracts and no problems had occurred to date.

The agent and trust accounts were administered by a local bank. There had been dramatic growth in these accounts in recent years. There were two sources for growth. First, donations had increased. The second and more important source of fund growth, however, was related to the increase in value of the portfolio holdings. The holdings were revalued to current market levels at the end of each period. Although the portfolio was diversified, the account balances were sensitive to changes in financial markets.

Environmental Analysis

There were two competing continuing care retirement communities in the home's primary service area. Mueller-O'Keefe's entrance and maintenance fees are lower than the others (see Table 7). There were also nine nursing homes in competition for residents at that level of care (see Table 8). The most significant finding was that the home's rates at all levels of care were the lowest in the county. Cantwell noted with some concern the differences in monthly maintenance fees among the retirement communities. He had discussed this informally with Clark on first reviewing the internal rate structure. Clark recognized that the fees were nowhere near adequate to cover costs. However, he stated that the board was more concerned about those living in the retirement village who could not afford the $120 per month that other communities charged. Clark thought that $120 was outrageous and that the other communities could not justify that amount. Cantwell also noted that the home's physical plant was more modest than those of the competitors' facilities.

The demographic analysis revealed several things that explained, to some extent, the competitive advantage of the home. First, there were few vacant beds in the county. Even those patients capable of self-pay for extended periods of time were having difficulty finding a nursing home bed. The home was located in an area characterized by a rapidly expanding elderly population. Housing values and elderly income, however, were below the state and national averages. Also, a higher percentage than expected of the oldest old lived alone—a situation that resulted in heavy demand for nursing home care. In the adjacent city, close to 50% of those

Table 7. Continuing care retirement community fees (in dollars)

Community	Entrance fees		Maintenance fees (monthly)
Mueller-O'Keefe (church-related)	Cottages:	55,000	20
	Apartments:	25,000	20
The Woods (church-related)	Cottages:	70,500	130
	Apartments:	47,500	130
Luther Village (church-related)	Cottages:	60,000	120

Table 8.   Licensed nursing homes–primary service area

Facility	Beds		Nursing care rates (per diem, in dollars)
	Nursing care	Personal care	
Mueller–O'Keefe (church–related)	102	40	Semiprivate: 46 Private: 47–49
Andover Manor (for-profit)	221	0	Semiprivate: 57–59 Private: 59–64
Clifton Home (for-profit)	49	0	Semiprivate: 50
County Home (government)	51	0	Semiprivate: 50–60
The Court (for-profit)	160	0	Semiprivate: 71–74
Greywood Memorial (for-profit)	37	17	Semiprivate: 49
The Woods (church-related)	100	45	Semiprivate: 51 Private: 51
Luther Village (church-related)	88	0	Semiprivate: 58–60 Private: 61
Methodist Home (church-related)	150	0	Semiprivate: 58–65 Private: 68
Advent Home (church-related)	97	0	Semiprivate: 53–56 Private: 61
Total	1,055	102	

older than age 75 lived alone, compared to approximately one third on a national basis. The demographic and economic profiles also explained the slow growth that was experienced by the retirement village.

Interviews

The committee interviewed several key participants. Following are their ideas, compliments, and concerns, in their own words:

Mr. Clark, Administrator "The retirement village residents are taking an increasing amount of my time. Without an assistant administrator, it is becoming more difficult to deal with problems caused by increasing age and decreasing independence. They pay a $20 per month maintenance fee. I can't provide all of the services that they expect on that amount.

"We emphasize excellent basic care in the nursing home. We intend to be the highest quality, lowest cost home in the county. Our philosophy of care is based on Christian principles. I don't want to deplete our residents' hard-earned savings. We figure that they will be on Medicaid soon enough, so why hurry the process. That is why we don't set self-pay rates above the Medicaid rate. We also aren't tempted to treat residents any differently based on payer status.

"Relations with the church have not always been smooth. The ladies' auxiliary, consisting largely of area church members, has made significant contributions, both financially and in volunteer time. Some pastors, however, have been reluctant to become involved in the activities that we sponsor for the ladies' auxiliary, such as an annual barbecue and periodic breakfast meetings. We would like to have more involvement from the church.

"In the past, funds were severely limited. Construction was not always the highest quality. Maintenance costs are going up as a consequence. We may need to replace certain facilities in the future. The farmhouse may not be considered safe for residents at some point. Because of the historical significance of the building, however, we would want to continue to utilize it."

Mrs. Hancock, Director of Nursing "Care requirements are increasing across the board. We have had to increase our R.N. staff as a consequence. Of particular concern are the retirement village residents. A few of them should be in nursing care now. We end up providing free care on an emergency basis when they can't get to their personal physicians.

"We don't know enough about their care requirements. This may be more of a problem in the future, especially if people are older when they first enter the retirement village or the personal care facility. We should be more aware of the medical care that they are receiving from their personal physicians. I don't have the time to make the contacts myself, even if the residents gave me permission to make contact."

Ms. Webb, Director of Social Services "People seeking admissions are generally older and sicker at each level of care. Nursing home beds are filled as soon as they are vacated. Most residents come from home or from other nursing homes. I seldom have a bed when the hospital social worker calls. She calls me anyway to see if I might have a bed, because the nursing home beds in this area are generally in short supply. The hospital has added its own skilled nursing care unit, but this isn't adequate to provide care for the many discharges who will require long-term care, rather than post-acute extended care.

"People only leave the retirement village when they absolutely cannot care for themselves and then go directly to nursing care. We are supposed to have two beds in reserve for the retirement village. It doesn't, however, always work out. Personal care would be better than remaining in independent living, but the residents don't care for the accommodations there."

Mr. Polk, Chairman, Board of Directors "The local congregation of the Evangelical Free Church, to which I belong, has generously supported the home. Most board and ladies' auxiliary members also belong to my congregation. I'm not sure how much benefit increased church involvement would have, because other congregations have not been as financially generous.

"We're not sure how we should set our priorities. In particular, we would like to know how we can best use our available funds. I don't think it is appropriate, however, to jeopardize our residents' security by incurring debt. I know of homes that have had financial difficulties as a result of overextending debt. If the board decides to finance growth through debt, I may need to reconsider my position on the board.

"I've suggested several mission statements, but the board has not decided which, if any, to adopt. Many believe that a mission statement might be too rigid. Obviously, our policies reflect the Christian mission of service on which this home was founded. We just don't have it written down."

Mr. O'Donnell, Chairman, Long-Range Planning Committee "We need your help in planning for the future. We don't know enough about the different approaches to growth. We do know that if we grow, it has to be slow and planned. I don't like debt, but if we need it to meet our goals, then we should do it. That's why we hired you. We also need to agree on our mission. We know that we want to serve the elderly and especially Evangelical Free Church elderly, but we also don't want to discriminate against those of other denominations.

"Our buildings may need to be replaced in the future and we need to be prepared for that. Also, growth in the retirement village needs to be better planned."

Mrs. Ruth, Board Member "We need to have closer ties to the Evangelical Free Church. It is not so much the financial support that they give, but the anchor that the church provides. That is, the church is where we go to ensure that what we are doing is consistent with Christian social teaching and allows us to share our experience with others who have similar concerns."

Mrs. Jones, Nursing Home Ombudswoman, Area Agency on Aging "I hear only positive things. This is the only nursing home in my territory from which I have received no complaints since I was hired into this position 2 years ago."

Mr. and Mrs. Miller, Retirement Village Residents "We love the single-family homes and the community spirit here. Nursing care is excellent. We know that if we really need care, the nursing home will provide good care. We are growing older and may need help with daily activities, such as shopping, food preparation, and cleaning. It's just not available, except from neighbors.

"The personal care facility is inadequate. There are a few nice rooms, but not many. That's why people wait so long before deciding to go to personal or nursing care. The home needs to have a better personal care facility and maybe provide more services in the home."

THE WORKING SESSION

Cantwell entered the final working session feeling confident in his recommendations, but uncertain about what the board's responses might be. Although committee members had talked freely during the interviews, they had been relatively quiet in the working sessions in which the analyses were presented. Cantwell did not know whether that was a positive sign or not. He had managed to elicit responses from Polk on relatively minor points related to financial position. Cantwell assumed that he had done a thorough and professional job and took their silence to mean concurrence with his analyses. Cantwell presented the following options:

1. Basic option—no facility expansion
   a. Upgrade the financial management system, especially the management of entrance fees and contingent liabilities for retirement village residents.
   b. Provide service contract options for retirement village residents that encourage continued independence. Such services may include transportation, onsite medical care, and housecleaning. Optional contracts would result in higher monthly fees to residents.

2. Expand and modernize current facilities
   a. Enlarge the Alzheimer's unit. This option would take advantage of the home's experience and allow for increased care of persons with later stages of the disease. It would also expand bed capacity and may ease problems with the waiting list.
   b. Expand and modernize the personal care unit. This is one of the most rapidly growing programs among continuing care retirement communities. The current units are inadequate. Bathing facilities in particular need to be upgraded. An enhanced personal care unit may also make retirement living more attractive and result in growth in the retirement village. Replacement of the personal care rooms in the farmhouse may become necessary if the facility cannot continue to meet safety codes.

c.   Develop a master plan for the retirement village. Growth has been unplanned to date. Future growth should be planned, including roads and sewage treatment plant improvements. Prospective residents should be given fewer options with new houses. The current system has discouraged sales in the past, especially to older persons who are not willing to expend the effort necessary to retain and supervise a builder.

In order to pursue this option, the board would need to hire an architect to lay out alternatives and estimate costs. Financing arrangements will depend on the options selected. A total marketing effort should be undertaken to support any program development effort.

3.   Program initiatives

Provide adult day care for persons with Alzheimer's disease. This has been identified as a need by the Area Agency on Aging and the health systems agency. It could be done on-site and would complement the residential Alzheimer's unit. It would involve minimal investment.

As at previous meetings, few questions were raised. Polk disagreed that the current financial management system was inadequate. The other options appeared to be acceptable. Following this meeting the recommendations were to be presented to the board for approval and action.

At the conclusion of the meeting, Cantwell became uneasy. As he left for home, he wondered what went wrong. How could he further help the committee to decide or to take action? He could not help but think about Polk's faith in "seat of the pants" decisions. He had done the best job he could. He hoped to be able to assist the board in implementing the selected strategies. The waiting had begun.

4

Electronic Child Health Network (eCHN)

Carol Anne Brothers

Murray J. Bryant

The University of Western Ontario, London, Ontario, Canada

Richard Ivey School of Business

The University of Western Ontario

Ivey

In September 1999, as Andrew Szende prepared for the Electronic Child Health Network's (eCHN) upcoming board of directors' meeting, he wondered how he could expand the scope of eCHN's services and membership in a financially profitable way. The Hospital for Sick Children (HSC), in partnership with IBM and four member organizations, designed eCHN to provide both the public and registered health care providers with Web-based access to children's health information and services. In particular, HSC, eCHN's most prominent partner, saw the Network's development as a major step toward fulfilling HSC's objective of being a "hospital without walls" and a leader in the delivery of health care to children. Szende envisioned eCHN as a not-for-profit organization committed to improving health care delivery to children. Szende, therefore, felt that he needed to present the eCHN's board of directors with a plan that would allow the Network to grow in a financially profitable way that would benefit both eCHN's member organizations and children's health.

HOSPITALS IN ONTARIO

Hospitals in Ontario were struggling. Fiscal constraints, technological advancements, and increasing public scrutiny of the health care system were forcing hospitals to find new ways to provide high quality, accessible health care at a lower cost. In addition, initiatives implemented by the Health Services Restructuring Commission (HSRC) were changing the nature of health care delivery in Ontario. The HSRC had a four-year mandate to restructure hospitals in Ontario and develop policies that increased the level of coordination and cooperation among health care providers. The HSRC estimated that hospitals could avoid spending $900 million annually on acute care services that were being used inappropriately.

THE HOSPITAL FOR SICK CHILDREN

In 1875, the Hospital for Sick Children was first opened in an 11-room house in Toronto, Ontario, "for the admission and treatment of all sick children." In its first year of operation, 44 patients were admitted to the new six-bed hospital, and another 67 children were treated in outpatient clinics. In 1951, the HSC moved to its current location where it has developed into one of the largest pediatric teaching hospitals in the world, with a 1998 operating budget of $305 million and 383 beds in service. In its mission statement, HSC identified itself as a "health care community dedicated to improving the health of children" that would "provide the best in family-centred, compassionate care, lead in scientific and clinical advancement, and prepare the next generation of leaders in child health." As a children's academic medical center, the HSC served as a: 1) resource to the local, regional and international communities in managing highly specialized children's health care problems; 2) site for training of specialists and primary care providers; and 3) site for clinical research.

The HSC envisioned itself in the new millennium as a "hospital without walls," and through its collaboration with others, aimed to become the "best pediatric academic health science centre in the world." As a "hospital without walls," HSC would serve not only the health needs of those children who visited the hospital, but also children around the world. The HSC developed seven strategic imperatives that would allow the hospital to achieve its vision (Exhibit 1).

THE CHILD HEALTH NETWORK

In 1994, HSC first described a new systems approach to the provision of child health services. This approach recommended the development of a seamless continuum of child health services. In 1997, the HSRC mandated the development of a Child Health Network for the Greater Toronto Area (CHN).

The CHN had a vision. Its goal was to provide an integrated and consistent system of maternal, newborn and child health services that would improve the health and quality of life for children independent of geographic location. The CHN's services would be provided through the alliances and partnerships among its members. The CHN was organized on a regional basis, with Regional Pediatric Centres (RPCs) designated in each region of the Greater Toronto Area to coordinate the provision of children's health services. RPCs worked with associated hospitals, other

---

The Hospital for Sick Children—Strategic Imperatives

1. We will lead in the delivery of exemplary patient care and the development of new forms of treatment so that children who come to HSC continually experience the best results.

2. We will become the preeminent research enterprise for children's health worldwide, continually generating new ideas and innovations for patient care.

3. We will build an outstanding education and knowledge dissemination capability that allows what we have learned to improve children's health around the world.

4. We believe passionately that our greatest resource is the people who choose to work at HSC and we will develop new ways to support, develop, and retain staff and attract the best results.

5. We understand that success in this new world will not be possible alone and so we will lead and work cooperatively with viable responsive networks and partnerships.

6. We will continually challenge ourselves to improve by measuring and evaluating the value and effectiveness of what we do and then sharing our results with others.

7. To become the best, we will need to enhance existing and develop new sustainable sources of funding so that our horizons will not be limited by our financial barriers.

Exhibit 1. Strategic imperatives to achieve HSC's vision. *Source:* The Hospital for Sick Children Strategic Plan, 1999.

health care providers and consumers to ensure that the unique health needs of their region were being met. The development of a communications infrastructure would, therefore, be a critical enabler of the CHN's goals.

THE ELECTRONIC CHILD HEALTH NETWORK

In 1998, the Electronic Child Health Network (eCHN) was developed from a partnership between HSC, IBM Canada and four other health facilities with significant pediatric components in Ontario (St. Joseph's Health Centre, St. Elizabeth Health Care, Orillia Soldiers' Memorial Hospital and Centenary Health Centre of the Rouge Valley Health System). The eCHN, a not-for-profit organization, provided the communications infrastructure that was required to support the development of the CHN. This communications infrastructure consisted of two web sites that allowed health care professionals, parents and children to access children's health information 24 hours a day. In addition, eCHN provided a secure system (not connected to the Internet) that allowed eCHN-associated health care providers to electronically share a child's medical records stored on a common database. Both the HSC and the Ontario Ministry of Health provided funding ($7.5 million each) for the $15 million eCHN, and the products and services supplied by IBM were provided at cost.

The eCHN provided both public and registered health care providers with web-based access to children's health information and services. While other telehealth networks had been developed in Canada and the United States, eCHN was unique in its focus on children. Andrew Szende, eCHN's chief executive officer (Appendix 1) envisioned eCHN playing a key role in the development of a common standard of care for children among its member organizations, no matter where those services were delivered. Szende said that eCHN's goal was to "electronically link hospitals, local pediatricians, home care agencies and other organizations that provide child health services in Ontario."

The eCHN enabled not only its member organizations to exchange secure, electronic patient information but also children to receive the right care at the right time as close to home as possible. For example, a young cancer patient in Orillia, Ontario, would no longer have to travel to Toronto for regular chemotherapy treatments. Instead, the child could go to a local hospital where a physician could access the patient's clinical data on-line that included radiographic images (e.g., x-rays), laboratory data and medical chart notes. Physicians would also be able to share in clinical protocols and obtain the latest information on a wide variety of health issues related to their patients' care. It also meant that parents would not have to retell their child's painful medical history every time they saw a new doctor and would have easy access to information related to their child's health.

Michael Strofolino, president and CEO of the Hospital for Sick Children, emphasized the importance of communications technology in the future of health care. Strofolino said that the necessity for a system such as eCHN became clear about five years ago, when hospital administrators realized that many children were not getting the medical services they needed. "When we looked at the symptoms, it became clear that there were many, many services out in the community that we had yet to utilize. In fact, many patients were showing up at the hospital, and while it was very complimentary, they were not appropriate to be seen here; they could have been seen in other locations."

The eCHN's services were provided in three separate components (Exhibit 2): 1) a web site designed specifically for parents and children ("Your Child's Health"); 2) a web site that allowed Ontario health care professionals to share resource materials and exchange opinions ("PROFOR"); and 3) IBM's "Health Data Network," a secure electronic database that allowed health care providers in different facilities to share children's health records.

"Your Child's Health"

"Your Child's Health" provided parents and children with web-based access to health information prepared by health care professionals from eCHN's member organizations.

The "Your Child's Health" web site was divided into three components:

"For Parents": This section provided parents with health information on common childhood illnesses such as asthma and the basics on tonsillectomy.

"For Kids": This section provided children from three to 18 years of age with health information (e.g., asthma, tonsillectomy) in formats appropriate to specific age groups. Interactive games and stories were developed to allow children to participate in the discovery of health information, and parents to work with their children to help them understand a visit to their physician or hospital.

"My Child is Sick": This section provided parents with information that would help them decide whether a health problem was really an emergency. In order to avoid long waits in emergency, parents could review information about common childhood illnesses (e.g., asthma, diarrhea, fever, febrile seizures, ear infections) at home. Parents could then decide whether their child required emergency help or could wait for their family physician or pediatrician to be available. If emergency help was needed, the locations for all of the emergency departments in the greater Toronto area were listed.

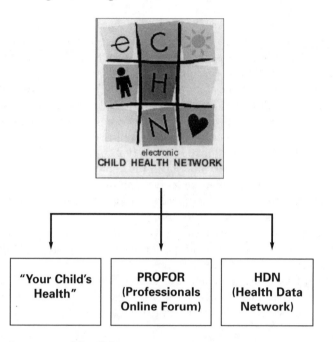

Exhibit 2. Components of the eCHN.

In 1998, "Your Child's Health" was awarded a Canadian Online Product Award for the Best New Consumer Product in the category of Health/Medicine. Shala Aly, vice president and general manager, e-business and ERP, IBM Global Services, said that "the site [was] an excellent example of how health care organizations [could] effectively use the web to better serve their community. Combining the Hospital's medical expertise with IBM's e-business capabilities—in designing, building and hosting the site—has produced a valuable online resource for children and parents alike."

Szende was aware of the public's concern over the availability of high quality health care wherever and whenever it was needed. He saw "Your Child's Health" as a valuable resource for both parents and children that could be accessed free of charge. Szende knew, however, that the maintenance costs for this web site would be high. The health information available through "Your Child's Health" had to be updated and new information added on an ongoing basis. Szende wanted to look for ways in which "Your Child's Health" could generate revenues that would offset the costs associated with site maintenance, and generate the profits that would allow the eCHN to grow.

"PROFOR"

PROFOR was a secure web site that was designed to facilitate communication and collaboration among health care professionals affiliated with eCHN's member organizations. The PROFOR web site offered opportunities for dialogue on child health issues, updates on current research projects, bibliographies on health topics, and parent education information that could be provided to parents after consultation with a health care professional. The information available on PROFOR's web site was provided by health care professionals from eCHN's member organizations and reviewed by the PROFOR Editorial Board prior to posting. The information was then organized by clinical discipline, e.g., dentistry, anesthesia, and posted on the PROFOR web site.

To access the site, health care providers needed a password that could only be provided through the PROFOR User Coordinator at one of the CHN's member facilities. Once health care professionals logged into PROFOR, they could access any of the following sections:

Presentations: This section provided health professionals with access to video presentations and discussions including rounds for medical, nursing and other professional services.

Collaboration: This section allowed professionals on the network to share information and ask questions on-line.

Standards: This section provided health care professionals with immediate access to "Standards of Patient Care" and "Clinical Practice Guidelines" for a variety of specialty areas including anesthesia, bioethics, and critical care (Exhibit 3). Health care professionals used these standards and guidelines to treat common childhood illnesses. Health care professionals could compare the clinical outcomes associated with their treatment methodologies to the standard approaches used by colleagues in member organizations.

Research: This section provided information about ongoing research projects involving eCHN members. This section also presented the status of clinical trials and other research being undertaken by eCHN members.

Journals: This section provided brief bibliographies of current literature on selected topics in pediatric medicine, surgery and related child health fields. Some of the bibliographies were annotated to indicate the reason the article was chosen and its strengths and limitations.

Parent Education: This section contained parent educational material that could be printed off PROFOR and given to parents and children for their reference after their office or hospital visit (Exhibit 4). Being able to print materials on demand ensured that up-to-date information was available to parents and children at low cost.

Szende knew that physician buy-in was required for PROFOR to be successful. Physicians functioned with considerable autonomy, and their

PROFOR Clinical Practice Standards for Physicians

Management Guidelines for Children Having Tonsillectomy and/or Adenoidectomy on the Same Day Discharge Basis

Tonsillectomy and/or adenoidectomy with the patient being discharged home the same day of surgery may be completed safely. Guidelines for this format of management are not intended to either replace a physician's clinical judgment or to be applied to all patients in a rigid fashion.

A. Eligibility Guidelines

1. Patient greater than two years of age at the time of surgery.
2. Absence of history of bleeding disorder in patient and immediate family.
3. Absence of systemic disease disorder or airway abnormality that increases preoperative risk for the patient.
4. Absence of significant obstructive sleeping disorders.
5. Absence of extended travel time, weather conditions, social/economic factors that will make return of the child to the hospital for possible emergency care difficult.
6. Parent has insight and understanding of recommended surgery and care required in the postoperative periods. Parent has no barrier (i.e., language, no phone) if emergency assistance is required in the home during the first 24 hours following surgery. It is recommended that patients remain in hospital for a minimum of six hours of nursing observation following surgery. Under certain circumstances, it will be appropriate to admit patients for overnight observation.

The following guidelines for discharge or admission are not intended either to replace a physician's clinical judgment or to be applied to all patients in a rigid fashion.

B. Discharge Guidelines

1. Patient able to drink and not vomit.
2. Absence of significant bleeding.*
3. Clinical signs stable and normal.
4. Discharge instructions understood by parent.

C. Admission Guidelines

1. Blood loss during surgery exceeds 5% of blood volume.
2. Significant bleeding during the period of observation following surgery.
3. Patient has vomited more than three times or less than two hours prior to the scheduled discharge time.
4. Patient febrile (>39 degrees Celsius) or abnormal clinical signs.
5. Excessive parental anxiety.

*It is recommended that a child with any evidence of bleeding postoperatively be examined by a physician prior to discharge from hospital.

Source: Company files.

Exhibit 3.   PROFOR Clinical Practice Standards for Physicians.

primary concerns focused around the efficient and effective delivery of high quality patient care. From the physicians' perspective, eCHN's effectiveness rested on its ease of use and the availability of updated, relevant health information. In addition, many physicians felt that the practice of medicine could not be achieved through the standardized protocols and guidelines that PROFOR offered. In contrast, sections such as "Parent Education" and "Presentations" provided physicians with reference material that they could integrate into the way they provided patient care. Szende knew that he would have to sell PROFOR to physicians based on the web site's value as a clinical tool that could be used to improve clinical outcomes and avoid unnecessary health care costs.

Health Data Network

IBM's "Health Data Network" (HDN) system provided health care professionals from eCHN's member organizations with access to children's medical records. Unlike "Your Child's Health" and "PROFOR," the HDN was not connected to the Internet and all information remained private within eCHN. The child's medical history that appeared on the screen looked much like a standard medical file with tabs for lab results, medical imaging reports and other documentation. The information contained in these electronic patient records included laboratory results, doctor's notes, x-rays, visit information and personal information such as addresses and contact persons. The information was presented in the same format regardless of where it originated. Data could be input into the system directly or collected from multiple legacy systems from different institutions and organizations.

The HDN provided eCHN members with instant access to patient records when a patient arrived in their location. Paper files were no longer required to follow a patient from location to location, where the opportunity for loss and misplacement existed. Szende felt that the HDN ensured the security of children's confidential, and sometimes highly sensitive, health information. Szende also felt that the Network's goal to expand membership to include health care organizations other than hospitals made the material available on HDN broader than information on any individual hospital record. Szende also felt that health care providers would have faster access to patient records, and more opportunities for research studies of children's illnesses and treatment.

Szende knew that the HDN site had the potential to generate significant revenue. eCHN's partners agreed upon a membership fee of $150,000 per organization per year. Most of the network's costs were fixed costs associated with the network's maintenance. As a result, Szende figured that the network's costs would be modestly incremental once membership in the

PROFOR Clinical Parent Education Guideline

Croup
Contents:
What is Croup?
Signs and symptoms to watch for
How to help your child get better
Follow-up arrangements

What is Croup?
Croup is a throat infection, caused by a virus that results in swelling and narrowing of the breathing passages. It usually begins quite suddenly and often at night when the child is asleep. The most noticeable symtoms are a barking, seal-like cough and a hoarse voice. Children continue to cough for four to seven days.

Signs and Symptoms to Watch For
1. Breathing
   • some difficulty breathing
   • noise with each breath taken in (stridor)
   • chest indents (caves in) with each breath (indrawing)
   • breathing faster than normal for your child
2. Cough
   • a congested, "barky" or seal-like cough
   • frequent and/or troublesome coughing
3. Behaviour
   • your child is sleepy, lacks energy or your child is cranky, fussy, restless, or crying a great deal (this may be a sign of increasing difficulty in breathing)
4. Drinking
   • your child is not drinking normally, for example less than $\frac{1}{2}$ oz. in 8 hours.

How to Help Your Child Get Better
If the sound of the cough frightens you, remember it is important to remain calm. There are things you can do to help.
   First, try turning on the water in the shower or tub until the bathroom is steamy. Close the bathroom door and sit with your child for about 10 to 15 minutes. You should see a big improvement in your child's breathing during this time but if not, then try taking your child outdoors for the same length of time. In winter, it will be necessary to wrap your child in a warm blanket, but often the cold air is of great benefit.
   Your child should be kept as quiet as possible. Hold your child upright sitting on your knee. When in bed, elevate the head of the bed by placing books or newspapers under the legs of the bed—this helps make breathing easier and helps to lessen the cough while sleeping.
   In winter, when our homes are heated, a cool mist vaporizer is helpful at your child's bedside, while sleeping at night and during daytime naps. Extra humidity is very important to help your child breathe easier.
   Making sure that your child is drinking well will help his/her temperature remain normal. Any increase should be recorded and brought to your doctor's and/or nurse's attention. Keep your child comfortably dressed. If your child is shivering or complains of being cold, add warmth with a sweater. Remove extra clothing if your child becomes too warm.

When Should I Call the Doctor?
Call your child's doctor if you observe any of the following:
   • your child's breathing has not improved after the bathroom steaming and/or the time out in the cold air
   • your child is upset and breathing fast
   • your child is fussing, restless, or more tired than usual
   • your child's chest caves in with each breath
   • breathing is noisy with each breath taken

When Should I Take My Child to the Hospital?
Take your child to the nearest hospital if he or she has any of the following symptoms:
   • is still having difficulty breathing after you have tried the actions described above
   • has a very sore throat and is unable to drink
   • is drooling and unable to swallow his or her saliva*
   • begins to look blue or grey around the lips, toenails or fingernails*

*The last two conditions require immediate attention. Call 9-1-1 if you feel the distress is such that you cannot make it to the hospital without help.

Source: Company files.

Exhibit 4. PROFOR Clinical Parent Education Guidelines.

Network moved beyond 10 institutions. Szende knew, however, that the membership fee would represent a significant portion of the operating budgets of many community hospitals, long-term care agencies and rural health facilities. These were the facilities that Szende hoped the Network would eventually include. The administrators in these facilities needed to be convinced of HDN's value. Value for them would be defined as an improved quality of patient care and ability to avoid the health care costs associated with the unnecessary duplication of laboratory and diagnostic tests. Szende knew, however, that the administrators' definitions of "value" were not always aligned with the physicians' or patients' perspectives of value.

Szende also knew that hospitals and other health care facilities in Ontario were at various stages in implementing new or updating existing information technology (IT) systems. Although the HDN could easily interface with many different legacy systems, many hospitals would have to modify their existing systems if they wanted to become Network members. These IT costs were not included with the $150,000 eCHN registration fee. In addition, Szende wanted to expand eCHN's membership to include physicians' offices, community hospitals, homecare organizations and teaching hospitals. Unfortunately, less than 10 per cent of physicians had electronic charts, and there was no real economic incentive for them to do so. Szende felt that the current membership fee and IT requirements might prove to be prohibitively expensive for some of the health care organizations he hoped eCHN would expand to include. Szende was also uncertain how quickly it would take for HDN expansion to occur.

eCHN'S STRATEGIC CHALLENGES

Szende knew that the eCHN could be an integral part of Ontario's health care system. He did not want the Network to be viewed as a luxury item tailored to physicians' ongoing professional development. Rather, he felt that eCHN would play a key role in allowing hospitals to avoid unnecessary health care costs, and in improving patients' access to high quality, efficient health care. Szende knew that he would have to present a strategy that would allow him to achieve buy-in from health care administrators, physicians and the public.

Szende also knew that there were many ways in which eCHN could grow both in the scope of its membership (i.e., hospitals, physicians' offices, and long-term care facilities) and the geographic locations of its member organizations. At the same time, although Szende wanted to ensure that this growth was financially profitable, he did not want the current membership fee to limit access to the Network to only those organizations that could afford to pay this fee. He, therefore, felt that the membership fee might have to be changed to make the Network accessible to a wider range of health care organizations.

In addition, Szende knew that eCHN's current governance would have to change to reflect the Network's growth. For example, HSC was a major partner in eCHN and Szende wondered if this arrangement should last as the Network grew. Szende knew that he needed to determine the most appropriate structure and composition for eCHN's board of directors. In addition, he needed to identify performance measures that would determine whether eCHN's mission and strategic goals were being met. Szende also knew that the board's structure would have to ensure representation, participation and collaboration with the medical staff of eCHN's member organizations.

As Szende prepared for eCHN's upcoming board of directors' meeting in September, he knew that he needed to present the board with a clear plan that outlined his strategy for eCHN's growth. More specifically, he knew that the board would want to know who eCHN's "customers" were, how Szende planned to access them and achieve buy-in, who would be paying for access to eCHN's services, and how he would price eCHN's services. Szende also knew that the board would want to know if and how he planned to expand eCHN's scope of its membership and the Network's geographic reach. As Szende reviewed a recent consultant's report, he knew that he had the next 90 days to prepare his own strategy for eCHN's growth.

APPENDIX

Andrew Szende

Prior to joining the eCHN, Andrew Szende, CEO of the eCHN, was a management consultant specializing in health services. Szende facilitated the creation of the Rouge Valley Health System, considered by professionals in the health care industry to be one of the HSRC's restructuring success stories. He also worked for other hospitals, the Ontario Hospital Association, and the HSRC. Szende was formerly an assistant deputy minister and head of the Health Economic Development in the Ministry of Health. In addition, he served as the associate secretary of the Ontario Cabinet and the province's chief economic and trade representative in Asia. He obtained a bachelor of arts degree from the University of Toronto and a master of social science from the National University of Singapore.

5

Caregivers

Randi Priluck
Pace University, New York, New York

Beginning in 1997, Caregivers, a nonprofit agency that provides care to patients in need, faced a series of cutbacks in state funding that led to a deficit in its budget. The CEO of the agency, Don Arnold, was concerned that Caregivers would be unable to continue its mission of caring for older adults in need if the agency did not find a way to raise revenue.

In March 1998, Arnold set up the New Business Group to explore ways for the agency to convert some of the services that it currently offered for free to a profit-based system for those who could afford to pay. Included in the group, which met every Tuesday at 9:30 A.M., were Arnold, Beverly Slater (chief operating officer), Roslyn Warner (director of marketing mid-development), Gilda Newburgh (director of housing), Colleen Confit (marketing manager), Pamela Tilden (housing manager), and Emily Furley (social services manager).

Used by permission from *2000 Annual Advances in Business Cases*, the Society for Case Research (SCR). All rights reserved to the author and SCR. Copyright © 2001 by Randi Priluck.

This case was prepared by Randi Priluck of Pace University, New York, and is intended to be used as a basis for class discussion. The views represented here are those of the author and do not necessarily reflect the views of the Society for Case Research. The author's views are based on her own professional judgments. The names of the organizations, individuals, and locations have been disguised to preserve the organizations' request for anonymity.

69

A number of new business areas were explored. It was critical for Caregivers to assess the potential of these areas of business, set goals and objectives, and implement a plan of action. The expenses for the agency were divided among three basic areas: home care, housing, and social services (see Table 1).

Staff within the organization did not fully support top management's efforts to require clients to pay for services. This was particularly true of social workers. Social workers were trained as advocates of people in need and did not recognize the difference between a client in need and one who could pay for services. They often did not recommend Caregivers to their clients for home-care services; they would recommend lower-priced alternatives instead.

THE ORGANIZATION

Caregivers' mission was to care for the needy in instances when they could not care for themselves. The agency operated exclusively in the Boston metropolitan area and offered a variety of services related to the mission. One main focus of the agency's effort was caring for the elderly, and this area was expected to grow because of the aging population in the United States (see Table 2). By 2040, more than 20% of the U.S. population will be 65 years of age or older.

Table 1. Caregivers agency budgeted revenue and expenses ($ in thousands)

	Amount	%
Revenue		
Social services	$31,037	58
Home care	13,882	26
Housing	5,807	11
Philanthropic	2,342	4
Total	$53,068	
Expenses		
Home care	$41,630	78
Housing	8,084	15
Social services	3,350	6
Total	$53,064	

Source: Caregivers Strategic Plan, 1998.

Table 2. Population by age (in thousands)

Year	Age 65–74		Age 75–84		Age 85+	
	Number	%	Number	%	Number	%
1990	18,045	7.3	10,012	4.0	3,021	1.2
2000	18,551	6.7	12,438	4.5	4,333	1.6
2010	20,978	7.0	13,157	4.4	5,969	2.0
2020	30,910	9.5	15,480	4.7	6,959	2.1
2030	37,984	10.9	23,348	6.7	8,843	2.5
2040	33,968	9.1	29,206	7.9	13,840	3.7
2050	34,628	8.8	26,588	6.8	18,893	4.8

Source: U.S. Bureau of Census, 1993, 2000–2050 projected data, middle-series assumptions.

DIVISIONS

The agency consisted of three divisions: Home Care, Housing, and Social Services. Each of the divisions operated independently with its own budget. The director of home care was responsible for both licensed and certified home-care programs as well as private-pay home care. The housing director ran senior centers and residences for older adults, and the director of social services managed the programs for the older adults in need.

Home Care

The Home Care division was a licensed home health care agency. It trained home health aides, homemakers, and housekeepers and placed them in positions. Home health aides were specially trained to assist older clients with personal care such as bathing, dressing, and toileting. They also served as companions for their older clients. Homemakers were trained to act as caregivers for children in the homes of incapacitated parents. Housekeepers cleaned and performed other household tasks for people incapable of doing so.

Within the Home Care division, services were provided through government contracts and Visiting Nurse Services (VNS), which billed Medicare or Medicaid. Alternatively, Caregivers billed the client directly, a payment system known as "private pay," which served about 10% of the home care business. Nationally, the private pay home-care market was smaller than the Medicare and Medicaid home care markets (see Table 3). Because Caregivers was a licensed agency, not a certified agency, it could not bill Medicare or Medicaid directly for services. Therefore, Caregivers

Table 3.   National home-care market

Home-care market agency receipts	1997
Medicare	65.2%
Medicaid	9.6%
Private pay*	7.0%
Private insurance	6.6%
HMOs, PPOs, state and local government, and bad debt	11.6%

Source: Standard and Poor's industry surveys, 1997.

*The National Home Care Association places the private-pay market at 30%.

had to align itself with a certified home health care agency that could bill in this manner (as did VNS).

In 1996, Caregivers had entered into a strategic alliance with VNS to provide home health aides in eastern Massachusetts exclusively, and by 1998 the VNS business represented 90% of the home health aides dispatched. Because approximately 26% of the agency's revenues were generated by VNS contracts, the agency was highly committed to this business and was very careful not to jeopardize it. One issue was whether, and to what extent, Caregivers could compete with VNS, particularly in Brookline, Massachusetts, where Caregivers did contract work for VNS. Some staff members of the agency were very concerned about attempting to increase private-pay services while trying to maintain VNS contacts.

Housing

Caregivers operated five buildings in Framingham, Massachusetts (a town 30 minutes from downtown Boston), which altogether housed 1,000 older adults. Most of the buildings offered subsidized housing, and only one of the buildings, known as F3, rented at market value. Residents were charged $800 for one-bedroom apartments that had a very basic decor. In addition, Caregivers operated a senior center two blocks from F3 that served 7,000 older adults and provided many services, including a social program and meals. As of July 1998, 14 units were vacant in F3, and Gilda Newburgh had devised a plan to provide assisted living in those 14 units. Assisted living is a care plan for elderly residents that includes three meals daily, day and evening social programs, personal care, and medication management. The cost to the resident for assisted living was $3,000 a month. Attempts to use promotional efforts to fill vacancies in F3 at market value had been limited prior to the decision to provide assisted living.

Social Services

The Social Services division was primarily responsible for the care of individuals in need. The division managed a number of programs. The Community Guardian program assisted people who did not have families to care for them. A Caregivers social worker acted as the person's guardian in legal and care matters. There was also a Case Management program, which helped individuals who needed assistance with their care but did not require total guardianship. Finally, the Financial Management program assisted clients with paying their bills.

Social Services also managed Elderlink, an information and referral database that contained information on a variety of eldercare services in the Boston area, including home health care, senior centers, meal programs, assisted-living facilities, and nursing homes. Elderlink was part of a national network of information providers that was used by Statler Referral, a firm that provided the employees of Fortune 500 companies with a national system of information and referral on aging. Employees of these firms could call a national number and be connected directly to Caregivers' Elderlink service. A Caregivers social worker would provide information to help the employee care for an elderly relative in the Boston area. Referrals from Statler, however, had been dwindling lately.

ALTERNATIVE PLANS OF ACTION

The New Business Group consisted of managers from each of the three divisions: Housing, Social Services, and Home Care. Through a series of brainstorming sessions, the New Business Group identified a number of potential businesses that would build on Caregivers' skills in the three divisional areas. However, the managers were unsure how to allocate resources among their ideas and which businesses were the most viable. They chose three areas to explore more fully: real estate development, real estate property management, and private-pay home care.

Real Estate Development

The New Business Group proposed the development of a 200-unit assisted-living facility somewhere in the Boston area and determined the costs for providing services to such a facility (see Table 4). Though Caregivers did not have any expertise in real estate development, top management felt that its expertise in providing services and its nonprofit status would attract a developer who needed Caregivers' assistance with the particulars of providing assisted-living services to the elderly. As of July 1998, top management had met with a few developers, but Caregivers was not

Table 4.   Service Costs for Assisted-Living Facilities of
100 and 200 Units

Cost Category	100 Units	200 Units
Food	$ 547,500	$1,095,000
Linens	100,000	200,000
Household supplies	54,750	109,500
Recreational supplies	15,000	30,000
Office supplies	6,000	9,000
Printing, duplication	6,000	9,000
Postage	24,000	48,000
Telephone	15,000	30,000
Marketing materials	50,000	75,000
Contracts machines	10,000	10,000
Transportation	68,000	68,000
Emergency response system	100,000	200,000
Consultants	36,500	54,750
Insurance, professional	35,000	40,000
Legal	20,000	20,000
Audits	20,000	20,000
Information services	47,758	72,419
Human resources	95,517	144,839
Finance	98,928	150,012
Administration	98,928	150,912
Management	252,000	504,000
Total	$1,700,881	$3,039,532

Source: Caregivers internal documents, 1998.

happy with the quality of the sites and did not feel comfortable lending the
Caregivers name to a poorly located facility.

Real Estate Property Management

The New Business Group determined that older inner-city residents
would not be likely to leave their apartments as they aged because many of
the day-to-day maintenance issues in a rental unit, co-op, or condominium
were handled by the building management. Caregivers' management,
however, saw an opportunity to market eldercare services to building managers who had large percentages of elderly residents in their buildings.
The marketing department began to identify buildings built prior to 1965

in the Boston area with 300 or more apartments. Letters and brochures were sent to building managers emphasizing the dangers of leaving older residents without care. For instance, an older person might leave the gas stove on and start a fire, hoard garbage in the early stages of dementia, or forget to pay maintenance fees. On the phone, many managers expressed interest in the problem. They felt that they could use some assistance with their older residents but did not see spending up front to avoid potential accidents. They felt that caring for older adults was the responsibility of the family. A few meetings were set up with larger complexes, but in such instances, co-op and condo boards were reluctant to spend money on this matter.

The New Business Group developed the Property Management program, which consisted of two services: an on-site model and a consultation model. The on-site model was designed for large buildings (more than 400 total residents) with at least 30% of elderly residents. Caregivers would conduct a survey to determine where the elderly residents lived and would then place on the premises a part-time social worker who would provide social programs and assistance to the elderly residents. The social worker would also intervene in difficult cases and assist building employees in identifying problem situations. The price would be $2,800 per month for the building. The consultation model provided many of the same services, but operated out of Caregivers' offices and did not include a part-time social worker on the premises. The price would be $1,000 a month.

Private-Pay Home Care

Private-pay home care clients pay for their own home care rather than relying on Medicare or Medicaid for payment. Caregivers' license allowed the agency to provide home health aides to those who could afford to pay out of pocket for the service.

In July 1998, the exact size of the private-pay market in the Boston area was unknown, but national information on older adults with disabilities was available (see Table 5), as was information on the older population in the Boston area (see Table 6).

Competition was intense in the private-pay home care market. One important competitor was the "gray market" for home care services. Since home care services for older adults were often an ongoing expense, many adult children chose to hire home care workers who were untrained and did not demand that their employers pay Social Security tax. Aside from the gray market, a number of other agencies competed for the private-pay business (see Table 7).

The New Business Group discussed their concerns regarding how to furnish home health aides under a private-pay system, when Caregivers

Table 5. Percent of elderly with functional limitations

Functional Limitation	Age 75–84	Age 85+
Walking	18.8	34.9
Getting outside	22.3	44.8
Bathing or showering	11.3	30.6
Transferring	11.6	21.9
Dressing	7.0	16.1
Toileting	5.7	14.2
Average	23.5	40.4

Source: U.S. Bureau of the Census, Survey of Income and Program Participation, Functional Limitations and Disability File, 1991, non-institutional persons.

also provided aides through VNS. As of July 1998, most of Caregivers' aides were working under VNS contracts and could not be switched to a private-pay case. Caregivers' management considered not pursuing the private-pay market because of the fear of losing the VNS contract. They also considered pursuing private-pay in areas that VNS did not serve.

The target market for home care services is the elderly population 75 years and older with one or more difficulties in the activities of daily living and incomes higher than $35,000 per year.

The New Business Group discovered some difficulties in marketing the private-pay home care business. First, home health aides were paid $6.50 an

Table 6. Older adults by income, selected Massachusetts counties

Income	Age 75–84	Age 85+
Under $5,000	11,013	13,938
$5,000–$9,999	32,477	49,706
$10,000–$14,999	24,539	24,354
$15,000–$24,999	39,353	25,708
$25,000–$34,999	28,410	14,670
$35,000–$49,999	26,546	11,009
$50,000–$74,999	22,294	8,549
$75,000–$99,999	8,746	3,055
$100,000+	8,286	2,823

Source: U.S. Bureau of the Census: Norfolk, Suffolk, Middlesex, Bristol, Essex, and Plymouth counties.

Table 7. Competitor data

Home care agencies	Number of private-pay cases	Weekday rate per hour
U.S. Home Care	400	$15.00
All Metro	150	$13.75
Caring Hand	150	$9.50
Allen	100	$14.00
COHME	100	$14.00
Select	100	N/A
Partners in Care	100+	$14.00

Source: 1998 Caregivers competitor survey, completed in-house.

hour, which did not provide much incentive for them to deliver exceptional service. Second, there were no home health aides available exclusively for private-pay cases, and sometimes an aide could not be found to service a particular case. Finally, most of the clients wanted service in the morning from 9 A.M. to 12 noon, but aides were often already working on morning jobs and only had afternoon hours available. Not only were clients not able to receive care when they wanted it, but aides did not receive a full day's worth of hours and often got only morning work.

There were, however, some positive aspects of Caregivers' services that would appeal to the target market. Caregivers always sent a nurse to a client's home to assess the case prior to dispatching an aide (this was a requirement under its license). Caregivers also provided health and drug screening of aides, background checks, and training. If an aide was sick or unable to provide service on a particular day, a replacement was sent. A 24-hour telephone assistance line was available for home health aides to call in emergencies.

Caregivers charged an individual client $12.75 an hour for home care services during the week and $14 an hour for weekend service. The gray-market rate was between $9 and $11 an hour for care. The New Business Group determined that Caregivers earned 75 cents of profit on every hour of care they delivered. In other words, it cost $12 an hour to provide service to clients during the week and Caregivers charged $12.75. The median number of hours per case was 20.

Caregivers had also identified a number of possible niche markets within the larger home care market:

- *Specialty diseases:* The niche of specialty diseases was considered because people with certain diseases require a significant amount of care. Though aides were already trained to provide Alzheimer's care, other diseases would require additional training.

- *Skilled nursing:* Skilled nursing was another potential niche market. Pursuing this market would require that Caregivers hire more nurses and obtain a special license to offer such services in order to be able to bill Medicare and Medicaid directly. The size of that market was substantial, as shown in Table 3.

- *Difficult cases:* Over time, Caregivers had developed a reputation for being able to handle difficult cases. These cases, which had been rejected by other agencies because the client was disruptive and disrespectful to the aide, often ended up at Caregivers. Caregivers was better able to handle such cases because of the special training that was provided by the agency and the support that the aides received from the home office. However, it was more expensive to service a difficult case because it required more managerial time to arrange for proper care.

- *Long distance:* Another possible niche market was the long-distance market, which consisted of adult children who lived more than an hour's drive from Boston but who had an elderly relative to care for in the Boston area. It was believed that adult children who were not available to care for a parent would be a better target market because they would need to purchase more home care hours to make sure that the parent was well cared for. They might also be willing to pay a premium for such services. Though the actual size of the long-distance market was unknown, the number of adults over the age of 75 living in the Boston area was more than 300,000.

CONCLUSION

With the fall approaching and a board meeting scheduled for early October, Don Arnold needed to nail down a plan of action for the agency. He looked at the data on the home care market, considered developing an assisted living facility, and thought about bringing services to existing buildings. Which would be the most profitable enterprise to pursue, and how could that be done without alienating VNS or staff members?

6

Merck's Crixivan

Kimberly A. Rucker
Health Care Consultant, Washington, D.C.

Kurt Darr
The George Washington University, Washington, D.C.

ORGANIZATIONAL BACKGROUND

Merck & Co., Inc., is a research-driven pharmaceutical products and services company headquartered in Whitehouse Station, New Jersey. Merck's activities can be broken down into the following four major product groups that are aimed toward improving human and animal health:

Research—Discovery and development of human and animal health products at eight major research centers in the United States, Europe, and Japan.

Manufacturing—Chemical processing, drug formulation, and packaging operations are carried out in 31 plants in the United States, Europe, Central and South America, the Far East, and the Pacific Rim.

Product marketing—Products are sold in the United States, Europe, Central and South America, the Middle East, the Far East, and the Pacific Rim.

Services marketing—The Merck-Medco Managed Care Division manages pharmacy benefits for more than 65 million Americans, encouraging the appropriate use of medicines and providing disease-management programs.

Merck's mission statement[1] reads as follows:

"The mission of Merck is to provide society with superior products and services—innovations and solutions that improve the quality of life and satisfy customer needs—to provide employees with meaningful work and advancement opportunities and investors with a superior rate of return."

In addition, Merck states that it embraces the following values:

- Preservation and improvement of human life

- Commitment to the highest standards of ethics and integrity

- Dedication to the highest level of scientific excellence and commitment of their research to improving human and animal health and the quality of life

- Expectation of profits, but only from work that satisfies customer needs and benefits humanity

- Recognition that the ability to excel—to most competitively meet society's and customers' needs—depends on the integrity, knowledge, imagination, skill, diversity, and teamwork of employees, and we value these qualities most highly

George W. Merck, the company's founder is quoted as saying, "We try never to forget that medicine is for the people. It is not for the profits. The profits follow, and if we have remembered that, they have never failed to appear."[2] In 2000, Merck booked $6.822 billion in net income.[3]

THE SITUATION

The History

Merck had spent several years and several hundred million dollars to develop an acquired immunodeficiency syndrome (AIDS) drug called Crixivan, a promising treatment for HIV infection in adults when antiretroviral therapy is warranted. "It's the largest research and manufacturing project we've ever undertaken," said Raymond Gilmartin, Merck's chairman and chief executive.[4] AIDS was first diagnosed in 1981 in the United States among homosexual men. HIV, the virus that causes AIDS, was later identified in 1983. AIDS is late-stage HIV infection. The overwhelming majority of HIV-infected individuals eventually develop AIDS. Individuals with AIDS have severely weakened immune systems that can no longer defend against opportunistic infections and cancers. Deterioration of the immune system is the reason for most deaths associated with AIDS.

Merck began its search for an antiretroviral therapy in 1986, but several years elapsed before it discovered indinavir sulfate, the active ingredient in Crixivan. During those years, Merck experienced several setbacks, none of which was as devastating as the death of Irving Segal, Merck's leading scientific investigator on the project, who died in the bombing of Pan Am flight 103 in 1988. Yet the project continued and indinavir sulfate was discovered in 1992. By 1995, Crixivan's clinical trials had progressed to Phase III. Completing Phase III clinical trials is the last step required by the Food and Drug Administration (FDA) prior to requesting approval for a drug's public distribution. In January of 1996, Merck's Emilio Emini presented some of the initial data from Phase III studies on protocol 035 at the Third Conference on Retroviruses and Opportunistic Infections. Protocol 035 showed that Crixivan alone caused HIV levels to drop to undetectable levels in four out of nine (44%) patients after 6 months of treatment. When Crixivan was combined with AZT and 3TC (two previously discovered, less effective anti-HIV drugs), the percentage of patients with undetectable blood HIV levels was even more dramatic. Patients receiving the triple-combination therapy displayed undetectable virus levels in 86% of the cases (six out of seven patients), nearly doubling the effectiveness of the drug. These results marked the first instance where an AIDS drug was shown to decrease the level of HIV to such an extent that it was undetectable. Never before had such promising AIDS treatment data been presented. The drug marked a breakthrough in AIDS treatment.

Crixivan's success was an enormous relief to Merck's management. Two months prior to obtaining the approval to begin Phase III trials, and before knowing with certainty that the drug would be successful, Merck's management team had taken an immense risk by beginning expansion efforts on two facilities that would be entirely dedicated to the production of Crixivan. Management was therefore elated when the drug passed successfully through Phase III clinical trials. The company could now obtain approval to begin distribution of Crixivan under the FDA's accelerated approval process. The approval came just 42 days after Merck submitted the FDA application and was the fastest approval in FDA history. After obtaining approval, Merck was eager to begin Crixivan sales, and the company was sure that the public would respond positively to the introduction of the drug that could extend so many lives.

The Competition

AZT and 3TC were the antiviral predecessors to Crixivan and the group of anti-HIV drugs that emerged in the mid-1990s. AZT in combination with 3TC was an effective drug therapy for its time. However, the class of drugs known as protease inhibitors, of which Crixivan is one, is much more potent. By the time Merck obtained FDA approval, Crixivan was one of three protease inhibitors approved by the FDA and available to the public. Merck's competitors, Abbott Laboratories and Roche Holding, LTD, produced the other two drugs, Invirase and Norvir, respectively. All three drugs interrupt the HIV virus's life cycle. Crixivan had an advantage over the other two drugs in that Crixivan was considered more potent than Invirase and had less severe side effects than Norvir.

Because the FDA's approval to distribute Crixivan was 6 months earlier than its executives expected, Merck was still months away from having production plants ready to produce the drug at levels that would satisfy demand. Yet, the competitive pressure was mounting since both Invirase and Norvir were already on the market. Crixivan's clear advantages in potency and decreased side effects would not be enough to gain a substantial foothold in the market if the competing drugs had a significant lead time in their distribution to the public. Merck felt it essential to introduce Crixivan as soon as possible and was committed to introducing the drug closely following Invirase and Norvir. Merck's limited production capability, however, would prove difficult to overcome.

The AIDS Epidemic: The Number of Patients to Potentially Benefit from Crixivan

Based on information from the Joint United Nations Program on HIV/AIDS, the number of new HIV infections worldwide in 1996 was 3.1 million and the number of people living with HIV/AIDS was 22.6 million.[5] It was estimated that from the start of the epidemic until 1996, 1.0 to 1.5 million cumulative HIV infections had occurred in North America. At the time, HIV infection was one of the major causes of death for individuals between the ages of 25 and 44. Among men in this age group, it was the leading cause of death in the U.S. In 1994, HIV infection was the third leading cause of death among 25- to 44-year-old women in the U.S., with an additional estimated 12,000 children living with the virus. The characteristics of those infected with HIV were also changing. AIDS cases related to heterosexual contact represented an increasing proportion of newly diagnosed cases in North America. The Centers for Disease Control and Prevention estimated that there were more than 1 million Americans who were HIV-positive, and could thus benefit from taking the medication.[6]

With such a large number of persons requiring drug treatment for AIDS, there would be a high demand for Crixivan once it was learned that the drug could substantially extend life without the high dosage and adverse side effects associated with the other two drugs on the market. High demand for the drug would pose a difficult problem for Merck on many levels. The difficulties were due to the limited production capacity and the medically disastrous consequences that could result if Crixivan patients could not continue their treatments due to limited supply.

Production Capacity

Crixivan is a difficult drug to mass-produce because of its complicated molecular structure. Whereas most Merck pharmaceuticals are made in about four steps over 2 weeks, Crixivan requires a 6-week process that entails 15 steps. Seventy-seven pounds of 30 raw materials are needed to produce just 2.2 pounds of the drug, which is only enough to supply one patient for 1 year.[7] The huge quantities of Crixivan that would be required to meet patient demand made matters worse. Patients are required to take six 400-milligram pills a day, in combination with other AIDS drugs to achieve the desired reduction of HIV in the blood. Due to the above factors, the supply of Crixivan would be temporarily very limited. Initially, Merck could only produce enough Crixivan to treat 25,000 to 30,000 patients. Yet thousands more would be likely to demand the drug because of its efficaciousness.

Due to the lack of available capacity, Merck could have outsourced the manufacturing of the drug to other companies. However, Merck had earlier decided to use its own plants in order to control quality. On previous occasions, for less complicated drugs, Merck had outsourced drug production and was displeased with the quality. The company feared the outcome if it used an outsourced supplier for its most complex production activities to date.

FDA's Conditions

Due to the drug's limited availability, the FDA made its approval of Crixivan contingent on Merck's ability to monitor how Crixivan was supplied or made available to AIDS patients. This requirement was added as a result of the serious consequences if patients discontinued taking the drug or took fewer than the 2.4 grams a day as prescribed. "If therapy is discontinued, the virus will likely re-emerge, perhaps in a form resistant to the drug.... Then the drug will be useless to the patient.... Worse, that raises the risk that a drug-resistant strain could cross over into the general population," said a researcher at the Aaron Diamond AIDS Research Center in New York.[8]

Selection of the Distributor: Stadtlanders Pharmacy

To quell the concerns surrounding the serious consequences that could result from interrupted drug treatment, Merck assured the FDA it would take precautions to monitor supply and ensure that an adequate volume of the drug was available to treat patients who started the Crixivan regimen. To guarantee an adequate supply for those who started Crixivan, the majority of prescriptions were to be channeled through a single distributor, a major mail-order seller named Stadtlanders. In the spring of 1996, Merck spokesperson Jan Weiner explained that the limited distribution was a temporary measure: "We intend to use Stadtlanders as a primary distribution outlet until we have adequate supplies. ...We believe we will have adequate supplies in the fall."[9] Once full production was achieved, Crixivan would be available through retail pharmacies, wholesalers, and other sources.

Stadtlanders Pharmacy (formerly Stadtlanders Drug Distribution) provides mail-order pharmaceuticals for customers with special needs, including those with HIV and AIDS or with organ transplants or those undergoing fertility treatments who need assistance in complying with drug regimens. Stadtlanders' services include customer monitoring and counseling and working with insurance plans and assistance programs to help customers with paperwork and billing.[10] Based on Stadtlanders highly specialized services in providing drugs to high-risk patients and the tailored services that the pharmacy could provide AIDS patients, it was decided that Merck's limited production volume would be monitored primarily through Stadtlanders. Also a limited amount of Crixivan would be sold to the Department of Veterans Affairs hospitals and some managed-care organizations that Merck determined would track and control the number of patients on the drug.

Merck executives reportedly agonized over the decision of how to distribute Crixivan. One of the alternatives considered was holding back the drug until the plants could reach full production. However, in light of the pressure from AIDS activists to provide the drug to HIV-positive patients as soon as possible in addition to the competitive pressures from Abbott and Roche Holding, that option was not pursued.

Nor could Merck pursue a broader distribution system. A broader distribution might have led to a disruption in patients' drug schedules. In coming to the decision to use a single distributor, Merck officials sought a distribution system that would allow the company to control the number of patients who started the drug and guarantee refills for them. Merck representative Michael Watts explained the reasoning behind the selected distribution strategy: "We selected to go through a single distributor on a temporary basis because the drug is so difficult to make. With a limited supply to work with, Merck needed to make sure that people who began the therapy had a sufficient supply." Watts added, "Going through one distributor is not just a matter of tracking who's on it...but [in addition], we can track the amount of drug we have."[11] Merck made the decision to use a single distributor in an effort to monitor the number of patients on the drug in the most efficient, effective, and controlled manner.

In effect, however, Stadtlanders Pharmacy would be given a temporary virtual monopoly since it was the only pharmacy permitted to distribute the drug. Those interested in obtaining Crixivan were required to register with Stadtlanders, or had to belong to one of the few VA hospitals or managed-care organizations that had obtained distribution rights. Stadtlanders, being the primary distributor of the drug, was responsible for controlling the number of new patients when there was not enough Crixivan to maintain current patients.

Pricing of Crixivan

When Crixivan was introduced, pharmaceutical prices were already a hotly debated issue. The Working Group on Pharmaceuticals and National Health Care Reform, an independent committee of academics, advocates, and policy makers, had pushed for government controls on pharmaceutical pricing. The group acknowledged that research and development costs could not be ignored, but that the pharmaceutical industry as a whole was too profit-oriented when lives were at stake. The pharmaceutical industry is one of the nation's largest profit makers. According to *Fortune 500* listings, it was the most profitable industry every year from 1988 to 1994.[12] It had been ranked as first or second most profitable in 30 of the last 38 years. Merck alone enjoyed a net income of more than $3 billion in 1995, up 11% from the previous year.[13] The rate of return on equity in the same year was 14%.[14] According to a 1994 United Kingdom Department of Health study, drug prices through much of Europe averaged 4%–78% lower than in the United States.[15]

Analysts believed that Crixivan could generate half a billion dollars or more in annual sales in a few years, but Merck initially priced the drug far lower than the industry expected. Crixivan was 24% less than Invirase and 33% below Norvir. A Merck spokesman said the price was set to be "competitive, to facilitate access, and to assure usage of the product."[16] Jules Levin, who directs the National AIDS Treatment Advocacy Project in New York, praised Merck for its pricing of the drug saying, "Merck has done a very humane thing with the price it's charging."[17]

Stadtlanders, however, was imposing a 37% mark-up on the price of the drug to consumers. Stadtlanders paid Merck $365 for a patient's 1-month supply of Crixivan that had a list price of $501.88. Stadtlanders stated that its actual profit was closer to 14% because most customers received discounts under various health plans. Stadtlanders claimed that the profit from Crixivan would be further decreased because it had to hire 400 additional employees to monitor distribution of Crixivan. However, AIDS activists were angered by the fact that non–health plan patients were required to pay the full retail price. Merck's lawyers determined that negotiating a price with Stadtlanders or pressuring it to lower its price would be vertical price fixing, because the producer and the distributor involved in the sale of the product negotiated its price. This is a *per se* violation of Section 1 of the Sherman Anti-Trust law, which deems every "contract, combination in the form of trust or otherwise, or conspiracy, in restraint of trade or commerce... illegal."[18]

Uncompensated Care Provisions

Merck's philosophy is that its overall business mission is to enhance health. Merck has stated that it believes that an essential component of its corporate responsibility is to provide support to charitable organizations that benefit society.[19] In keeping with its corporate philosophy, Merck developed a patient assistance program called SUPPORT™ that specifically assisted patients who needed Crixivan and provided free Crixivan to those who were unable to pay for it if certain conditions pertaining to third-party payers were met as described below. Merck realized the difficulty that many patients had in identifying and securing drug coverage, and therefore wanted to help find resources to pay for Crixivan. Using a toll-free number, physicians and their patients could obtain assistance on many levels. The SUPPORT™ program assisted insured patients in obtaining maximum reimbursement for Crixivan and assisted uninsured patients in locating and applying for alternate coverage sources. Program counselors were assigned to individual cases and provided the following services:

- Answered questions regarding insurers' policies, regardless of whether one had private insurance, was part of an HMO, or had insurance through public programs, such as Medicaid or AIDS Drug Assistance Programs (ADAPs)

- Assisted patients in identifying and applying for alternate insurance coverage for Crixivan

- Assisted physicians, their patients, and patients' families with the application process for patient assistance

- Arranged for eligible patients to have Crixivan sent to the prescribing physician's office

- Assisted physicians with billing, claim form completion, and coding for Crixivan

- Worked with physicians or patients to resolve specific issues related to payment, reimbursement, or claims denials for Crixivan

For patients with no alternate insurance, the program could provide Crixivan at no cost when medically indicated and certain conditions were met such as having an income of less than $20,000 per year. In addition, Merck planned to offer Crixivan free of charge to those who had participated in most of its Phase II and one of its Phase III studies.

There were, however, limitations to the SUPPORT™ program. Merck had implemented a policy which stipulated that if a state ADAP or private insurance company chose not to cover Crixivan, Merck would block all patients in that state's ADAP or insurance program from entering its patient assistance program, regardless of financial need. Merck believed that otherwise payers would refuse to pay for Crixivan because Merck would pick up the costs for people who could not pay out-of-pocket.

The Public Outcry

Merck believed that it had acted in good faith to make decisions that would benefit Crixivan users and, accordingly, had developed a fair and comprehensive distribution plan. During the early years of Crixivan's development, Merck had built what it thought was a strong, positive relationship with AIDS activists. A community advisory board was created to keep the AIDS community informed on the drug's development process and, after receiving increasing pressure from the AIDS activist community, Merck created a compassionate use program that was implemented to allow access to Crixivan to patients who were dying. In addition, Merck had cooperated with AIDS activists when they accused Merck of conducting the Crixivan development process too slowly. Merck responded by allowing an independent drug-manufacturing consultant to evaluate Merck's production efforts. The consultant later reported to AIDS activists that Merck was doing all it could to make the drug ready for public consumption. Despite Merck's efforts, the company has received a great deal of bad press.

Distribution and Pricing

Once Merck's plan to distribute Crixivan primarily through Stadtlanders was known, AIDS activists called for public protests against Merck and Stadtlanders. A spokesman for a prominent AIDS activist group said that it has made the restricted distribution of Crixivan one of its "target issues" in its meetings with legislators and with the Federal Trade Commission. The group is seeking to have a provision added to the FDA reform bill that ensures that all FDA-approved drugs will be available to all licensed pharmacies in the United States.[20] The group is calling for a review of the Crixivan distribution system and an investigation as to why the FDA approved it and how the Crixivan approval was obtained so quickly.

The National Alliance for the Restoration of Democracy (NARD) called the decision to distribute the drug through a single distribution agent "anticompetitive," "ill-conceived," "ludicrous," and "cynical and preposterous." NARD's president has asked Merck to dismantle the program and to immediately open the distribution of Crixivan to all community pharmacies that wish to dispense it.[21] NARD's president feels that if Merck wanted to encourage accountability, it could have set out clinical guidelines as was done for other drugs that require limited distribution. Yet, Merck feels that there is a critical difference between the two situations; in earlier cases of limited drug supply, having continuous drug treatment was not as crucial.

Furthermore, AIDS activists and pharmacists accused Stadtlanders of using its virtual monopoly to price-gouge AIDS patients. Kate Krauss, the spokesperson for the AIDS activist group ACT UP Golden Gate, commented, "We want to send a message to Merck, Hoffman La Roche and Abbott that price gouging is unacceptable....Boycotting Stadtlanders, which survives because of the goodwill of the AIDS community, would be easy for us to do."[22] The group accused Stadtlanders of imposing a 37% mark-up on the drug when the average profit on drugs sold in pharmacies is 15%. Moreover, local pharmacies feel that Stadtlanders has an unfair advantage in that it has a mailing list of HIV-infected patients that it can use for direct marketing. As noted, Stadtlanders acknowledged that Crixivan is marked up 37%, but added that most patients would not pay full price because they had discounts under various health plans.

To a lesser extent, Merck is also receiving criticism for its decision to prevent entry into its indigent-patient program if a person's insurance plan or state ADAP program won't pay for Crixivan. Opponents feel that it is unfair to block entry into the program on this basis regardless of a person's financial need. Many believe that this policy prevents the already vulnerable HIV-positive population from obtaining a drug that could extend their lives. Patients are caught between Merck and health care payer organizations that are disputing who should pay for drug treatment.

The accusation that the limited distribution system is in violation of anti-trust law seems unfair to both Merck and Stadtlanders. Some AIDS activists agree. Martin Delaney, founding director of the AIDS activist group Project Inform, defended Merck by saying that "People should understand that the reason they [Merck] did it this way was a patient-oriented one: to guarantee that no patient would be cut off. Everyone agrees there had to be some tracking method. I don't know if this was the only way to do it or not."[23] Merck has received similar support from other AIDS activists who say that the company is trying to be responsible. Negative press has been more prevalent, however.

Pharmacist/Patient Relationship

Merck is being accused of insensitivity to how heavily AIDS patients rely on their local pharmacists to counsel them about taking their medicines properly and to provide allowances for price breaks when patients have financial problems. The editor and publisher of the *Journal of the International Association of Physicians in AIDS Care* stated that AIDS patients "rely on their pharmacists as much as they rely on their doctors. Merck wasn't sensitive to this at all."[24] Critics do not believe that a single, mail-order pharmacy across the country can provide the same amount of support that neighborhood pharmacies provide. Yet, in Merck's opinion, that view is untrue.

As to the accusation that Merck has not been sensitive to the needs of AIDS patients for a relationship with their local pharmacists, none of the critics seems to mention that Stadtlanders is unique in providing specialized support services to its customers. Stadtlanders specifically provides mail-order pharmaceuticals for customers with special needs, including those with HIV and AIDS. Although a mail-order pharmacy, Stadtlanders provides support that caters to the needs of HIV/AIDS patients by providing medical counseling as well as assistance with financial issues. Stadtlanders' mission is to be a partner in the successful management of high-risk disease.

In addition, AIDS activists feel that not enough information is being provided to the public about Crixivan and its dosage requirements. This accusation is particularly distressing to Merck because its publications department has written the literature about the drug, but the documents must be approved by the FDA and have been delayed by the approval process. The literature gives specific instructions on usage of the drug and how it can be accessed.

Retail Pharmacy Industry

Retail pharmacists are fearful that pharmaceutical companies that grant exclusive distribution rights to single pharmacies could be the beginning of a trend that threatens them. Pharmacists are particularly wary of drug chains that obtain exclusive rights to AIDS drugs because the profit that can be obtained on HIV-inhibiting drugs is substantially greater than most other common drugs sold by pharmacies. In response to the limited distribution of Crixivan, pharmacy trade groups have initiated a letter-writing campaign to federal regulators and have begun lobbying Congress to prohibit pharmaceutical companies from being able to restrict drug distribution. Lobbyists argue that exclusive distributorship agreements are unlawful if they decrease competition and do not include other pro-competitive justifications.

NEXT STEPS

Merck's mission and vision statements seem to prohibit the actions of which the company is accused. Its philosophy includes the following:

- Merck's mission is to provide innovations and solutions that improve the quality of life and satisfy customer needs.

- Merck is committed to the highest standards of ethics and integrity. "In discharging our responsibilities, we do not take professional or ethical shortcuts. Our interactions with all segments of society must reflect the high standards we profess."

- Merck has an expectation to make profits, but only from work that satisfies customer needs and benefits humanity.

Merck cannot believe that such a public outcry has erupted over a temporary measure that will last only until Merck's plants are able to produce sufficient supplies of Crixivan. Merck has called an emergency meeting of the board to discuss how it should handle the situation.

ASSIGNMENT

You are the CEO and have been asked to brief the board on the situation by summarizing the facts, giving your opinion as to how the public relations debacle should be handled, and providing suggestions as to what should be the company's next steps. In addition, although the public relations dilemma is the most immediate problem, consideration must be paid to other issues such as:

- Addressing the board's concern over public policy changes that may result from this controversy and that may influence the manner in which drugs are introduced to the public

- Deciding whether changes should be made to the decision-making process when introducing drug products to the public in the future to avoid the problems that resulted from this situation

- Identifying other countervailing groups that may find fault with the way in which Merck conducts business in an attempt to proactively address the potential concerns that those groups may raise

REFERENCES

AIDS Activists/Merck-4-: HMOs could negotiate lower cost. (1996, April 11). Message posted to *Dow Jones News Service*.

AIDS Activists/Merck-2-: Stadtlanders main distributor. (1996, April 11). Message posted to *Dow Jones News Service*.

A Program of Reimbursement Support and Patient Assistance Services. Retrieved from http://www.crixivan.com/indinavir_sulfate/crixivan/consumer/patient_ resources/support.jsp.

Barnett, A.A. (1996). Protease inhibitors fly through FDA. *The Lancet, 347,* 678.

Breu, J. (1996). AIDS drug distribution eases—By a crack. *Drug Topics, 140*(9), 30.

Breu, J. (1996). R.Ph.s steamed over AIDS drug's limited distribution. *Drug Topics, 140*(8), 32.

Gottschalk, K. (1996). Protease inhibitors—The cost of AIDS drugs. *Consumer News, 1*(5). Retrieved September 1, 2001 from http://cidronline.com/cnews_/healthcare/9605.html.

James, J.S. (1996, April 5). *Indinavir (Crixivan®) access and distribution.* Posted to http://www.immunet.org/immunet/atn.nsf/page/a–244–03.

MacPherson, K., & Silverman, E.R. (1996, February 27). Business makers chase profits in quest for AIDS drug. *The Plain Dealer,* p. 4C.

Tanouye, E. (1997, November 5). Medicine: Success of AIDS drug has Merck fighting to keep up the pace. Posted to http://www.pulitzer.org/year/1997/national-reporting/works/6.html.

Tanouye, E., & Waldholz, M. Pharmaceuticals: Merck's marketing of an AIDS drug draws fire. (1996, May 7). *The Wall Street Journal,* p. B1.

Womack, A. AIDS activists may boycott pharmacy over sale of Merck product. (1996, April 11). Posted to *Dow Jones News Service.*

ENDNOTES

1. Merck's corporate web site. 01 September 2001 http://www.merck.com/about/mission.html.
2. Merck's corporate web site. 01 September 2001 http://www.merck.com/about/cr/.
3. Merck's corporate web site. 01 September 2001 http://www.anrpt2000.com/financialhighlights.htm.
4. MacPherson, K., & Silverman, E.R. "Business makers chase profits in quest for AIDS drug." *The Plain Dealer.* 27 February 1996, 4C.
5. HIV/AIDS Global Epidemic Fact sheet. Online Posting. Retrieved 1 September 2001: http://www.unaids.org/publications/documents/epidemiology/estimates/situat96kme.html
6. Womack, Anita. "AIDS activists may boycott pharmacy over sale of Merck product." *Dow Jones News Service.* 11 April 1996.
7. Tanouye, Elyse. "Medicine: Success of AIDS drug has Merck fighting to keep up the pace." Online posting. 5 November 1997. The Pulitzer Board. 1 September 2001 http://www.pulitzer.org/year/1997/nationalreporting/works/6.html.
8. Tanouye, Elyse and Michael Waldholz. "Pharmaceuticals: Merck's marketing of an AIDS drug draws fire." *The Wall Street Journal.* 07 May 1996, B1.
9. "AIDS Activists/Merck-2-: Stadtlanders main distributor." *Dow Jones News Service.* 11 April 1996.
10. Stadtlanders Pharmacy Profile. 21 September 2001. The Industry Standard. http://www.thestandard.com/companies/dossier/0,1922,264504,00.html
11. Gottschalk, Kurt. "Protease inhibitors—The cost of AIDS drugs." *Consumer News.* 1.5 (1996). Retrieved 1 September 2001 http://cidronline.com/cnews_/healthcare/9605.html.
12. Ibid.
13. Ibid.

14. Merck's corporate web site—1997 Financial Highlights: http://merck.com/ overview/97ar/p3.htm.
15. Gottschalk, 1.
16. Waldholz, Michael. "Merck's newly approved AIDS drug is priced 30% below rival medicine." *The Wall Street Journal.* 15 March 1996, B5.
17. *Ibid*
18. Greenberg, Warren, *The Health Care Marketplace* (New York: Springer-Verlag, 1998) 103.
19. Merck's corporate web site. 01 September 2001 http://www.merck.com/ overview/philanthropy/13.htm.
20. Breu, Joe. "AIDS drug distribution eases—By a crack." *Drug Topics.* 140.9 (1996): 30.
21. Breu, Joe. "R.Ph.s Steamed Over AIDS Drug's Limited Distribution." *Drug Topics.* 140.8 (1996): 32.
22. "AIDS Activists/Merck -2-: Stadtlanders Main Distributor." 1996.
23. "AIDS Activists/Merck -4-: HMOs Could Negotiate Lower Cost." *Dow Jones News Service.* 11 April 1996.
24. Tanouye, et al., B1.

PART II

Administration, Medical Staff, and Governing Body

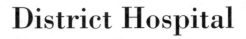

District Hospital

A Lesson in Governance

Cynthia Levin
Kaiser Permanente Medical Group

Kurt Darr
The George Washington University, Washington, D.C.

HISTORY

Barclay Memorial Hospital (BMH) has enjoyed a reputation for excellent medical care in an affluent community for more than 50 years. In the mid-1940s the community was mainly agricultural, but it was becoming urbanized. Hospitals in the area were operating at capacity. Community members and physicians proposed a solution: Form a hospital district that would be supported by the community through a tax. Voters approved the district in 1945 by a 5-to-1 margin. Its first decision was the selection of a 15-acre construction site. In 1947, the voters approved a $7.3 million bond issue to finance construction and operation of a 300-bed hospital. The tax district spans seven townships that elect five district community members to a governing board for the district hospital's four entities, which include the hospital, a joint venture operating an urgent-care center, and a hospice, and the hospital foundation.

THE PHO

About 10 years ago, the district hospital board and the CEO devised a strategic plan to form a physician–hospital organization (PHO) with Valley Physician Group (VPG). VPG was formed in 1951 when a group of physicians agreed that they could provide better care to their patients by sharing resources and ideas. Over the years, VPG expanded as more physicians and physician groups joined. Currently, VPG is composed of more than 140 physicians in 28 medical specialties and subspecialties. VPG provides services to 325,000 patients and delivers 2,500 babies each year. It employs 600 full-time equivalent (FTE) staff, and enjoys gross revenue of $120 million.

Joining with VPG to form a PHO required that BMH change its legal classification from a public (governmental) hospital to a private, not-for-profit hospital. The new governing board was responsible for the PHO, which included the Barclay Hospital and the VPG. Within 2 years, it became apparent that the PHO was going bankrupt because of poor management and a lack of focused leadership. In-fighting among VPG and non-VPG physicians began as the hospital deteriorated financially and employee morale plummeted. With the help of consultant Gregory Schilling, the district board, which had not disbanded, fought against the PHO's governing board and successfully brought the hospital back under the district's control. As a tax district (governmental) hospital, BMH has several advantages: it is a public hospital and a political subdivision of the state, which gives it certain legal advantages; board members are elected by voters in the tax district; financial surpluses are put back into the hospital; and it has authority to levy a tax on homeowners in the district. Schilling was asked to become the new CEO immediately following the dissolution of the PHO (see Exhibit 1).

MARKET POSITION

Currently, BMH is licensed for 400 beds, but last year operated only 275 beds with an average daily census of 249 patients. This number reflects a decrease in volumes in many service lines. Discharges totaled 26,731. The average length of stay for all inpatients was 3.4 days. This has increased somewhat due to changes in the law allowing new mothers to stay in the hospital longer than 24 hours for normal deliveries. Deliveries last year were at an all-time high with 3,216 and will most likely increase because BMH is the desirable maternity hospital in the area. The nurses are particularly attentive and the nursing units have only private, newly renovated patient rooms. Outpatient visits totaled 232,363, which should continue to

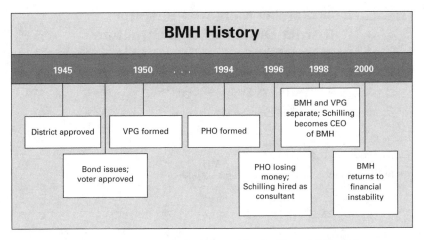

Exhibit 1. Timeline of major events in the history of Barclay Memorial Hospital.

rise as technology allows for less invasive treatments. Surgeries totaled 6,201. Projections show a potential for increases in occupancy if more surgeons admit at BMH and the processes for delivery of services become more efficient, which, in turn, would make them more profitable. Transplant surgery, however, should be generating more revenue. Orthopedics is another service that could be expanded; it has only 60% of the estimated market. Total full-time and part-time employees were 2,705, giving the hospital a higher than average FTE ratio compared to other hospitals in the area, which, in turn, is reflected in the high percentage of revenue used for salaries and benefits. There are 654 physicians on staff, reflecting a decade-long downward trend. The number of hospital volunteers also has decreased from 804 last year. The operating budget was $200 million for the last fiscal year. Managing to budget has been difficult. A hiring freeze mid-year showed some positive results, but after three months some nursing departments were concerned that nurse–patient ratios were too low (see Exhibit 2).

THE DISTRICT BOARD

The BMH district board has five members that are elected by residents in the district to serve three-year terms. The CEO is hired by the district board and is a voting member of the board. The chairman of the district board, Dr. Larry Harvey, is an orthopedic surgeon with privileges at the hospital. His responsibility and authority within the hospital have raised

Barclay Memorial Hospital
District Organizational Structure

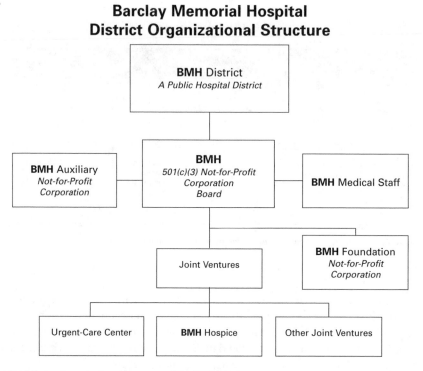

Exhibit 2.   Organizational structure of the BMH District.

questions of conflicts of interest. He used this power to disregard requests from the operating room supervisor that he arrive on time for his cases. His patients waited unnecessarily for their procedures; highly paid staff were also idle. Harvey threatened to have the orthopedic surgery department manager fired because she tried to control excessive use of supplies and pressed him to keep to his schedule. According to the estimates of demand shown in marketing reports, the orthopedic surgery service should be producing a profit; instead, it has continued to lose money. When the subject was broached by Schilling, Harvey threatened to admit his patients to a competing hospital. He would often become emotional in meetings, accusing Schilling of yelling at him. Eventually, Harvey stopped returning Schilling's phone calls. Compounding these problems was Harvey's difficulty in separating his anger about health care reimbursement reductions and the hospital's rocky relationship with the VPG physicians from his work in the hospital.

Dr. Ray Brandon is also an orthopedic surgeon. Brandon was on the district board during the PHO, where he took a more introverted role.

During a closed-door meeting of the board, however, he did not hide his animosity towards the VPG physicians who formed the PHO with the hospital. He is also frustrated about health care reimbursement. Symptoms of the breakdown in communications with the CEO were also becoming apparent with Brandon. Occasionally, Brandon appeared to disregard state law that applied to tax-district hospitals and their governance. The law requires that two or more board members of a district hospital must discuss hospital issues only in a public meeting. Meetings where proprietary information is discussed are exempt from the state's "open meetings" requirement. At one orthopedic surgery committee meeting, he spoke privately with Harvey, for example. On another occasion, in a board meeting where proprietary matters were being discussed, Brandon wanted to legally challenge physicians who refused to take ER call. He was frustrated about the breakdown in the relationship between physicians and hospital governance. After the open board meeting which followed, Brandon pulled aside the hospital legal counsel and asked him to research taking legal action against the physicians who refused to take ER call. Schilling had advised all board members to approach this issue more diplomatically and not attract media attention. Schilling undertook a more politically acceptable solution by gathering benchmarking data from surrounding hospitals and offering to pay on-call physicians the average of the market. Physician groups were then asked to bid for taking ER call.

Dr. Karl Pearl, a neurologist with privileges at the hospital, is the third district board member who was on the district board during the years of the PHO. He is the board member who was most bitter about how VPG "ruined" the PHO, and he publicly criticized them. Pearl's resentment toward the decrease in health care reimbursement is a topic he often pontificates on at board meetings. Like the other physician board members, his clinical privileges at the hospital have been perceived as a conflict of interest. He has publicly criticized the large size of the management staff. The CEO took this as a personal affront and a blow to morale.

The fourth member of the board is also a clinician. Aaron Travis is an osteopath with privileges at a competing community hospital. He respects Schilling and accepts his advice. Travis boasts of "saving" the hospital during the PHO by asking "a few simple questions" about the hospital's performance that, at the time, nobody could answer. This led to other questions and the eventual financial turnaround of the hospital. Unfortunately, Travis has his own limitations that affect his ability to be an effective district board member. He is openly angry about his experiences during the PHO when his car was vandalized and he received threatening phone calls.

The fifth board member, Stephanie Stewart, is a businesswoman in the community. She has a lot of respect for Schilling and is willing to work with him. Stewart had a difficult time grasping the complexity of the hospital's operations and its finances when she first became a board member. The reality that what the hospital charges for services is not what the hospital is paid was an illogical way to do business in her mind. She wants to be a team member and at times becomes frustrated with the physician members' negativism. She and Travis have often asked the physician board members to "move on from the past."

THE NEW CEO

Three of the five district board seats were up for election. Before the November elections, the board asked Schilling to become the new CEO. Schilling was the former CEO of a not-for-profit hospital and had spent his entire 45-year professional career as a hospital administrator. Schilling has a history of back problems. When he arrived on the job, however, he appeared to be in good health. He was originally hired by the district board to help the hospital dissolve its relationship with the physician group in the PHO. He successfully returned the hospital to district control. He eliminated the hospital's $2 million per month deficit. The number of FTEs had been decreased to very low levels during the affiliation with the PHO. Although this kept expenses for salaries and benefits to a low percentage of hospital revenue, Schilling wanted to increase morale by hiring more staff, reinstating salary increases, and providing better benefits to the employees. He also began to put resources back into the hospital by making desperately needed upgrades to the facility. These changes greatly increased employee trust and respect for Schilling and his warmth and caring attitude toward his employees helped him gain their loyalty.

LEADERSHIP STYLE

The board members, physicians, and employees gave Schilling accolades for returning the hospital to profitability. Schilling's leadership style, however, was quickly criticized when later financial projections showed a $24 million loss for the next year. The physicians described his leadership style as patriarchal and paternalistic. The physicians, nurses, and managers were accustomed to a culture of teamwork that had been supported and fostered by the former CEO. Schilling became frustrated when his authority was questioned, not only by the medical staff and nurses but also his own executive team. Schilling actually felt his team was sophomoric. Most were good at taking direction from him and his COO, but they felt that the absence of a strategic plan impeded their ability to focus on a common goal. Schilling delegated the authority to run all executive team meetings to his COO, Daniel Porter. Porter was not well respected by the team because of his authoritarian leadership style and his lack of listening skills. The dynamic in the executive meetings would either break down into arguing or nobody would contribute ideas. A lack of leadership was becoming apparent throughout the organization.

LOSING SUPPORT

By increasing morale, renovating the facility, and bringing in some of his own executive team, Schilling was able to stabilize BMH. A strategic plan had been developed and presented to the hospital board. Schilling's approach to keeping the strategic plan confidential until it was ready to be launched, however, made many of the management, physicians, and hospital staff uneasy. Unfortunately, because of the politics involved when physicians felt that their turf was threatened, it was impossible to increase market-driven, revenue generating services. Orthopedic and open-heart surgery were two such services. When pressed to expand the orthopedic surgery service by recruiting new surgeons, the physicians threatened to go to neighboring hospitals. The orthopedic surgeons had been there for many years and were comfortable with the department's current status. Added to the equation was the physician board members' reluctance to make enemies. The PHO experience had left a bitter taste in the board members' mouths; they appeared to be paralyzed by past events. Schilling began to lose support.

The board criticized even highly successful decisions made by the CEO. The last major decision the board made at his recommendation was to get out of risk pool agreements with the insurance companies. Schilling presented two options to the district board: increase revenue or decrease expenses. The board had agreed to decrease expenses by renegotiating the hospital's insurance contracts, but later claimed Schilling waited too long to present this information to the board. In fact, Schilling had been trying to persuade the board to get out of risk pool agreements for more than 2 years.

A TROUBLED PHYSICIAN

The vice chief of staff, Clara Mavory, M.D., was a practicing anesthesiologist during this time. She was praised for her commitment to BMH's survival as a freestanding facility. Mavory had helped lure Schilling from a neighboring hospital to help bring the hospital back to district ownership. Mavory had a troubled history with VPG; she was asked to leave the VPG after being disciplined for disruptive behavior seven years prior to establishing her own medical practice. A year after Schilling became CEO, Mavory began to demand confidential files, including legal records and peer review files. Mavory disagreed with many sections of the medical staff bylaws and recommended revisions. This caused a slowdown in preparation for the Joint Commission on Accreditation of Healthcare Organizations (Joint Commission) survey because the quality department had to refocus its energy on legal counsel's approval of the revisions. The Joint Commission requires all bylaws changes to be in place a year before a survey. When Mavory did not receive all the confidential files she demanded, she criticized Schilling publicly and began to persuade other physicians to distrust his administration. She had done the same thing to the prior administration.

The board members began to feel bullied by Mavory. The three physician board members with hospital privileges disagreed with Mavory's demands, but found it easier to acquiesce. A peer review file on Mavory's clinical performance prepared by the quality department showed several instances of questionable clinical judgment. Also in this file were complaints about Mavory's inappropriate behavior toward patients and hospital staff. Schilling had felt protective as a friend and obligated to Mavory for his position as CEO at BMH. Although her peer review file had gone to a peer review committee, no disciplinary action had been taken against her. Schilling kept her file locked away in a file in the clinical quality department's office. According to the hospital's attorneys, the only way to remove a physician's privileges is to substantiate evidence of poor-quality medical practice in accordance with the medical staff bylaws.

Schilling later realized how critical the information in her peer review file could have been in stopping Mavory from causing a rift between the medical staff and the administration. The file still existed and could be acted upon. Because his relationship with Mavory had become adversarial, however, reporting Mavory might have appeared vindictive considering the time lapse from when the events originally occurred. Schilling's only recourse had been to persuade the board to support him in blocking her demands for confidential information. Over the last year, however, Schilling received no support from the board in disciplining Mavory on her behavior towards the hospital staff. Schilling's numerous attempts to telephone Harvey had been futile. Harvey would not return his calls.

Schilling also wrote memoranda to all the board members when Mavory demanded information. These memoranda often included responses to Mavory and explanations to the board as to why certain information was confidential or not appropriate for Mavory to see. Schilling's weekly memoranda went unanswered by all of the board members. Verbal communications had become infrequent and were limited to the board meetings. Harvey, along with the other board members, felt Schilling was not healthy enough to continue in his role as CEO. Their attitude toward his health clouded their ability to trust Schilling's decision making. They also preferred to ignore Mavory instead of dealing with her. As fellow clinicians, the four physicians on the board felt obliged not to criticize Mavory.

REORGANIZING THE BOARD

Schilling trusted his intuition and 45 years of experience as he tried to make better use of two board members who still supported his ideas and remained loyal to his leadership. He developed a plan to organize the board into subcommittees to better use the support of these two board members to sell ideas to the other three members. The subcommittees included strategic planning, finance, emergency room on-call coverage (which was a short-term commitment), and governance. The membership on each subcommittee consisted of two board members, the CEO and other designated administrative staff. The proposal for the new subcommittees was presented at an evening public board meeting and passed unanimously by the board. This restructuring was the first step towards solving the communication problems and increasing the level of trust the other three board members had in him.

SUCCESSION PLANNING

Schilling's contract was to end next fall. Should he retire or should he seek to renew his contract? As much as he did not want to admit it, his health was deteriorating and maintaining relationships that were in turmoil was becoming too demanding. Major surgery relieved a back condition but his general health improved only minimally. Schilling had succeeded in what he had been hired to do—getting the hospital back into district control and stabilizing the organization. Continued success depended on regaining support from his board and the trust of the medical staff. After adding staff and upgrading the facility, however, the hospital's expenses now exceeded revenues. Financial projections showed that the hospital would soon repeat history by losing $2 million a month. Patient volumes were very low in most services. Nursing ratios were high, but the culture of the organization demanded lower patient ratios in return for not increasing salaries, a compromise that a strong in-house nursing union supported.

Unfortunately, almost all of the board members were less interested in following the CEO's advice to improve the numbers because they no longer believed that he knew what he was doing. As the date for his contract renewal loomed closer, employees, too, began to question Schilling's continuation as their leader. Morale declined further as employees began to fear the instability of a possible change in leadership at the hospital. Employees feared that a for-profit hospital system would buy the hospital. This would completely change the culture of the BMH, and possibly cause lay-offs. During the PHO period, employees had been laid off, salaries frozen, and benefits cut. The employees did not want that to happen again. The local branch of a statewide union brought in their leadership to organize the nonnursing employees after receiving a phone call from a BMH employee. The nurses and facility engineers were already unionized. Schilling did not have the motivation to stop the infiltration of the union, which could ultimately unionize all hospital employees.

CHIEF OF STAFF

Mavory was elected vice chief of staff after successfully running against several opponents. The medical staff bylaws provided that the vice chief of staff would automatically become chief of staff if the election was uncontested. Mavory had stated that she would refuse to take the salary usually paid to the chief of staff because she considered it a conflict of interest. As the election drew near, her only opponent withdrew after she confronted him by telling him that his candidacy was causing a rift in the medical staff. His withdrawal made an election unnecessary and Mavory became chief of the medical staff.

In response to Mavory's criticism of Schilling's power over the board, Schilling recommended that the hospital change its bylaws to make the CEO a nonvoting member. As Schilling's presence waned due to health problems, Mavory requested that the hospital board make her a voting member because she was chief of staff. This action would require a change in the hospital and medical staff bylaws. The board members did not act on her request.

TERMINATION FROM VPG

Seven years ago Mavory had been forced out of VPG because of disruptive behavior. This appeared to be the only possible motivation Schilling could think of for Mavory to make enemies of the VPG physicians by publicly attacking them in the medical staff's newsletter and at the medical staff executive meetings. This group was 50% of the hospital's physicians and they were essential to its continued financial health. Schilling thought her disruptive behavior would wane if she were not confronted. He hoped that by ignoring her behavior Mavory would lose her audience. Unfortunately, this did not prove to be the case. On a weekly—and sometimes daily—basis, she would demand access to computer files, legal correspondence between the medical staff office employees and the hospital attorney, and files on malpractice cases. Mavory demanded the right to attend confidential department meetings and verbally abused physicians who disagreed with her. She constantly tried to pit the medical staff against administration. She appeared to want the physicians to become a unionized bargaining unit.

OBSTRUCTING PREPARATION FOR JOINT COMMISSION

In one meeting that focused on Joint Commission preparation, Mavory demanded a change in an organizational diagram that showed the flow in communications throughout the hospital. During the last Joint Commission visit the surveyors had actually praised the hospital on this excellent tool for representation of how all hospitals should expedite communications through the layers of bureaucracy. Mavory felt that the chart appeared to show the medical staff reporting to the CEO.

As soon as she became chief of staff, Mavory tried to dissolve the medical executive committee and change most of the membership of the physician committees. She wanted most representatives of administration removed even if they served as support staff to the committees. These would be violations of the medical staff bylaws and could compromise the Joint Commission accreditation survey only six months away. The only Type 1 violation the hospital had received in the previous survey was the medical staff's failure to comply with its own bylaws. Mavory wanted the vice president of quality, Harold Fredrick, removed from all meetings and eventually fired. Mavory said she did not like Fredrick because they had a personality conflict. Mavory thwarted changes to many policies and procedures that also were reviewed and approved by the medical executive committee. She added and removed appointments to joint medical staff and administrative committees and stalled bylaws revisions for months and even as long as a year. According to the VP of quality, this jeopardized Joint Commission accreditation because all approvals by the Medical Staff Chiefs' Committee (MSCC) that must also be approved by the board should be in place for at least a year before a Joint Commission survey (see Exhibit 3). The manager of the medical staff office quit, citing high levels of stress over the last year.

Mavory made it clear to all hospital employees and physicians that she was everyone's boss. When the copy room informed her that she could no

REMOVAL OF COMMITTEE MEMBERS
....A committee member appointed by the chief of staff may be removed by a two-thirds vote of the Medical Staff Chiefs' Committee. A committee member appointed by the department chief may be removed by a two-thirds vote of the department medical staff membership or the Medical Staff Chiefs' Committee...

Exhibit 3.   Proposed medical staff bylaws provision thwarted by Dr. Mavory.

longer make personal copies at the hospital's expense, she told one of the mail room supervisors, "Do you know who I am? I am the most powerful physician in the hospital. I am your boss. You will do as I say!"

COMPENSATION FOR ER ON-CALL PANEL

It appeared that Mavory searched for issues or problems to pit physicians against administration. Knowing that physicians were demanding pay for being ER on-call, she coached one plastic surgeon to take this issue to the MSCC to be discussed. When some members of the MSCC asked the plastic surgeon for benchmarking data on what other hospitals are paying for ER on-call physicians, the physician claimed he was "too busy" to conduct research on this issue. The plastic surgery group became the most frustrated with not being paid for being on-call in the ER. They gave the administration a deadline to begin on-call payments that the hospital could not meet. None of the physicians would agree to do research or benchmark how much other hospitals were paying physicians for on-call service. Some board members wanted to report some of the physicians to the state authorities for writing an ultimatum to administration saying they would refuse to take call. Patients not seen in the ER because there were too few physicians would have to be transported to other hospitals. Some board members were concerned that this could be a violation of the Emergency Medical Treatment and Active Labor Act, which could become very expensive in fines for the hospital and bad public relations. Administration thought this was unlikely, however. The two board members on the on-call subcommittee came to the MSCC meeting to show their willingness to resolve the issue and to get feedback from the physicians as to what they believed the solution to be. They were well received by the physicians attending this meeting after the board members encouraged the physicians to help find solutions to the problem. Ultimately, the CEO proposed a solution that was accepted by the physicians. Physicians would be paid $300.00 for carrying an ER pager; physicians called in to the ER would be paid $1,000.00 per 8-hour shift.

NO STRATEGIC PLAN IMPLEMENTED

The board would not sell or close the money-losing cancer unit because the physicians providing that service might take their other patients to a competing hospital. They also were worried that these VPG doctors would become wealthy because of the financial arrangement. Schilling believed that the board was uneasy about a change in the hospital's services. After the PHO, they seemed reluctant to cut services that could possibly make even one hospital physician angry or add services that could make one of them "wealthy."

Dr. Mavory's replacement as vice chief of staff was the secretary/treasurer of the medical staff, Dr. Barry Landon. He was the only open-heart surgeon at BMH. This violated state law requiring hospitals performing open-heart procedures to have a two-surgeon team. When the director of strategic planning, Kelly Nelson, approached Landon about recruiting another cardiovascular surgeon, Landon wanted to have her fired. Landon felt threatened by Nelson's recommendation. He wanted full control over the open-heart surgery. Mavory supported Landon in efforts to remove Nelson, calling her "no good."

SCHILLING'S RESIGNATION

Schilling decided to resign. He did not want to be blamed for the demise of the hospital and felt responsible for solving its financial problems. His attempts to rebuild his relationship with his board and the chief of staff, however, seemed futile. He did not have the energy because of his poor physical health to strengthen his relationship with employees, managers, and physicians. Schilling agreed to stay until the district board hired a consultant as the interim CEO.

CONSULTANT HIRED

Jena Carson agreed to take the interim CEO position. Carson's 20 years of experience as a "turnaround" expert made her an obvious choice. She had many decisions to make in her new role. How would she approach improving the financial position of the hospital? How would she approach increasing patient volumes? Could she use the old strategic plan or would she need to develop a new one? Would the board support her decisions? Could she stop other hospital employees from unionizing? How could she control the chief of staff's divisiveness? Could she focus the organization on completing its preparation for the Joint Commission? How would she manage her board members and executive team into becoming effective leaders to assist her in turning the hospital around and perhaps making the hospital a market leader? Most important, what priority should be assigned to these problems?

8

The Day After

Richard L. Johnson
Physician Management Resources, Inc.,
Clarendon Hills, Illinois

Charlie Jones opened his eyes and looked at the clock, which stood at 7:40 A.M., then gazed up at the ceiling asking himself if he had just had a nightmare or if he really had been—terminated... let go... fired... relieved of his administrative responsibilities—whatever it was that Russell Adams, the board chairman, had said to him at 8:13 P.M. last night. It was then he had been informed that his services as the chief executive of Riley Memorial Hospital were no longer needed.

Automatically, after 23 years as the chief executive, his thoughts turned to the hospital. For the first time in more than 2 decades he realized that his day's activities no longer included the hospital, but were concerned with what he wanted to do for Charlie Jones. Getting out of bed, he realized that he could dress leisurely this morning and not have to hurry to get to work—there was, for him, no work to go to.

As he adjusted the hot water faucet in the shower, he began to ask himself why this had happened. Mentally reviewing various aspects of the hospital operation, he knew that the cost at Riley per patient day was next to the lowest of the seven hospitals in the area, so productivity was not a factor. The physical plant certainly was in A-1 condition. During the past

Adapted and reprinted with permission from "The Day After," by Richard L. Johnson, in *Hospital & Health Services Administration*, 30, no. 6 (November/December 1989): 106–117.

4 years, $3.5 million had been spent on bringing the mechanical and electrical systems up to date, and he had paid for those improvements out of operating surpluses. No board member, that he could recall, had ever taken exception to this.

Certainly he and the board had been concerned that the average occupancy had fallen to the mid-60s in the last 18 months. This had forced the hospital to lay off 134 people to keep the hospital from going into the red. That had caused some problems with a few trustees; several physicians had gone to them and complained about the closing of two specialized nursing units and the commingling of their patients with those on the general medical and surgical floors. On balance, he concluded that the board had understood the necessity for taking these steps and that there had been general support for doing so.

As he stepped out of the shower, he directed his thoughts toward his relationships with the board and the medical staff and asked himself how the two had changed. What immediately came to mind was his inability to control the number of matters of importance that he had had to bring to the board. Because of the speed with which matters were changing in the external environment, he had lost the ability to time decision making with the pace at which the board could comfortably handle the items.

As he dressed, he realized that his greatest concern about the governing board was its lack of understanding of the medical staff and individual physician relationships to the hospital. He had known for well over a year that this was the most likely arena to give him problems. As the surplus of physicians had grown, coupled with the downturn in use of physicians and hospitals by the public, he had watched the medical staff become fearful of their economic futures. He had been particularly surprised by some of the older, well-established practitioners, who had been telling him that they had been experiencing a downturn in the number of patients they were seeing. He had instinctively known that this would inevitably lead to difficulties with these physicians because the hospital would be economically forced to compete for revenues on the same turf as the physicians on the medical staff. What bothered him the most was that he had seen this conflict coming, had tried to prepare the governing board for dealing with this kind of situation, but had had little success because of resistance from the four physicians on the governing board.

Pausing to look out the window, he let his eyes follow the path of the youngsters on their way to school as he recalled the difficulties he had encountered in a recent board meeting when he had attempted to review a proposed contract submitted by a health maintenance organization. Rather than reviewing the contract, as he had expected, the physicians had taken the position that the hospital's responsibility was to be supportive of private practitioners engaged in fee-for-service medicine and that the hospital should not be a party to any payment scheme that deviated from what was already in place. He remembered thinking, at the time, that the four physician board members probably regarded his actions as the first step in an attempt to take over the medical staff. After the board meeting, he had walked with the board chairman out to the parking lot, where they talked for almost an hour about what had happened, and the chairman had assured him that he knew those physicians and that they could be counted on to keep the hospital's needs and interests above those of the medical staff. Although he only half-believed what Russell Adams said, Charlie mentally conceded that this might indeed be true, given time and the changing events going on in the hospital field.

Charlie sat down to breakfast, staring out of the window, lost in thought. Thinking back over the last 6 months, he began to appreciate that his naming of Bill Handy as chief operating officer and turning over all of the internal operations to him, an action that had been fully endorsed by the board, had really never been understood or accepted by many of the physicians. They considered Charlie's role to consist primarily of serving the interests of the medical staff. The fact that he had little familiarity with the parking problem of physicians, which had surfaced at a general medical staff meeting, had led to comments being made in the corridors by physicians that Charlie Jones really didn't care whether Riley Memorial had a medical staff or not.

As he finished his cup of coffee, Charlie thought about the straw that broke the camel's back. All too vividly the events of the last 3 weeks rushed through his mind. On Monday, 3 weeks ago, Bill Handy told Charlie that he had received a call from a local real estate broker, with whom he was friendly, stating that the hospital's three radiologists had purchased a 2-acre site across the street from the hospital and were planning to build an ambulatory imaging center. Hearing this, Charlie had reached into a file drawer in his desk and quickly scanned the hospital's contract with the radiologists. Although there was no provision preventing them from investing in this kind of activity, the contract did specify that their full-time professional services were to be devoted to the hospital. The contract further specified that only the chief executive of the hospital could make any exceptions.

Armed with the contract, Charlie had gone to the radiology department and looked up Dr. Ralph Kemper, the chief, whom he'd known for the last 15 years. Sitting in Ralph's office drinking coffee together, he had asked him about the broker's information. Dr. Kemper, without hesitation, said that it was true, that they had the schematics in hand from the architect, and had a preliminary understanding with the largest local bank about a loan. When Charlie asked about the hospital's contract, Ralph indicated that the three radiologists had agreed they would not divert ambulatory patients from using the hospital and went on to add that the three planned to staff it on their days off and bring in one additional radiologist, who would be completing his residency in 3 months. They did not plan on bringing him into their partnership that served the hospital but planned to employ him by the new company, "Imaging Center, Inc.," the vehicle they'd created to undertake this venture.

Charlie finished his cup of coffee and left Ralph's office with a sinking feeling in the pit of his stomach that the wheels were now set in motion for a confrontation that could not be avoided. He knew that the three radiologists were regarded by their colleagues as the best in the city, and that any attempt made by the hospital to enforce its contract with them would create a real storm with the entire medical staff. Yet, to do nothing would lead to a significant loss in revenue; in spite of the assurances of the radiologists, it was clear that building an imaging center across the street from the hospital was no coincidence. Charlie knew he was caught in the middle without any workable alternatives. He remembered he had listed possibilities in his mind:

- Go along and do nothing.

- Threaten to terminate their contract.

- Have the board hold a session with them.

- Bring it up at the joint conference committee meeting.

- Find an alternative radiology group and give notice of cancellation of contract.

As he had mulled over the list, Charlie realized that the board would be willing to hold a meeting with the radiologists, but when the chips were down they would not force the issue. Instead, they somehow would expect the hospital management to develop a program that would compensate for lost revenues. At that point Charlie had smiled to himself; the safest way out for him was to make no waves and get along by going along. If he followed the course, it would be about 3 years before the impact would be felt in the financial statement of the hospital; in the meantime he could look around for another CEO position at his leisure and be out long before the hospital faced serious financial problems. He quickly rejected this notion, saying to himself that this was not in the hospital's best interests, yet he knew that he would be exposed if he took any other course. Although he hadn't anticipated his dismissal, he realized he had known that something like this was bound to occur, sooner or later. In fact, he had raised the question of a long-term contract for his services with the executive committee of the governing board 6 months earlier.

Charlie had pointed out at that meeting that the hospital field was undergoing rapid change that was adversely affecting the financial picture and that he could foresee a time ahead when he would be coming to the board with recommendations that would be highly unpopular with the medical staff but would be necessary to the financial viability of the hospital. His comments were politely received and it was indicated that this would be studied. He had heard nothing further on the subject and had found himself reluctant to again raise the issue.

As he looked back from his perspective of this morning, Charlie realized that he should have been much more forceful about a contract, but he'd been afraid that if he had brought up the subject a second time, he would have been turned down and then forced to decide whether to stay or to look seriously for another hospital. Had he looked around and received an offer from another hospital, he knew that one of the conditions of employment would be a contract. He knew this was becoming routine in CEO positions filled in the last couple of years. He also knew that CEOs with long tenure, such as he had, were seldom able to achieve the same results. Boards usually had to go through replacing one CEO for another in order to learn that competent executives were no longer willing to take chances with boards seeing issues realistically and were therefore seeking to protect themselves financially for taking on a job that had become increasingly risky in the last few years.

As he reviewed the contract situation, Charlie recalled two other instances in the past 3 years when he'd thought about the desirability of having a contract. The first had taken place during consideration of the hospital's constructing a medical office building 5 miles away in a newly developing area of the city. At that time he had discussed the idea with the medical executive committee, who had agreed with him about the timing and location of such a facility but had taken the position that this was a physician activity and the hospital should not be involved. They had been so adamant that Charlie had backed off without pursuing it. To this day he regretted not having gone ahead with the project.

The other incident had occurred about a year ago when Charlie had wanted to develop three off-site primary care centers. Again he had discussed it with the medical executive committee, as well as the executive committee of the governing board. Both groups had seen the desirability of this program, but as before, the physicians had taken the position that the hospital should not be involved. They had added a wrinkle to their argument that had led the board to agree with their position. The physicians claimed that, if the hospital went ahead, this would be the corporate practice of medicine. Charlie thought to himself, if I had a contract I would have pushed harder in both of those situations. Thinking back over those two instances, he realized that the physicians wanted to keep the hospital as an economic neutral in the health field and certainly did not want competition from hospitals in addition to what they already encountered from their own colleagues.

The difference between those two situations and this last problem with the radiologists was that this latest incident no longer kept the hospital neutral. As Charlie saw it, it would lead to a significant drop in radiology revenue, and therefore was a step beyond what had previously been the case. If he had had a contract, he would not have been forced to accept the political pressure so readily, but would have had more organizational flexibility to protect the best interests of the hospital. Looking to the future, he knew that his successor, whoever it might be, would need a contract if the hospital was to remain financially viable.

Grudgingly, Charlie had to admit to himself that, on "the day after," he sure wished he had had a contract. Knowing the board members as he did, he figured that they probably would give him 3 months' severance pay and the title to the hospital car he drove and wish him well.

At 54 years of age, he knew he had to find a position. He didn't have enough money saved to retire, nor did he want to, but he was concerned that his age would be a barrier to employment. Thinking about retirement, he suddenly realized that when the hospital had altered its pension plan 6 years ago, vesting had been an important issue but had ultimately been resolved by establishing a 10-year period and that prior employment in the hospital would not be counted. Thinking back on those discussions, he knew that, as of today, he would receive no pension benefits even though he had been at the hospital for 23 years. Ruefully, he admitted to himself that he had looked out for the interests of the hospital for a long time but he surely had ignored his own.

As he thought about the radiology problem that had brought everything to a head, he realized that physicians today were concerned with the growing surplus and the decline in the use of medical services by the public. They would take whatever steps they could to protect their incomes, even at the expense of the hospital. He admitted to himself that, if he were in their shoes, he would do the same.

After breakfast, Charlie decided to go for a walk and think about his own future. As he put on his jacket, he couldn't help but wonder what lay ahead for him and Myra, his wife. At his age, he speculated that he might not be too saleable in the marketplace, given the difficulties of managing a hospital in the last few years; he wasn't too sure that he wanted to go back to a hospital. He had been thinking for the last year or so that he ought to go into some kind of business for himself. As he thought about that possibility, he knew that any step in a new direction would require remortgaging his house; and, at his age, with one son still in college, he wasn't sure that taking such a risk was advisable. If the business failed, he would have nothing for the rest of his life. Turning the corner and starting to walk down the next block, he wondered what other kinds of work he might consider. Given his knowledge of a hospital, he wondered if he should go into consulting. This would be a field where he would be able to help others gain from his experiences and he'd also earn an excellent income. He thought he might look into that possibility, even though he wasn't sure how one goes about getting clients.

Another idea occurred to him—what about becoming president of an HMO? This was certainly a growing field that would need leadership. He knew the health field, had served for 6 years on the board of the Blue Cross plan, and always had an interest in prepayment. As he thought on, he concluded that claims management wouldn't be much different from the way accounts receivable are handled in the hospital, and marketing should be easy if the plan offers a good package of benefits.

Once again his thoughts turned to the events of the last few days. He knew that what had taken place was not a reflection on his administrative skills; he ran a good hospital and he knew it, but he had just gotten trapped by circumstances. When he had recommended to the board that they terminate the radiologists' contract by giving the required 90-day notice, because they were dead set on moving ahead, the board had assured him that they were all in accord that this was the proper course to follow. He remembered that he'd carefully drafted the letter to the radiologists clearly indicating that this was a board decision and that, acting as their agent, he was transmitting the action to them by letter. As a courtesy, he had sent a copy of the letter to the president of the medical staff. Although he knew the letter would create a problem, he had not been prepared for the storm that ensued.

For the 3 days following the receipt of the letter, the radiologists spent the majority of each day buttonholing as many members of the medical staff as possible, telling the physicians that Charlie Jones was taking steps to move them off of their percentage arrangement with the hospital to a salary basis, and that this was the reason behind his opposition to their building a new facility across the street.

By the end of the week, the president of the medical staff had called a special meeting of that body to discuss the hospital's intrusion into the private practice of medicine, which was held the following Wednesday evening in the hospital's cafeteria. Charlie recalled the meeting vividly—it was one of the worst he had ever attended. It started off with the president reading the copy of the letter to the entire medical staff. Charlie remembered looking around the room and thinking to himself that this was the largest turnout in the history of the hospital. When the president finished, a dozen hands shot up in the audience. The first one to his feet was a physician who seldom admitted a patient but was an outspoken critic of the administration. He quickly pointed out that the radiologists had as much right as others on the staff to go into another business for themselves, even if it was the same one in which they were engaged in the hospital. He, for one, would refer all of his ambulatory patients to them for imaging.

From the other side of the room, another physician stood, was recognized by the chair, and said that the real trouble with the hospital was not the medical staff but the administration. He said that the physicians had been asking for a private dining room for 3 years and it was still only a hope, that not enough parking spaces were provided for doctors, and that in his eyes Charlie Jones wanted to run the medical staff just as he did the rest of the hospital. What was really needed, he said, was a motion to terminate the administrator. This was immediately seconded, passed by a substantial majority with only a scattering of nays. The meeting was adjourned shortly thereafter.

At the next meeting of the board, Charlie had been excused after the routine matters had been disposed of, and he had gone back to his office knowing that the physician board members were going to present the staff recommendation. Although he had mentally counted noses during the time between the special medical staff meeting and this board meeting, he had made no attempt to meet individually with selected board members because he had told himself that after 23 years of service, the board had long ago come to a decision about his abilities and that they would therefore vote accordingly, if the question of his continued employment came to a vote. As far as he could tell, of the 13 board members, the 4 physician board members would vote in accordance with the wishes of the staff, the two lay board members would automatically vote with them as they always did, and the others would be in Charlie's corner. He thought it would be tight, but that he would win. When at 8:13 P.M. Russ Adams came to his office and informed him that he had been terminated, Charlie had been shocked. He knew he'd heard incorrectly. However, Russ had repeated the statement when he had asked him again.

Returning from his walk, Charlie slowly hung up his coat and began to recount the board vote of the previous evening. Russ Adams had told him that the vote had been close and he had lost by only the narrowest of margins. He took this to mean the vote had been 7 to 6 for terminating his services. That meant that one vote he had counted on had swung against him. As Charlie reviewed the possible swing votes, he realized that it really didn't matter. What he hadn't fully appreciated up to now was that a bloc of votes, even if less than a majority, can be effective in swaying a group decision. When the governing board had decided to include four physicians of the medical staff in their group 8 years ago, Charlie had not objected because the size of the board had been increased from 9 to 13 at the same time. He'd concluded that, because the physicians would only be one third of the votes, he really didn't have to be concerned. Now, in retrospect, he knew that it really did make a major difference, as he had witnessed on innumerable occasions when the four had voted together. He could recall no instance in which the board vote had been against the position of the physicians when they all voted alike. When the physicians had voted 3 to 1 on issues, Charlie remembered several times when the board would vote with the one and not the three, but, when the physicians all stood together, the rest of the governing board had always gone along with their thinking.

Having picked up the daily newspaper on his way into the house from his walk, Charlie sat down in his rocking chair in the living room, determined to take his mind off of the events of the previous day. Finishing the sports section, he casually turned to the help wanted pages and scanned the columns, wondering if he would shortly be reading them carefully every day. The ringing of the phone interrupted his thoughts. Answering it, he found himself talking with an old friend, the chief executive of a large hospital in an adjoining state. He had just heard about Charlie's termination from Bill Handy, the COO at Riley. Charlie's friend had gone through a similar experience not too many years before and had found it traumatic. Like Charlie, on the day after, he wished he'd had a contract. When he took his present position he had been firm on the necessity for one, and, looking back, he told Charlie that, as the CEO of a hospital, he thought it to be the only prudent course to follow. He told Charlie that, before he had a contract, he had never realized the advantages of having one. He considered the recommendations he now made to his board to be more open and frank because of it. He was comfortable in this because of the economic safeguards that protected him in the event he had to make a choice between telling it like it is and providing the politically palatable answer or recommendation. He then asked Charlie if Charlie intended to retain an attorney.

Charlie admitted the thought had crossed his mind, and he was considering calling the hospital attorney. They had worked together for more than 15 years and had a warm, personal relationship. Charlie's friend immediately reacted to this comment by pointing out that Charlie should not do that because the attorney represents the hospital as his client, and Charlie has to appreciate that he may well become an adversary of the hospital, so he needs to discuss the matter with an attorney who is not associated with the hospital or any of its governing board members. Charlie acknowledged this made sense and thanked his friend for calling.

As he put down the telephone, Charlie began to consider more seriously the question of whether or not to discuss what had happened with an outside attorney. He recalled hearing in corridor conversations at the last meeting of the state hospital association that three chief executives had recently reached settlements of several hundreds of thousands of dollars each, after encountering similar situations with similar results.

He wondered if they had experienced any difficulties in finding a new position because they had sought legal remedies. Charlie thought about how he would answer the question, "Have you taken, or are you contemplating, any legal action against your former employer?" Would such an admission rule him out of further consideration? He wasn't sure, however, that he was still marketable, having crossed the 50-year mark a while back, in which case he wouldn't have to worry about answering such a question.

Then there was the question of whether or not it was ethical to sue the hospital. Not long ago, Charlie had terminated 134 employees because of the decline in census and not one of them had threatened to take the hospital to court. Was his situation so different? Yet, didn't his 23 years count for something? The more he thought about it, the more he thought he should at least sit down with an attorney experienced in this field and get an opinion as to what course he should follow. Having dealt with attorneys for years, he appreciated that seeking counsel didn't mean he would sue the board, but that he really needed to understand his current situation. Never having been fired before, he thought he might benefit from such a conversation.

With that, Charlie began considering calling Russ Adams and suggesting that the board may have overreacted the previous evening and might want to reconsider the action they had taken. Because the vote had been so close, one person changing positions would be enough to reverse the decision. Yet, the more he considered doing this, the more he realized that neither he nor the board members would forget what had taken place, and that it would color any situation that might be encountered in the future. Furthermore, suppose no one did change his vote in his favor? Suppose one or more of those who had voted for him elected to change their votes? All things considered, Charlie concluded, the best for all concerned would be not to contact Russ Adams. For better or worse, what was done was done, and he realized he needed to get on with his life. But, he vowed, I am not going to make the same mistakes in the future that I have in the past.

9

Hartland Memorial Hospital

An In-Basket Exercise

Kent V. Rondeau
University of Alberta, Edmonton, Canada

Jonathon S. Rakich
Indiana University Southeast, New Albany, Indiana

Hartland Memorial Hospital, established 85 years ago when wealthy bene-factor Sir Reginald Hartland left an estate valued at more than $2 million, is a 285-bed, free-standing community general hospital located in Westfield, a ski resort community of 85,000 people. Ridgeview Hospital is the only other hospital in the area, situated some 18 miles away in the village of Easton. Hartland Memorial is a fully accredited institution that provides a full range of medical and surgical services. It has an excellent reputation for delivering high-quality medical care for the citizens of Westfield and the surrounding area.

YOUR ROLE

You are Elizabeth Parsons, B.S.N., M.S.N., R.N., Vice President–Nursing Services at Hartland Memorial. You accepted this position 17 months ago

Used by permission of the authors. Copyright © 1995 by Kent V. Rondeau.

and have been instrumental in introducing a number of innovations in nursing practice and management. In particular, these innovations have included the establishment of job sharing, self-scheduling, and a compressed work week for all general-duty nurses. In addition, you have also developed a new performance appraisal system and are contemplating using it to create a merit pay system for the nursing staff.

Your secretary is Wilma Smith, who handles all of your correspondence as well as schedules your meetings and conferences. Each morning she opens all of your mail and places relevant items in your in-basket, along with any telephone and personal messages that have been received in your absence.

Your assistant is Anne Armstrong, who is Assistant Director–Nursing Services. She has worked at Hartland Memorial for 7 years and is very competent. She has only recently returned to work, however, after spending some time in the hospital recovering from the suicide of her husband. A list of the key personnel at Hartland Memorial is presented in Table 1, and selected biographical sketches can be found in Table 2.

Having just returned from a 3-day seminar on total quality management (October 2–4), you must go through all of the items contained in your in-basket and determine what action should be taken. It is now 9:00

Table 1.   List of key personnel

Name	Position
Allan Reid	President and CEO
Scott Little	Assistant to the President
Elizabeth Parsons	Vice President–Nursing Service
Anne Armstrong	Assistant Director–Nursing Service
Cynthia Nichols	Vice President–Human Resources
Clement Westaway, M.D.	President–Medical Staff
Janet Trist	Nursing Supervisor–3 East
Sylvia Godfrey	Weekend Supervisor
Jane Sawchuck	Clinical Nurse Specialist
Norm Sutter	Vice President–Finance
Marion Simpson	Auditing Clerk
Fran Nixon	Staff Relations Officer
George Cross	Nurses' Union Representative
Bernard Stevens	Chairman of the Board
Wilma Smith	Personal Secretary

Table 2.   Brief biographical sketches

Elizabeth Parsons	A professionally trained and degreed registered nurse (B.S.N.,M.S.N.). Age 40, with 15 years of progressive management and nursing experience. Married, one child.
Allan Reid	CEO at Hartland Hospital for 2 years. Age 35, with 6 years experience as an administrative assistant at a 100-bed rural hospital. Married, two children.
Bernard Stevens	Retired army (infantry) colonel. Chairman of the Hartland Board for the past 12 years. Age 70. Widower, four grown children.
Clement Westaway, M.D.	Medical degree from the University of Pennsylvania. Internist. Member of the Hartland medical staff for 30 years and president of medical staff for the past 10 years. Age 64. Divorced, two grown children.
Anne Armstrong	Assistant Director of Nursing Service at Hartland for the past 5 years. Age 35. Recently widowed, two children.
Janet Trist	Diploma R.N. Interrupted career at age 26 to raise her children. Resumed working 2 years ago. Age 41. Married.
Wilma Smith	Personal Secretary in her present position for the past 15 years. Has worked at Hartland for 28 years. Age 50. Single, no children.

A.M. on Monday, October 7, and you have just 1 hour until your first meeting of the day with Norm Sutter, Vice President–Finance. A schedule of your appointments appears in Table 3.

YOUR ASSIGNMENT

For each item found in your in-basket, identify the various alternative courses of action that you may pursue. For each alternative identified, state its underlying rationale. Select the course of action that you believe is most appropriate. If delegating authority to act, identify who should be responsible for each item. (See Exhibit 1 for an analysis form. Twenty copies of this form will be needed for use with this in-basket exercise.)

Because this case study may not contain all of the information needed to make a decision, please make any assumptions that you believe are needed to justify your actions. Make notes of those assumptions on the analysis form.

Table 3. Schedule of appointments

	Monday, October 7
9:00 a.m.	
9:30	
10:00	Meeting with Norm Sutter
10:30	
11:00	Meeting with Clement Westaway
11:30	
12:00 noon	Lunch with Anne Armstrong
12:30	
1:00	
1:30	Orientation talk to new nursing recruits
2:00	
2:30	Meeting of infection control committee
3:00	
3:30	
4:00	Meeting with Allan Reid
4:30 p.m.	

Alternatives	Analysis/Rationale	Choice
1		
2		
3		
4		
5		

Exhibit 1. Sample analysis form.

ITEM 1

MEMO

To: Elizabeth Parsons, VP-Nursing Service
From: Scott Little, Assistant to the President
Date: October 3

Subject: Wandering patients—IMPORTANT!

On Thursday evening, Mrs. Grace O'Brien, a patient with diabetes and Alzheimer's disease, was missing from her room when her daughter came to visit her. It took the staff more than 3 hours to finally locate her. She was found naked and comatose in the basement washroom of the Stuart Annex. Her daughter is extremely upset and is threatening to sue the hospital. We don't need another lawsuit!

ITEM 2

September 26

President
Hartland Hospital
Westfield

> To: E. Parsons 10/2
> From: A. Reid
> What is the
> problem?
> Please see me about
> this right away.
>   Allan

Dear Sir,

    I have been a patient in your hospital on three
different occasions over the last 4 years. In the
past I have been very satisfied with the nursing care
that I have received; however, my last stay there
has left much to be desired. For the most part I
have found that many of your nurses are very rude
and arrogant. On a number of times when I asked
these people for assistance, they would either
refuse to help me, tell me they were too busy, or
ignore me altogether.

    I have great respect for Hartland Hospital and I
trust that you would want to correct this problem.
My late husband, Horace, was once a trustee at your
hospital and would never have allowed this to happen.

Sincerely,

Mable Coleman Westfield

Mable Coleman Westfield

ITEM 3

MEMO

To: Elizabeth Parsons, VP-Nursing Service
From: Allan Reid, President/CEO
Date: October 4

Subject: Employee-of-the-Month Program

I have heard that a number of other hospitals have been very successful at motivating their staff by implementing employee recognition programs. These programs can go a long way toward increasing employee commitment and morale. I would like to institute an "Employee-of-the-Month" award here at Hartland. I have a few ideas and would like to discuss them with you at your earliest convenience.

ITEM 4

MEMO

To: Elizabeth Parsons, VP-Nursing Service
From: Sylvia Godfrey, R.N., Weekend Supervisor
Date: October 6

Subject: Insufficient staffing

Again this weekend we had a number of nurses call in sick and we were subsequently short staffed. I had to call in nurses from the "availability list" that was provided by the Temp Placement Agency. I don't really think these nurses are any good because they are poorly trained and make too many errors. I am sick and tired of having to go through this hassle every week!

ITEM 5

MEMO

To: Elizabeth Parsons, VP-Nursing Service
From: Janet Trist, R.N., Supervisor-3 East
Date: October 4

Subject: Scheduling problems

    I am really having a problem with this new self-scheduling system that we adopted last month. A number of my senior nurses are refusing to go along with it and are threatening to quit unless we go back to the old system. It's affecting the morale on my unit and making my life miserable. We need to discuss this right away.

ITEM 6

WESTFIELD HIGH SCHOOL

September 28

Elizabeth Parsons
Vice President-Nursing Service
Hartland Hospital
Westfield

Dear Mrs. Parsons:
    The Future Careers Club of Westfield High School would like to invite you to be the guest speaker at our November meeting. The meeting will be held on November 14 at 8:00 P.M. in the school auditorium. We would like you to discuss "The Changing Role of the Professional Nurse."
    We believe that your presentation will be quite informative for us because several of our students are interested in pursuing a nursing career.
    We hope that you will be able to accept this invitation. Please call our sponsor, Mrs. Bonnie Tartabull, to confirm at your earliest convenience. Thank you.

Sincerely,
Kathy Muller
Kathy Muller
President, Westfield High Future Careers Club

ITEM 7

MEMO

To: Elizabeth Parsons, VP-Nursing Service
From: Marion Simpson, Auditing
Date: October 4

Subject: Hours of work for part-time nurses

Once again, many part-time nurses are working between 25 and 30 hours per week. If we permit this to continue, under the terms of the collective agreement, we must give full-time benefits to those involved. The agreement states that full-time benefits must be given to those working in excess of 25 hours per week. The actual number of hours worked per week for part-timers averaged 24.5 hours for the month of September.

ITEM 8

TELEPHONE MESSAGE

To: Elizabeth Parsons
From: Scott Little, Assistant to the President
Date: October 4
Time: 10:20 a.m.

Mr. Little called, but did not leave a message.

ITEM 9

MEMO

To: Elizabeth Parsons, Vice President-Nursing
    Service
From: Cynthia Nichols, Vice President-Human
      Resources
Date: October 2

Subject: Sexual harassment charges

STRICTLY CONFIDENTIAL

We have just received a notification from a nurse employed here at Hartland alleging sexual harassment by one of our physicians on staff. The charges, if verified, are extremely serious. I would like to appoint you, along with Fran Nixon, from our staff relations department, and George Cross, union representative for the nurses association, to form a committee to investigate these charges. I have been told that the individual claiming harassment has already begun legal action, so we need to proceed with haste.

ITEM 10

MEMO

To: Elizabeth Parsons, Vice President-Nursing
    Service
From: Marion Simpson, Auditing
Date: October 1

Subject: Reimbursement for travel

Further to your request for travel reimbursement for your upcoming conference, I regret to inform you that you have already used up this year's travel budget allocation and therefore will not be reimbursed from this account.

ITEM 11

TELEPHONE MESSAGE

To: Elizabeth Parsons
From: Norm Sutter
Date: October 4
Time: 3:05 p.m.

Mr. Sutter called and asked if the next year's budget projections for nursing have been finished. He needs these figures by Monday.

ITEM 12

MEMO

To: Elizabeth Parsons, VP-Nursing Service
From: Scott Little, Assistant to the President
Date: October 3

Subject: United Way Campaign

This is a follow-up to our discussion of last week concerning the appointment of someone from your department to serve as a representative for our hospital's annual United Way Campaign. I need to have the name of your representative by Friday, October 4th.

ITEM 13

FROM THE DESK OF WILMA SMITH

To: Betty Parsons
Date: October 4
Time: 2:12 p.m.

Mr. Stevens dropped in and was looking for you. He seemed quite upset and was muttering something about a lawsuit. He wants you to call him as soon as you get back from your trip.

ITEM 14

MEMO

To: Elizabeth Parsons, VP-Nursing Service
From: Jane Sawchuck, Clinical Nurse Specialist
Date: October 3

Subject: Nosocomial Infections

It has come to my attention that, again last month, we have recorded high levels of *Staphylococcus* and *Pseudomonas* in operating rooms B and C. It is becoming apparent that we need to review our standard procedures in this area before an epidemic breaks out.

ITEM 15

MEMO

To: Betty Parsons
From: Allan Reid
Date: October 2

Subject: Jennifer Reid

   My niece, Jennifer, just graduated from nursing school and will be in town just one day—Monday, October 7. She is looking for a job in her field and I have asked her to talk to you. She is a really delightful girl. Would you please see her? I would very much appreciate it.

ITEM 16

MEMO

To: Elizabeth Parsons, VP-Nursing Service
From: Scott Little, Assistant to the President
Date: October 4

Subject: Nurse working illegally

   Carmen Espinoza, the woman I talked to you about, was working illegally for us. She was using a stolen Social Security number. The Immigration and Naturalization Services (INS) contacted me yesterday and a representative will be coming Monday afternoon to inquire about the matter. Please give me a call right away.

ITEM 17

TELEPHONE MESSAGE

To: *Elizabeth Parsons, Vice President – Nursing Service*
From: *Bernard Stevens, Chairman of the Board*
Date: *October 7*
Time: *8:55 a.m.*

Mr. Stevens just called and says that he needs to meet with you and Allan Reid this morning at 10:00 a.m.

ITEM 18

MEMO

To: Elizabeth Parsons, Vice President-Nursing
    Service
From: Dr. Clement Westaway, President-Medical Staff
Date: October 2

Subject: Nurse-physician relations

Further to our discussion last week concerning the pressing need to improve communication between physicians and nurses at Hartland Memorial, I am hoping that the suggestions that I gave you will be successfully implemented by your staff. Remember, we are all trying to provide the best possible medical care for our patients.

ITEM 19

MEMO

To: Elizabeth Parsons, Vice President-Nursing
    Service
From: Cynthia Nichols, VP-Human Resources
Date: October 2

Subject: Firing Ms. Jean White, R.N.

As we discussed yesterday, it is important to conduct the termination interview of nurse Jean White as soon as possible. Her last day of work at Hartland will be October 18 and, according to our collective agreement, she requires 2 weeks' notice. Please call me when the deed is done.

STOP!

1. You must respond to all previous items (1–19) in your in-basket before continuing.

2. If this in-basket exercise is being completed in class, do not look beyond this page until told to do so by your instructor.

3. If this in-basket exercise is being completed as a homework assignment, turn the page and complete item 20 now.

ITEM 20

Telephone Call

Time: 9:45 A.M., Monday, October 7

Allan Reid calls and tells you that Mrs. Grace O'Brien, the patient with diabetes and Alzheimer's disease, is again missing from her room, apparently since late last night. He advises you that he was just informed of this by a local newspaper reporter who had gotten wind of the story. He instructs you to call Mrs. O'Brien's daughter to tell her of this recent development before she hears or reads it in the media. Reid gives you no opportunity to respond, saying, "I have the reporter on the other line and have to go." He then hangs up the telephone.

10

The Bad Image Radiology Department

Kurt Darr

The George Washington University, Washington, D.C.

HISTORY AND SETTING

MacMillan Hospital was established in a metropolitan area of the southeastern United States in the decade following the Civil War. It was named for Abner MacMillan, a successful lumber and hardware merchant whose business had prospered at war's end when there was a great need for rebuilding in his war-ravaged region. The hospital was originally located in a large, colonnaded antebellum home that was MacMillan's residence before his death. In addition to the house, MacMillan had donated the 40 acres on which it stood and $50,000—a large sum in the 1870s—for the charitable purposes to which the hospital was to be dedicated. Originally named for the city in which it was located, the board voted to change the name after MacMillan's death.

In the 125 years since MacMillan Hospital was established, it has undergone numerous building projects and renovations. By the late 1990s it was licensed for 350 beds, but operated only 250, which have an average occupancy rate of 75%. The parcel of land was large enough that construction and renovation could occur without the need to move the hospital. The original house had been restored and at present is occupied by the hospital's administrative offices.

MacMillan Hospital offers all primary and secondary acute care inpatient services. A few tertiary services are available: autologous bone marrow transplant services, neonatal intensive care, cardiac catheterization, and radiation oncology. Annual outpatient admissions exceed 50,000. Its busy emergency department has more than 25,000 admissions annually. The hospital has just over 1,000 full-time equivalent (FTE) employees. MacMillan has no bargaining units, but there are occasional rumors that union organizers have talked to employees.

MacMillan's service area has two hospitals of similar size that offer similar services. Many area physicians have privileges at all three hospitals. MacMillan has several advantages, however. It has enjoyed a good reputation in its service area and its competitors face natural barriers that include two rivers and a range of foothills. MacMillan's competitors are not served by public transportation; the road system favors it, as well. The service area has several physician-owned, freestanding centers that offer urgent care, imaging, and ambulatory surgical services. A small psychiatric care facility offers inpatient alcohol and drug detoxification services and rehabilitation. MacMillan and its competitors refer complex cases to the university hospital, which is 75 miles distant.

In terms of hospital-based physicians MacMillan has contracts with five different physician groups that independently provide anesthesiology, cardiology, emergency medicine, clinical and anatomical laboratory, and medical imaging (radiology) services. These concessionaires use equity-owner physicians as well as physician employees to provide services. As is true in most hospitals, these clinical departments at MacMillan are closed—which means that only physicians in the group or employed by the group may have privileges in them. Nonetheless, physicians must go through the usual credentialing process. Nonphysician staff in these five clinical areas are employed by the hospital, but their work is directly supervised and evaluated clinically by physicians in the group. This split between supervision and employment is common in health services delivery. The resulting matrix-type approach facilitates delivery of services by improving coordination and communication, but divides employee loyalty, blurs lines of authority and reporting, and violates Henri Fayol's principle of unity of command. MacMillan has been continuously accredited by the Joint Commission on Accreditation of Healthcare Organizations. The "deemed" status provided by Joint Commission accreditation is important for reimbursement of Medicare and Medicaid patients, which represent 35% of admissions.

BOARD OF TRUSTEES

MacMillan Hospital is governed by a 21-member board of trustees, who are true trustees because they are responsible for the trust originally established by Abner MacMillan. The board is self-perpetuating, which means that it nominates and selects replacement trustees. Trustees serve 3-year terms, and they may be renominated for two additional terms. One third of terms expire each year. The hospital CEO is an *ex officio* member of the board, but has no vote. Board committees include executive, professional staff organization (PSO), human resources, strategic planning, budget and fiscal, quality evaluation, and nominating. The executive committee meets monthly and is comprised of the chair of the board and the chairs of the seven committees. The board bylaws require that committees meet at least quarterly, but they are subject to call of the chairs.

The board chair is Harriet Buchanan, a retired schoolteacher and community leader. She recently started her second 3-year term as chair and is seen by other board members and management as dedicated, well intentioned, and reasonably effective. The board is comprised of interface stakeholders who are social and economic leaders in the community and who are of various ages and ethnic backgrounds. Three are physicians who are members of the active medical staff at MacMillan and not part of a contract group. The board has been active and successful in strategic planning and fundraising. It emphasizes the hospital's financial performance and uses that as a major basis for judging management's success. Implementation of board policy decisions (resolutions) is left to senior management and there is no review of day-to-day performance. The PSO committee makes recommendations through the executive committee after it reviews credentialing recommendations of the PSO, which have come to it through the PSO credentialing and executive committees.

THE PROFESSIONAL STAFF ORGANIZATION (PSO)

The professional staff at MacMillan Hospital is organized, self-governing, and quasi autonomous; like the overwhelming majority of hospital medical staffs, it has chosen not to be a separate corporation. Although legally subordinate to the board of trustees because its bylaws (and revisions), as well as PSO appointments and clinical privileges must be approved by the board, the PSO sees itself as a partner in the full range of hospital activities. As is typical in private (nongovernmental) hospitals the PSO has bylaws that describe its organizational structure, including officers, committees, and policies. There are also PSO "Rules and Regulations" that include specific procedures and rules. In addition to the vice president for medical affairs (VP/MA) who is appointed by the CEO (with approval of the board) and is part of administration, the PSO elects a president who represents the PSO to administration and the board. PSO standing committees include executive, credentials, bylaws, technology, nominating, quality assurance, and medical records. The chairs of the standing committees serve on the executive committee, whose presiding officer is the president of the PSO.

There are 920 physicians on MacMillan's PSO, of whom 200 are active. In addition to physicians, the PSO bylaws allow doctors of podiatric medicine (DPM), certified registered nurse anesthetists (CRNAs), and certified nurse midwives (CNMs) to be members of the PSO. Podiatrists privileges are determined individually. Privileges for the CRNAs and CNMs are determined as a group; they have a vote on the PSO, but may not hold office. The PSO bylaws define "active" as physicians who admit five or more inpatients per year. For purposes of defining active, three outpatient admissions are considered equal to one inpatient admission. Only active members of the PSO are allowed to hold office or chair committees. All members of the PSO may vote on general matters such as elections; the vote on matters such as amending the bylaws, however, is limited to active staff.

Hospitals commonly use *locum tenens* physicians to temporarily staff hospital-based physician clinical departments. The PSO bylaws at MacMillan allow appointment of *locum tenens* physicians and state in part:

> All appointments to the PSO shall be reviewed by the PSO department, which is to be the applicant physician's primary department.... The department chair shall make a recommendation to the credentials committee as to the appropriateness of the appointment and the suitability of the clinical privileges requested by the applicant, in consultation with such members of the department as are deemed appropriate. All appointments shall be subject to approval by the board of trustees.

Historically, this provision has been interpreted to include *locum tenens* appointments and temporary physicians have been processed consistent with this provision. Ultimately, as is universal practice for hospitals, the board at MacMillan approves all appointments to the PSO and the specific privileges of each individually credentialed member of the PSO, or the credentials held by groups such as the CRNAs.

ADMINISTRATION

MacMillan's chief executive is Jack Gargon, who was appointed 15 years ago. Gargon is 60 years old and holds a master's degree from an accredited health services administration program. He is a Fellow of the American College of Healthcare Executives and has more than 25 years of senior-level experience. A first task on assuming his duties at MacMillan was to reorganize the management hierarchy. One of the goals was to reduce the number of middle managers in anticipation of reduced reimbursement because of implementation of the federal Diagnosis Related Groups payment system. The resulting structure was much flatter and had fewer middle managers. The board was very pleased with the reorganization and other efficiencies Gargon implemented and concluded that he was a capable and technically proficient manager. Mr. Gargon's elimination of middle management, however, caused significant grumbling among surviving middle managers who had seen friends and colleagues fired. Satisfied that its internal operations were under control, the board increasingly turned its attention to external responsibilities. Gargon's reputation in the hospital is that of a capable and technically proficient manager who gives his management team wide latitude in decision making. He expects them to solve problems on their own and not to bother him unless his specific assistance or intervention is needed.

Gregory Halton is Gargon's vice president for clinical services (VP/CS). Halton is 27 years old and has been at MacMillan since he completed a postgraduate internship there five years ago. Prior to being promoted to VP/CS 2 years ago, he was responsible for strategic planning and marketing. He holds a bachelor of science in health services management and is working part-time on his master's degree; his areas of responsibility include medical imaging. Halton is seen by his hospital colleagues as enthusiastic, hardworking, and work-oriented. He can be stubborn, however, and occasionally peers have questioned his judgment.

The guidelines for managers who are responsible for clinical departments are general and unwritten, but reflect long-standing custom at MacMillan. Managers are expected to focus on the nonphysician staff and to leave the review of physicians' activities to the VP/MA and the PSO. The chief technologist in medical imaging, for example, reports to the clinical department head for clinical matters and to the VP/CS for administrative matters, which results in a matrix-type arrangement. The clinical chief and the responsible manager jointly do evaluations of the performance of support staff in clinical departments. Halton is administratively responsible for the department of medical imaging, which until recently was known as the department of radiology.

The VP/MA position has been vacant for 6 months, despite efforts to recruit a replacement for the previous incumbent who retired.

MEDICAL IMAGING

The chief of medical imaging is Harold Goodview, M.D., a board-certified radiologist. Goodview is the majority stockholder in Good Views Medical Imaging, LLC, the professional corporation that has had an exclusive contract to provide radiographic services at MacMillan for the past 15 years. Goodview's wife and her family are minority stockholders. Two years ago, MacMillan and Good Views signed a 5-year extension of the basic contract. Good Views employs all the radiologists, including Goodview, who is both an employee and an owner.

The Department of Medical Imaging is extraordinarily busy and has a volume of more than 100,000 cases per year. There are 40 FTE radiologic technologists and 27 FTE file room clerks, secretaries, receptionists, and transporters. The technologists include radiographers, cardiovascular-interventional technologists, sonographers, radiation therapists, and magnetic resonance imaging technologists. Each area of activity has a lead technologist. There is a chief technologist for the entire department who functions as the department administrator. The department performs a wide range of radiographic studies including plain film studies, contrast studies, intravenous pyelograms, magnetic resonance imaging (MRI), computed tomography (CT), needle biopsies, drainages, nuclear medicine, ultrasound, and interventional procedures such as angiograms and stent placements.

The terms of the contract between MacMillan and Good Views are typical for the field. MacMillan provides and maintains all capital and noncapital equipment. It provides and maintains the space and all supplies and consumables, including disposables. MacMillan employs the nonphysician staff. The hospital is paid for its work by budgetarily apportioning part of the DRGs for Medicare and Medicaid patients and by billing other third-party payers and the small number of self-pay directly. Good Views has a contract billing service which does the billing for the professional fee charged by the radiologists. Part B pays for Medicare beneficiaries; Medicaid, other third-party payers, and self-pay patients are billed directly. Primarily because of the high volume, this basic arrangement has generally been very financially rewarding for both parties.

Relationships with administration have generally been business-like, if distant. Goodview prefers "dealing with the top" and calls Gargon whenever there is a problem that needs attention. Even when there was a VP/MA, Gargon rarely involved her in any departmental problems. Being bypassed in this manner greatly annoys Halton, but the pattern was established before he came to MacMillan. Halton has mentioned the problem to Gargon several times, but Gargon has taken no action. Believing this reflects a lack of support in terms of his role in medical imaging, Halton has been reluctant to challenge Goodview's actions directly. Consequently, Halton has been embarrassed numerous times when he learned about decisions affecting his responsibilities in medical imaging from the chief technologist. Halton's efforts to develop a more effective working relationship have been rebuffed by Goodview.

Historically, Goodview has had difficulty keeping radiologists employed in his company and, thus, in staffing the department. When Good Views Medical Imaging first obtained the exclusive concession to provide radiology services, the group had four equal partners. Over the years Goodview bought them out when they wanted to leave. His long-term employed radiologists have become fewer and fewer; currently there are only two, Drs. Banda and Leipzig. In addition, there are several *locum tenens* radiologists.

The chief radiographic technologist is Sally Lebeau who has been employed in the department for 18 years, during half of which she has been the chief technologist. She is well-regarded by her staff and is seen as fair and reasonable, especially given the fast-paced and intense working environment. Lebeau has tried to implement Deming's quality principles and the methods of continuous quality improvement, but neither Goodview nor the administration supported her efforts, and they have come to nought. Lebeau is concerned with what she perceives to be a decline in the quality of work in medical imaging. She has unsuccessfully tried to discuss it with Goodview on numerous occasions. In the past several years she has seen other developments that have raised concerns. First is that there are fewer radiologists in total in the department, despite increased volume. Second, the constant turnover of radiologists, because of all the *locum tenens* physicians, is very disruptive to the department's work. Third, Goodview does more and more of the work himself—both because of the radiologists staffing problems and because of what Lebeau thinks is an increasing obsession with money. Fourth, without the knowledge of senior administration, Goodview ordered a cable connection so that he could follow the stock market and trade technology stocks on line. He is often distracted from reading radiographs by stock market developments and his reaction to them, especially in the volatile technology stocks, in which he invests heavily.

Lebeau's concerns were such that she went to see Halton. When Lebeau described how she saw the four problems, Halton frankly told her that he could do little about the first three, nor did he think they were his responsibility. The number of *locum tenens* physicians and the quality issues would have to be dealt with by someone else—probably the PSO. Halton seemed incensed, however, that Goodview would be so bold as to order installation of Internet access without clearing it with administration. While Lebeau was in his office Halton called maintenance, which reports to the vice president for support services (VP/SS). The head of maintenance confirmed that there was a cable hook-up and the hospital was paying the fee. While Lebeau waited, Halton called the VP/SS, Susan Williams. After a lengthy discussion in which Halton became quite agitated and began to shout, Williams finally agreed to have the cable disconnected the next day. This greatly pleased Halton who said to Lebeau, "I've been trying to get Goodview's attention; I bet this'll do it. He'll have to come to me to resolve this problem—I'm sure that, over the long term, it will help us develop a better working relationship."

Lebeau was disappointed by Halton's response, especially his feeling that he had no role in quality. She thought that the cable issue was the least of the problems, even though it was clearly a distraction and Goodview was using hospital resources for his private purposes. When Lebeau returned to medical imaging, she saw several of the staff standing as though transfixed outside the room where the radiologists read the films. They were listening intently to a heated conversation Goodview was having with an online broker who Goodview alleged had failed to make a trade in time to avoid a significant loss. The language was foul and was becoming so loud that patients waiting for procedures could hear it. Lebeau quietly shut the door to the reading room and told the staff to go back to work.

The next day Goodview's Internet connection suddenly went dead, just as he was trying to execute a sell order on a rapidly falling technology stock. He reacted violently and threw the monitor on the floor breaking the screen and chipping the flooring. Upon calling the cable company Goodview was told that the hospital had ordered it disconnected. Goodview stormed over to "management house" to see Gargon, who was only partly successful in calming him before Goodview left his office. After talking to Halton, Gargon basically agreed with his action, but chided him for how he had handled it. In the weeks that followed, Goodview brooded about the loss of his cable connection; he frequently cursed out administration. Several times he stated that if he had a bomb he'd blow up "management house."

Goodview's agitation was increasingly reflected in his work. For example, he read mammograms as quickly as he could put them up on the view box. He found virtually none that required more than a few seconds of study. When Dr. Leipzig raised a question about the speed of his readings, Goodview said, "Reading mammograms is so simple that a one-eyed first-year medical student could do it." To check Goodview's readings, Leipzig reread 100 randomly selected mammograms and found several that he thought warranted follow-up studies, including repeat mammograms and fine needle aspirations. He ordered them without telling Goodview.

Concerned about the mammograms and similar problems, Leipzig followed Goodview's custom and went "to the top" to see Mr. Gargon. Gargon was initially noncommittal and told Leipzig that he would have to undertake his own investigation. Gargon called Halton and asked him to speak to Lebeau. When their meeting began Halton asked Lebeau for her comments on the information relayed from Leipzig. Her response was a torrent: poor staff morale, low patient satisfaction, high turnover among the radiologists, and Goodview's continuing bad behavior was causing a great deal of stress. Alarmed, Halton met with Gargon, but they were unsure how to proceed and the meeting produced no plan of action. The following week, Dr. Leipzig resigned, citing in his letter the continuing and significant quality problems in medical imaging. This meant that Drs. Banda and Goodview were the only nontemporary radiologists in the department. The other radiologists were *locum tenens*, who usually stayed only 1–3 months.

The controversy between administration and Goodview and questions about the quality of work in medical imaging were common knowledge in the hospital. Their extent and duration were such, however, that admitting and referring physicians in the community were increasingly concerned about the quality of imaging services their patients would get at MacMillan. Gargon and several board members, including Ms. Buchanan, had received calls from prominent active staff physicians who said that they had become uncomfortable referring their patients to MacMillan for radiographic work and that they would use one of the competing hospitals or a free-standing imaging center. In the short term fewer referrals would affect hospital revenue from medical imaging; in the long term inpatient admissions would be affected, thus potentially affecting quality of care received by persons in the hospital's service area, but certainly causing a decline in hospital revenue.

Greatly concerned and prompted by a call from the board chair, Ms. Buchanan, Gargon scheduled a meeting with Goodview and Halton. As usual, Goodview arrived late. Looking at Halton he blurted out, "What are you doing here?" With little conviction, Halton replied that as the VP/CS he was administratively accountable for medical imaging and it was his responsibility to be present. Goodview proceeded to harangue Gargon about the poor support he was getting from administration, how the technologists were badly trained and disloyal to him, and the equipment was inadequate for a 21st-century radiology department. All the while he ignored Halton. Gargon began by expressing his concern that there were too few radiologists for the volume of procedures. Goodview said that radiologists were in great demand and that he was doing the best he could to recruit additional staff and in the meantime he, Banda, and the *locum tenens* radiologists could handle the workload. After 30 minutes of heated discussion, the meeting ended with no resolution.

After Goodview left, Gargon told Halton to contact physician search firms and determine whether Goodview was correct about the shortage of radiologists. A week later, in early July, Halton reported that the search firms had sent him information that radiologists were available in adequate numbers, but that they were being attracted to groups that paid better than Good Views was willing to pay. Goodview's salary offers were well known to search firms—one even called Goodview "a cheapskate." The search firms sent 10 résumés of radiologists who could be employed on a long-term basis by Good Views or who could be hired as *locum tenens*, if the salary offers were adequate.

Armed with this information, another meeting was held with Gargon, Halton, and Goodview. Goodview was adamant that he would not bring any more "traitors" such as Leipzig or other full-time radiologists into his company. He felt that all of his full-time radiologists had betrayed his trust and friendship over the years. He said, however, that he would consider more *locum tenens* appointments, but only if he really needed them. A week later, in mid-July, Goodview had done nothing about hiring more *locum tenens* radiologists. This prompted Halton to contact the search firms. He asked them to send applications from the 10 radiologists whose résumés they had been sent previously. Halton was sure this would force Goodview to take action. Applications received in administration were forwarded to Goodview, who stubbornly ignored them.

CONTRACT TERMINATION

When Gargon arrived at work on August 1st his secretary told him there had been a voice mail from the chair of the hospital board, which had been received at 5:30 A.M. Buchanan stated that she had slept little the night before because the problems in medical imaging were weighing on her mind. She ended her recording by stating that something had to be done and that she wanted Gargon to review the contract with Good Views to determine how to terminate it. By noon she had called twice to see if there was an answer to her request. Gargon had to put her off until early afternoon; by then he had checked with legal counsel and was able to speak to Buchanan in an informed manner. The relevant contract provision stated:

> Either party may, upon demonstration of adequate cause, terminate the contract with a 30-day notice. Cause is defined as either parties': inability to meet the clinical needs of the other; nonperformance of a significant provision of this contract; and actions that interfere with the ability of the other party to perform this contract.

After talking to Halton, who said, "It's about time!" Gargon called Buchanan and told her that legal counsel had informed him that there appeared to be adequate cause to terminate the contract. Buchanan instructed him to draft a letter advising Good Views Medical Imaging that its contract with MacMillan would be terminated as of September 1st.

Consistent with board bylaws, Buchanan polled the executive committee, which approved the action. The letter, which was signed by Gargon, was hand delivered to Goodview the same day. Goodview was performing a fine needle biopsy and he asked a technologist to read the letter to him. Upon hearing the contents he became enraged. He shouted for Banda, who was on a coffee break, to "get in here and finish up this patient." The patient became very agitated and had to be reassured by the technologist before Banda could complete the procedure. Goodview stormed over to "management house" and burst into Gargon's office without being announced. Gargon's executive assistant was so concerned about Goodview's rage and the potential for violence that she called security and asked them to send two officers to the administrative suite immediately. Goodview left shortly thereafter, vowing to get the "meanest, nastiest lawyer in town."

Goodview's attorney petitioned the court for a temporary restraining order (TRO), arguing that contract termination would cause irreparable economic harm to Good Views Medical Imaging and would also irreparably harm Goodview's professional reputation. The TRO was granted despite arguments by MacMillan's lawyers that focused on the need to provide quality radiologic services and maintain the quality of patient care. The TRO prohibited MacMillan and its management from interfering in the role of Good Views Medical Imaging and its agents and employees in the medical imaging department of MacMillan. Less than a week after the TRO was granted, Goodview filed suit against MacMillan for breach of contract and defamation of character. Gargon and Halton were named personally as having "conspired to deprive Goodview of his business and professional livelihood and of causing irreparable harm to his professional reputation." In addition to economic damages for breach of contract, the lawsuit asked that the court award punitive damages based on the alleged conspiracy and bad faith on the parts of Gargon and Halton, as agents of the hospital. Given the urgency of the situation, MacMillan was successful in gaining an early trial date on the breach of contract and defamation lawsuit. Trial was scheduled for December 1st, even as the TRO remained in effect.

BREAST CANCER AWARENESS MONTH

As it had for the past 8 years, MacMillan Hospital's "Health Promotion Promotion" program had designated October as breast cancer awareness month. The local radio and television stations aired public service announcements that urged women older than age 45 to go to MacMillan for a free screening mammogram. Special efforts were directed at MacMillan Hospital staff. The Health-Promotion Promotion used flyers, bulletin board notices, and public address announcements in the cafeteria to encourage women older than 45 to be screened. The extra workload seemed especially burdensome this year, both because of the continuing shortage of radiologists and the pending legal proceeding.

Cowed by the TRO and the pending lawsuit for breach of contract and defamation and concerned that there might be charges of harassment, which could result in being held in contempt of court or prompt another lawsuit, Gargon and Halton stayed as far away from medical imaging and Goodview as they could. Goodview was emboldened by the initial success of obtaining the TRO; he was even more critical of administration and his behavior became increasingly bizarre. Lebeau's stress level was so high that she sought medical attention and began taking a mild tranquilizer. To the technologists and other staff, the whole situation was overwhelming; morale sank even lower and there was talk of a mass resignation. Only the perseverance of Lebeau gave the staff some encouragement.

A MacMillan Hospital housekeeper, Amelia Tendo, presented herself at medical imaging early one morning in October for a screening mammogram. She said she had felt a small lump in her right breast and was concerned about it. Goodview read the mammogram in his usual fashion and diagnosed the lump as benign and "nothing more than a calcium deposit in an overly anxious female." Reassured, Tendo asked that a copy of the report be sent to her primary care physician.

THE FIRST TRIAL

In preparing for trial, attorneys for MacMillan and Goodview/Good Views took depositions (questions answered under oath) of the major parties in the case. Without exception, persons employed by the hospital, including radiologic technologists, stated in their depositions that Goodview's work in managing and providing radiologic services was well below acceptable limits and that his actions that effectively resulted in inadequate radiologist staffing had put and were putting patients at risk. Testimony such as this was necessary because the hospital had the burden of proving that the grounds for termination in the contract had been met. In addition, the hospital had retained two medical experts who stated, after reviewing Goodview's readings, diagnoses, and the depositions of the other witnesses that Goodview's work fell below the standard of care.

Except for tepid support from Banda and the *locum tenens* radiologists, Goodview had few allies in the hospital. He did have an expert witness who stated that his work and Good Views performance of the contract was at an acceptable level and within the range of performance for departments of radiology nationwide.

The trial commenced December 1st and lasted 5 days. The witnesses who appeared also had given depositions. Goodview could not restrain himself when he testified, and he proved to be his own worst enemy, even as he tried to present himself as a poor physician who was being bullied by an overwhelming bureaucracy. The jury found in favor of the hospital and against Goodview and Good Views Medical Imaging on both the breach of contract and the defamation claims. The findings caused the TRO to be vacated.

Hospital administration was jubilant and, with Good Views' contract terminating in 30 days, it immediately began efforts to find a new radiology group to staff medical imaging. Radiologists who had previously been part of Good Views were contacted. Dr. Leipzig indicated he was interested and he set about organizing a radiology group.

SECOND LAWSUIT

Ms. Tendo, who had had the screening mammogram done in October during breast cancer awareness month continued to be concerned by the lump. When she performed her intermittent breast self examinations over the next several months it seemed to be getting larger. Whenever her anxiety rose, she recalled Dr. Goodview's reading and diagnosis that it was only a calcium deposit and was reassured. Six months later, in April she had become convinced that the lump was substantially larger and she scheduled an examination with her gynecologist. He immediately ordered a mammogram at a free-standing imaging center, which led to a fine needle aspiration. After other tests, the final diagnosis was cancer of the right breast with metastases to one lung, nearby lymph nodes, and liver. She died less than 3 months later. Within a year, Ms. Tendo's estate sued Dr. Goodview, Good Views Medical Imaging, and MacMillan Hospital for medical negligence.

Questions

1. Identify the issues in the case.

2. Prepare a time line of major events in the case. Determine the points at which intervention by hospital administration or the board might have prevented the problems in medical imaging from developing as they did. For each intervention point, outline the intervention that you think should have been undertaken.

3. What is the role of hospital executives in monitoring quality and intervening, as needed, in the delivery and/or quality of clinical services?

4. Identify the points at which hospital administration should have intervened to lessen the probability of Dr. Goodview's failure to diagnose Ms. Tendo's breast cancer.

5. What steps should be taken by MacMillan to resolve the lawsuit brought by Ms. Tendo's estate? Is an apology part of an appropriate response?

6. What actions, if any, should be taken against Messrs. Gargon and Halton? Who should take these actions?

11

Westmount Nursing Homes, Inc.

Implementing a Continuous Quality Improvement Initiative

Kent V. Rondeau

University of Alberta, Edmonton, Canada

Shirley Carpenter took a deep breath and looked at her watch. It was 3:40 P.M. and just 20 minutes were left to get ready for her meeting with the board. She knew there was going to be a difficult confrontation and believed that many board members would call into question her leadership skills and administrative judgment. She felt that her well-earned reputation as a brilliant strategist and dynamic change agent would be put to a severe test. She needed to find a way to calm the widespread fear that the total quality management (TQM) initiative she had worked so hard to implement at Westmount Nursing Homes was badly off the rails. She wondered what had gone wrong and how it could be saved.

BACKGROUND

Shirley Carpenter came to Westmount 22 months ago to assume the role of president and chief executive officer. Westmount Nursing Homes,

Used with permission from *Cases in Long-Term Care Management* by Donna Lind Infeld and John R. Kress. (Chicago: Health Administration Press, 1995, pp. 85–95.)

Incorporated is a for-profit chain of seven nursing homes located in a northeastern state. Since 1953, it had grown from a single 42-bed residential facility for affluent seniors, to a dynamic company comprised of four divisions: 1) the Facilities Division, managing skilled nursing homes; 2) the Home Care Division, operating homemaker and nursing services for seniors in their own homes; 3) the commissary services division, operating a central kitchen preparing and distributing meals to four of its homes, two small local hospitals, and elderly people in their own homes; and 4) the consulting division, marketing management consulting and accounting services to a variety of clients in the long-term care industry. Westmount's statement of profit and loss for the past 3 years can be found in Table 1.

Westmount continues to search vigorously for opportunities to expand its core business. Last year it began a comprehensive day care program for seniors at five of its homes. Recently, discussions have been undertaken with Breton Funeral Homes to purchase its assets, including four family-owned funeral establishments. Westmount has also commenced negotiations with a regional chain of drug stores to lease them commercial space in its three largest homes. It also is exploring the establishment of a home care alliance with two other hospital-based home care programs in order to attract new managed care contracts and to improve referrals from existing contracts involving their parent hospitals.

Over the past 3 years, under the leadership of Shirley Carpenter, Westmount purchased two additional nursing homes, increasing its total

Table 1. Westmount Nursing Homes, Incorporated Statement of Revenue and Expense (years 200x–200z) (figures in thousands of dollars)

Year	200x	200y	200z
Facilities Division			
Revenue	15,640	18,622	26,453
Expenses	12,458	15,140	22,512
Profit margin (%)	20.3	18.7	14.9
Home Care Division			
Revenue	1,741	2,254	3,060
Expenses	1,360	1,752	2,493
Profit margin (%)	21.9	22.3	18.5
Commissary Services Division			
Revenue	1,382	1,940	2,188
Expenses	1,263	1,614	1,870
Profit margin (%)	15.9	16.8	14.5
Consulting Division			
Revenue	—	42	426
Expenses	—	16	230
Profit margin (%)	—	61.9	46.0

skilled nursing bed complement by almost 43%. A strategic planning process began last year. Out of this initiative came Westmount's formal declaration to pursue the goal of becoming the "home of choice" in the tri-state area. Its primary target market was identified as affluent seniors who desire a broad range of single access, high-quality health and social services. This strategy was based on the belief that to survive in a rapidly changing health care environment, customers require "one-stop shopping" for a wide variety of services outside of the acute care setting. Westmount firmly believes that future success will go to those proactive organizations that achieve a vertically and horizontally integrated delivery system.

SHIRLEY CARPENTER

Shirley Carpenter, R.N., M.B.A., came to Westmount Nursing Homes 2 years ago from Grasslands Community General Hospital, where she had been the vice president of nursing. Grasslands is a 325-bed acute care hospital located in a rapidly growing community in the Midwest. At Grasslands, Shirley was widely received as a dynamic and resourceful leader who was not afraid of making the difficult decisions that went with her job description. She was primarily responsible for Grasslands' radical redesign of its patient care delivery system toward a highly integrated patient-focused approach. The changes she had initiated saved the hospital more than $1.7 million per year on direct patient care services, while at the same time lowering hospital length of stay and improving patient outcomes. When the press got wind of Grasslands' successful reorganization, the hospital and Shirley received a great deal of local and national media attention. Grasslands became recognized as an innovative organization at the cutting edge of excellence in patient care delivery. It wasn't long before Shirley was being asked to speak at forums about a wide variety of health care issues. She also received additional recognition when she was selected as "one of the most outstanding young health care executives in the nation."

Although the changes Shirley had instituted were widely acclaimed as successful, she did have her detractors. Her direct, no-nonsense style was often seen as confrontational, and many found her to be intellectually intimidating. On several occasions she had openly chastised staff members with whom she took issue. Although she was greatly respected and even admired by her staff, people tended to give her a wide berth on most issues. Shirley demanded perfection from her staff but also held herself up to the very highest level of performance expectation. She once stated, "You've got to be visible and out front if you're are going to navigate an organization toward progressive change. This requires that you stand behind your words and accept the consequences of your convictions.

Complacency never got the job done. Too many people are attached to the status quo. You can't make an omelet without breaking a few eggs."

George Pearson had been the chief executive officer at Grasslands during Shirley Carpenter's tenure. George once stated that Shirley was "the daughter I never had." He had given her wide latitude and regularly deferred to her judgment in most areas related to running the hospital. Everyone had assumed that George had been grooming Shirley to take over the hospital upon his pending retirement. When he departed, the selection committee did the unexpected and chose another candidate. Shirley was devastated; 6 weeks later, she left Grasslands for Westmount Nursing Homes.

A NEW DIRECTION FOR WESTMOUNT

Shirley Carpenter's arrival at Westmount created a great deal of anticipation and excitement. Her reputation as a health care innovator and progressive change agent was now well established. Over the years, Westmount had languished through a series of rather bland administrators who lacked the vision that could move the organization forcefully into the 21st century.

The first year of Shirley's tenure at Westmount was marked by a number of bold initiatives on her part. Soon after arriving, she was able to dissipate the threat of loss of licensure and potential funding on two of its nursing homes that had been cited for a number of violations. Shirley also instituted a broad and sweeping reorganization at Westmount in creating the four operating divisions. In addition, after securing support from her board, Shirley began a very aggressive program of asset diversification because the firm had relied for too long on revenues from its affiliate homes. Declining reimbursement rates, coupled with full occupancy, meant that Westmount needed to broaden its base of revenue. This was partially achieved by expansion of its home care and food commissary services, and by establishing a consulting division to market management services to a variety of clients in the long-term care industry. In particular, the Consulting Division was thought to have significant growth potential due to a perceived lack of expertise by most local consultants on long-term care management issues. During this period, Westmount also purchased two additional homes with the option of acquiring three more. The firm spent more than $1.5 million on renovations to these facilities.

Within 18 months, Shirley had implemented a number of innovative programs at Westmount focused on providing augmented services to its seniors and, in addition, expanded employee services. Shirley formed and chaired a quality-of-work life committee aimed at improving conditions for Westmount's employees and staff. Morale in all of the homes had suffered after years of neglect. At the time of Shirley's arrival, the turnover level of staff nurses and nursing assistants at Westmount was among the highest in the state. To reverse this, a recognition and performance-based pay system was implemented identifying and rewarding outstanding individual and group achievement. A career planning and inventory program was developed to assist employees in identifying their career goals and charting a path toward these goals. In addition, the staff education and development program was greatly expanded. All employees were openly encouraged and received financial support to acquire their high school equivalency or to seek further education and skills enhancement. Westmount also established a progressive literacy program to address the intractable problem of illiteracy in the work place. The quality-of-work life committee estimated that about 35% of the workforce at Westmount had deficiencies in reading and writing. Shirley once stated, "Organizational excellence comes about only when people are sufficiently motivated and empowered to make a difference. The bedrock of staff empowerment is knowledge and education. This requires a significant investment in the intellectual potential of each employee. Our people are our most important asset."

THE TOTAL QUALITY MANAGEMENT INITIATIVE

Three months after arriving at Westmount, Shirley initiated a strategic planning retreat to identify Westmount's preferred future. One conclusion emerging from the retreat was that there was a need to find a way to better address quality-of-care issues in delivering services to seniors. Shirley latched on to the notion that TQM would be the vehicle through which Westmount could achieve the cultural transformation articulated in its vision statement, which included a statement that "Westmount Nursing Homes, Incorporated believes in striving for excellence in everything we do."

Shirley quickly became immersed in the burgeoning literature on TQM. Her interest in and passion for its possibilities grew. In fact, she was so determined to become an expert in its theory and application that she began to explore the possibility of focusing her doctoral dissertation in this area.

Her faculty advisor and mentor was Dr. Daylon Quinby, a sage yet crusty academic, now nearing retirement. Shirley asked the venerable professor if he would "lead the quality improvement journey at Westmount." Dr. Quinby readily agreed, and was soon found wandering around the grounds at all hours observing people at work or showing up quite unannounced at management committee meetings. Several staff members found Dr. Quinby to be "an odd old duck" whose presence was somewhat annoying, if not unnerving. Most people did not know why he was there; some speculated that it was management's way of spying on them.

One of Dr. Quinby's first activities was to evaluate the organizational culture in the seven nursing homes. Findings from the cultural audit, used to assess readiness to pursue organizational change, indicated that much work would be required to transform Westmount. In particular, the professor found that prevailing work practices at Westmount were, in many respects, antithetical to the philosophy of TQM. Dr. Quinby announced the findings of the cultural audit at the semiannual general meeting of board, management, and staff. He stated in his address that "if Westmount is to successfully implement total quality management, no less than a total and unequivocable repudiation of current work place values and norms needs to be achieved." Quinby further stated that "the management in the homes consistently demonstrates patterns of practice that are overly autocratic, rigid, and dysfunctional. All too often, management treats its employees like little children. Employees respond by behaving as if management believes they cannot be trusted. An overly confrontational atmosphere, based on suspicion bordering on paranoia, has created an element of fear surrounding and pervading work in many of the homes." Dr. Quinby cited several examples from incidents he had observed. Needless to say, the conclusions he rendered were not well received by a number of members of the staff and managers.

Soon after the cultural audit feedback sessions, Shirley Carpenter and 12 senior managers embarked on a 10-day educational retreat to learn the tools and techniques of TQM and the leadership skills needed to successfully navigate the cultural transformation it required. Although the retreat was located on a resort island in the Caribbean, Shirley impressed on her managers that the time spent was not a paid holiday, but an opportunity to acquire new leadership and management skills. When the news broke that management had gone to a resort for a "working retreat," many employees openly questioned why they needed to "go so far away to learn how to manage better at home."

When the senior managers returned from the retreat, many could scarcely contain their enthusiasm and set about immediately to apply the principles they had learned. A quality council was quickly formed, chaired jointly by Shirley Carpenter and Dr. Quinby. The quality council was charged with leading and directing the TQM transformation at Westmount. Its membership consisted of the directors of the seven homes and the divisional directors of home care, commissary services, and consulting services, along with senior representatives from human resources and strategic planning. Within 2 weeks, executives in each of the homes and divisions were busy holding educational seminars for their middle managers and supervisors on the philosophy, tools, and techniques of TQM.

Not long afterward, under the supervision of the quality council, the first quality improvement (QI) team was formed. Led by Shirley Carpenter and facilitated by Dr. Quinby, a seven-member multifunctional team of service providers suggested innovative ways to dramatically reduce the waiting period for nursing response to requests from bedridden residents. Within 2 months, 23 QI teams examined quality-related problems ranging from improving resident food to designing a new commercial exercise video program for seniors. Table 2 provides a list of these early quality improvement projects at Westmount.

Initial interest and excitement generated by many employees for the TQM initiative at Westmount convinced Shirley that she was on to some-

Table 2. Westmount Nursing Homes, Incorporated Quality Improvement Projects

QI Program	Responsibility
1. Client satisfaction survey	Headquarters
2. Family satisfaction survey	Headquarters
3. Nursing response times	Facilities
4. Seniors' exercise video	Headquarters
5. Staff retention study	Facilities
6. Guest relations study	Headquarters
7. Medication errors	Facilities
8. Suggestion system design	Headquarters
9. Resident fall study	Facilities
10. Wandering patients study	Facilities
11. Employee recognition program	Headquarters
12. Patient accounts	Headquarters
13. Food quality	Facilities
14. Food preparation	Headquarters
15. Pet therapy	Headquarters
16. Job redesign	Headquarters
17. Physician reimbursement	Headquarters
18. Physician satisfaction	Headquarters
19. Ethical review	Facilities
20. Grounds beautification	Facilities
21. Resident transportation	Facilities
22. Self-scheduling	Facilities
23. New ventures	Headquarters

thing big. Many of her junior managers, however, were privately expressing fear that the changes, which now were transforming Westmount's once
placid culture, were happening all too fast. Vice President of Finance Norm
Taylor's opinion was shared by many other managers at Westmount: "It's a
proven fact that people in the long-term care industry really can't absorb
organizational change as easily as those working in acute care settings.
People here just have too much respect for tradition and past practice."

For her part, Shirley was strongly convinced that these changes could
not occur fast enough. Shirley stated, "I don't believe in waiting around
and hoping that something good comes your way. That just never happens. I like to create success right away. One small victory produces
another, and soon you've won the war. The fact is people like to associate
with winners."

THE WESTMOUNT BOARD RESPONDS

The board of Westmount was never really very enthusiastic about Shirley's
TQM makeover. Explained to them as a tool to enhance productivity and
create a long-term competitive advantage in Westmount's chosen markets,
the board reluctantly gave its approval "to implement a TQM program, as
long as it wasn't too costly." The chairperson of the board was Dr. Ann
Howard, age 57, a highly respected family physician with a specialty in
geriatric medicine who was a long-time board member. Dr. Howard was
not convinced that TQM could work at Westmount, and stated, "Total
quality management might be all right for building cars, but I just can't
understand how it can work in a nursing home. Anyway, I read somewhere
that this TQM stuff is just an expensive fad, and that over 80% of health
care organizations who have tried to implement it have failed. Can we
really afford to try something with such a spotty track record? Perhaps
Shirley should be spending her time and the organization's money on
proven management methods."

Shirley knew that the turnaround at Westmount would not happen
overnight. She chalked up the board's indifference to ignorance, and
resolved that she would not be deterred from her quest to transform
Westmount. "Give me 3 years and you won't recognize this place," she was
heard to have said.

LABOR CONTRACT NEGOTIATIONS

Several months after the TQM initiative had begun, Westmount began
contract negotiations with the local chapter of the United Federation of

Nurses, representing Westmount's 214 registered nurses and nurse assistants. Shirley believed in taking a hands-on approach to dealing with the unions, and insisted on conducting all negotiations personally. In the beginning, management at Westmount felt that contract discussions would be straightforward and would proceed with little of the rancor that had characterized much of their collective bargaining in the past. In the earliest months of the TQM initiative, Westmount had witnessed a remarkable improvement in work place morale. It was hoped that improved morale would pay an important "peace dividend" with the organization, winning important concessions from the union.

In fact, all three of the unions representing nonmanagement employees at Westmount believed that the active participation of their membership in TQM demonstrated their steadfast commitment to finding new ways of working responsibly with management. For many years, the fractious nature of their contract negotiations had left both sides bitter after they had concluded.

From the union's vantage point, negotiations were aimed at improving the collective agreement by obtaining significant wage gains and achieving formal union representation on the Westmount board. Two issues were of particular significance during contract talks. First, the union sought to replace the merit pay plan for registered nurses with an across-the-board pay increase for all nurses. Most people felt the merit pay plan, conceived to reward top performers, was not working very well. Many viewed it as a complicated and subjective protocol that caused a great deal of confusion and bitterness in its application. Second, the union sought protection against what they felt was management's abhorrent practice of substituting RNs with certified nursing assistants (CNAs) and other personal care workers. The union claimed that management was using lower-paid nursing auxiliaries for tasks that legally should be done by RNs.

Early in the contract negotiations it became apparent that they would be very difficult indeed. In its opening address at the negotiation table, the union stated that its "price of compliance" with Westmount's total quality program was significant wage increases for its membership. Shirley countered by offering to provide job security and suggesting the formation of a committee to study questions of nursing labor deployment. She also stated that she was in favor of allowing union representation on the board. This was consistent with her idea of incorporating more vibrant forms of employee participation in the work place. Shirley insisted, however, that the merit pay plan must remain in place. As its architect, she felt a deep personal commitment to its consummation. Shirley stated, "You've got to have a way of rewarding those people who consistently perform above the call of duty. That's what quality service is all about. Pay is a great way to motivate people. To ignore the impact money has on the performance of employees is to remove a very powerful weapon from your arsenal." After several heated meetings, the negotiations seemed to be at an impasse.

THE BOARD STEPS IN

It was soon apparent to the Westmount board that contract negotiations with the nurse's union were not going well. The executive committee of the board met with Shirley to determine an appropriate strategy to help reach an agreement. After much heated discussion, they decided that management should take a more direct approach in dealing with the union. Dr. Howard summed up the attitude of the board in saying, "You can't allow a union to ruin the financial viability of your enterprise. The truth is 80% of our costs are direct expenditures for labor. If we are ever to reverse our fiscal problems around here, we need to get control of our labor costs. These people have to realize we're all in this thing together." The board also gave a thumb's down to the idea of allowing union representation on the board. Dr. Howard remarked, "You know, this move to democratize the work place is just a bunch of rampant socialism. You give these people an inch and they take a mile."

When Shirley returned to the bargaining table, she brought along Dr. Quinby to assist in discussions. Unfortunately, he was not able to expedite breaking the impasse. His abrasive and abrupt manner further alienated the union and created additional tensions at the table. With no new offer made by either side, no resolution on any of the major outstanding issues could be achieved. Shirley suspended negotiations by claiming that the union was being inflexible while "holding the residents of the homes ransom for a few extra pennies."

THE FLASH POINT

At this point the executive committee of the board began to make direct overtures to union representatives requesting an informal meeting to "determine if there were not avenues of mutual interest that could be explored." Dr. Howard and two other board members met in private with the union negotiators and suggested the possibility of major staff cuts if the union did not agree to make significant wage concessions. The union representatives countered by insinuating that the Westmount management was bargaining in bad faith. Robert Sawyer, the chief negotiator, said, "We will not be bullied into signing a collective agreement that does not have the best interests of our membership at heart. We have showed our willingness to bargain in good conscience by engaging in activities aimed at improving productivity. The participation of our members in these efforts is often unpaid and obviously unappreciated." The meeting ended with the union threatening to boycott further participation by its membership in future quality improvement activities. According to Robert Sawyer, "If we are going to be treated with such contempt, I can only recommend to my membership that we suspend our active participation in this program immediately."

As Shirley prepared for the 4 P.M. board meeting she was frustrated and angry that persons and events had conspired against her. She had always felt pride in her ability to control any agenda. Her record of achievement was one of soaring accomplishments. She wondered how she could regain control of her board and move ahead with the important reforms she had initiated.

12

Dr. Johnson, Network Medical Director

William Q. Judge
University of Tennessee, Knoxville

Curtis P. McLaughlin
University of North Carolina at Chapel Hill

Charles A. Johnson, D.O., M.B.A., reviewed his 6 months of experience as a network medical director for the Southeast region of Vigilant-Xtra Mile Healthcare located in Atlanta, Georgia. He was one of two physicians responsible for developing and managing the professional medical network of providers and hospitals serving this market, which included the states of Alabama, Georgia, and Mississippi. His duties involved recruiting providers, negotiating contracts, promoting the company's disease management approaches, credentialing physicians, maintaining NCQA (National Committee on Quality Assurance) accreditation, reviewing cost and quality data as well as provider report cards, arranging education efforts for outliers, and controlling the unit cost side of the firm's medical loss ratio in that market.

Dr. Johnson had a full plate of responsibilities that were new to him and his organization. Furthermore, he had limited staff to delegate duties

This case was prepared by Professor William Q. Judge, College of Business Administration, University of Tennessee, Knoxville, and Professor Curtis P. McLaughlin, Kenan-Flagler Business School, University of North Carolina, Chapel Hill, for use as a basis for class discussion rather than to illustrate the effective or ineffective handling of an administrative matter. Copyright © 1998 by the Kenan-Flagler Business School of the University of North Carolina, Chapel Hill, NC 27599-3490. All rights reserved. Not to be reproduced without permission.

to and there were overlapping responsibilities with two other medical directors in his office that needed to be coordinated carefully. Despite these challenges, he felt fortunate to have a supportive and powerful boss and he was convinced that Vigilant-Xtra Mile Health Care was the wave of the future. His immediate challenge was fundamentally a matter of time management. Although Dr. Johnson was highly organized, he felt he was constantly "putting out unexpected fires" and these urgent projects tended to push out longer-term strategic issues. In the past month, for example, his schedule had been consumed by several unexpected activities including 1) supervising a database cleanup, 2) addressing open enrollment adminis-trative glitches, 3) being available for audits of the Medicare program by CMS (Centers for Medicare and Medicaid Services) and the state of Georgia, 4) preparing for a mock NCQA audit, and 5) dealing with supervisory and human relations issues within his unit. These issues tended to get in the way of refining his network of providers and over-seeing quality, but they had to be addressed. Dr. Johnson hoped that with time things would settle down.

BACKGROUND

When Charles Johnson graduated in 1970 from Baldwin-Wallace College in Berea, Ohio, with double majors in zoology and philosophy, he went to work as a pharmaceutical salesman in Ohio and western Pennsylvania. He was successful there, but he wanted direct patient contact, so he decided to pursue a medical degree. In 1973, he entered the Midwestern University–Chicago College of Osteopathic Medicine. Graduating in 1977, he interned at HCA (Hospital Corporation of America) Northlake Hospital in Tucker, Georgia. In 1979, he founded the East Cobb Family Practice in Marietta, Georgia, and joined the staff of the Archway Hospital. He became board certified by the American Board of Osteopathic Family Practitioners and a fellow of the American Academy of Family Practice in 1986 and a diplo-mat of the American Board of Medical Management in 1997.

In the late 1980s, Dr. Johnson and his partner differed markedly over the importance of managed care. His partner did not want to participate, while he was convinced it was the wave of the future. When he witnessed the loss of 20% of his patients after Lockheed Marietta moved all of its employees to managed care, he was convinced that he needed to change his practice. He had been participating in management workshops pro-vided by the American College of Physician Executives (ACPE) and decided to enter Emory University's weekend executive MBA program. He found this to be a valuable learning experience, particularly his thesis project, which involved a study of methods of valuation for small medical practices. When he graduated in June 1991, he installed a total quality management effort in his family practice and asked his partner to leave within 90 days. After his partner left, Dr. Johnson increased the volume of the practice 83% within 12 months while accepting managed care patients and adding a new partner, two physician assistants, and a nurse practitioner. Dr. Johnson tried to start a group practice without walls in conjunction with other providers, but it failed within 6 months due to lack of capital and physician management skills and involvement. Then in late 1994, he received four offers to sell his practice. One of the offers came from an organization that was connected to the hospital where he practiced. Ultimately, he decided to harvest his practice to this organization and become involved in the management of the resulting organization. Thus, he became one of the founding members and chief of family medicine for Dominion Northwest Physician's Group, a group with 180 physicians and 60 locations with affiliations with 13 hospitals in the greater Atlanta region. There he spent half time in management and half time in patient care delivery.

The job with Dominion Northwest was a useful transition for him. He negotiated contracts for the physicians and was involved in developing methods for equitably dividing capitated payment among the specialists and primary care physicians. He was on the contracting committee of the Dominion PHO (physician-hospital organization) and the Physician's Group, and on the strategic planning and the informatics committees as well as the physicians' advisory board. He learned more about working in large organizations with hours spent in committee meetings and dealing with larger bureaucracies. With time, however, he became convinced that this organization did not have sufficient physician involvement in decision making to satisfy him in the long run, but he kept on learning about medical management and leadership.

Then one day an executive recruiter called him about the job at Vigilant-Xtra Mile Healthcare (Vigilant-XMHC). Dr. Johnson felt he had nothing to lose in looking at it, especially since it was in Atlanta. He concluded that it was the type of job that would allow him to make a difference at a higher level. Vigilant-XMHC was looking for a physician with management skills, with a good reputation and credentials, and well connected to the local network. Dr. Johnson had been very active in the Georgia Academy of Family Practice, was on the board of directors of Blue Ridge Area Health Education Center (AHEC) and of a couple of managed care plans in addition to his involvement with administrative duties within Dominion.

In 1994 Governor Zell Miller had appointed Dr. Johnson to the nine-member Georgia Joint Board of General Practice, which oversees the allocation of $50,000,000 in state residency and training funds. Dr. Johnson worked with the other members to formulate state policy on funding of graduate medical education and to redesign all state funding mechanisms for medical education. He was currently secretary/treasurer of the board. He had also served as a preceptor for Emory University and the West Virginia College of Osteopathic Medicine and on the 6th U.S. Congressional District (Newt Gingrich's [former] district) Medicare Advisory Board Task Force on Alternative Plans for Medicare. In short, his connections and experience were ideal for the job.

The job carried with it a salary comparable to a good primary care practitioner income with major upside potential in the long run. There were very good benefits and he would be part of the regional management team. Fortunately, Dominion Northwest allowed Dr. Johnson to opt out of the remaining 2 years of his employment contract and he joined Vigilant-XMHC in August 1997.

His counterpart, Chris Donovan, M.D., was a native of the West Indies who had previous experience as a medical director with Domina in Charlotte, North Carolina. He was also new to the organization as he joined Vigilant-Xtra Mile Healthcare about the same time as Charles Johnson did. Drs. Johnson and Donovan had a good working relationship. Their responsibilities were basically the same, but covered different parts of the market.

Corporate Background

Vigilant and Xtra Mile Healthcare merged in April 1996, bringing together two quite different firms. Vigilant was a traditional full-line insurance company founded in 1899 with 48 highly decentralized HMO operations and a rather conservative business outlook. It was headquartered in Boston. In contrast, Xtra Mile Healthcare was founded in Wheeling, West Virginia, in 1978. It was a highly centralized and entrepreneurial company developed and managed by physicians. Vigilant, for example, had 50 different claims processing centers, while XMHC had only one. In addition to structural differences, their growth strategies were also quite different. Vigilant had been buying primary care practices, while Xtra Mile Healthcare did not buy any practices.

The resulting merger was a giant company with revenues in excess of $17 billion, more than half of which were in health care products. It divided the nation into six regions, which are depicted in Exhibit 1. In 1998, Vigilant-Xtra Mile Healthcare provided health care services to 23 million Americans in 50 states through networks involving 300,000 physicians and 3,000 hospitals. Roughly 1 insured American in 12 was covered for health care by the resulting organization.

The merged company developed a number of strategies aimed at capitalizing on its extensive asset base and unique array of competencies. First

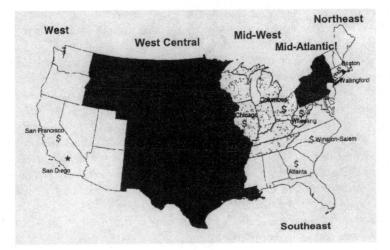

Exhibit 1.   Map of the six regions created by the merger.

and foremost, it would offer a full line of health care insurance products (e.g., indemnity, PPO [preferred provider organization], POS [point-of-service] plan, HMO, senior HMO) on a national basis to offer "one-stop shopping" to nationally based organizations. The firm would not purchase medical practices or facilities, but would maintain an open panel of physicians and nonexclusive contracts with hospitals and ancillary providers. Its basic HMO contracting model called for primary care physicians (PCPs) to serve as gatekeepers on quality-based capitation, with specialists paid on a discounted fee-for-service or capitated basis and hospitals paid at a negotiated rate by the case or *per diem.*

By 1997, Vigilant-XMHC had an approved HMO in 23 states and the District of Columbia covering 73% of the population and had applications pending in the rest. Each physician recruited to the network was expected to service all Vigilant-XMHC health care products under one contract. This consistent national presence and full range of health care products allowed the company to approach large national employers on a highly competitive basis. The fact that they could also supply disability insurance, group life, retirement plans, 401(k)s, dental insurance, and a variety of other products to the same benefits managers nationwide was considered a strong competitive advantage. The company was a leading provider of Medicare managed care services and could also service the company's retirees.

The two companies had been highly profitable in 1995 and 1996. Profit margins narrowed, however, and medical loss ratios rose sharply in 1997. The stock had dropped sharply from 1996 levels. The economies in operations and from scale that had been expected took much longer to achieve. Dr. Johnson talked about the loss of human capital during the reorganization that cost it dearly. According to Dr. Johnson, "In our efforts to reengineer the organization, a lot of administrative help was eliminated. In so doing, we let go of a lot of Ms. Smiths. You know, Ms. Smith was the one in the local office who knew that Dr. Jones never checked box 30 on the CMS 1500 form, but checked it for him rather than sending it back to his office."

The resulting delays and other glitches with new offices and employees slowed down claims processing and overstated initial earnings, with costs catching up later. The new organization, however, was now getting more integrated and claims processing was functioning better in 1998. The new Vigilant-Xtra Mile Healthcare organization was partially decentralized into six regions. The Southeast region consisted of four markets stretching from Mississippi to Florida to Maryland.

Organizational Structure

The overall corporate headquarters was located with Vigilant in Boston, while the health care operations were headquartered at XMHC in Wheeling. The six regional offices reported to the Wheeling corporate offices. There were three medical director hierarchies in the company. Network medical directors, of whom Dr. Johnson was one, reported to the general manager for each market who reported in turn to the regional manager. Patient management medical directors were involved with utilization management, pre-authorizations, length-of-stay reviews, case management development, retrospective reviews, and disease management enrollment. Patient managers came under the regional medical director who reported directly to the team at Wheeling. Finally, there was also a regional quality medical director who reported to quality management in Boston. A detailed comparison of these three types of medical directors is listed in Exhibit 2.

Dr. Johnson supervised a team of eight individuals: two provider-relations managers, who in turn led five professional service coordinators, and an administrative assistant shared with Dr. Donovan. The professional service coordinators were the ones out on the firing line with the providers. There were numerous dotted line relationships among the various medical directors. In fact, when he was hired, Dr. Johnson had only dotted line relationships and no direct reports, so he recommended a reorganization in which he took on budgetary and supervisory responsibility for a portion of the provider services staff. He also made a determined effort to be seen as a contributor to the management team of the market and the region. He hosted a weekend strategic planning session

Job characteristics	Patient management director & quality management director	Network medical director
Fundamental role	Develop and manage a health services organization focused on reducing medical cost and improving clinical outcomes, member satisfaction, and provider satisfaction	Develop and manage a health services organization focused on reducing medical cost and improving clinical outcomes, member satisfaction, and provider satisfaction
Central activities	Implement utilization and quality management programs through timely policy interpretation and local applications	Provide strategic and operational direction for the delivery of performance-based medical management
	Manage budget	Manage budget and risk drivers
	Provide marketing support through sales presentations, site visits, and support for requests for proposals	Analyze and report business performances data to customers and colleagues
	Render medical necessity determinations	Handle Vigilant funds as if they were his/her own
	Chair committees in accordance with market and contractual needs	Participate in internal and external health industry development efforts
	Participate in national, regional, local work groups as required	Participate in management of local profit and loss
	Serve as liaison between field organization, home office, and governmental agencies	Serve as liaison with regulatory and accrediting agencies and other business units within the company
	Develop local medical review and coverage policies	Develop and maintain strong provider relationships
Leadership	Maintain a customer-driven passion for excellence and commitment to action and change	Maintain a customer-driven passion for excellence and commitment to action and change
Direction setting	Make timely and high-quality decisions as well as implement them	Make timely and high-quality decisions as well as implement them
Selection	Hire, develop, and reward staff to effectively support the company's strategy	Hire, develop, and reward staff to effectively support the company's strategy
Communication	Excellent verbal and written skills as well as negotiation and conflict resolution skills	Excellent verbal and written skills as well as negotiation and conflict resolution skills
Business knowledge	In-depth knowledge of managed care, finance, business processes, and strategies and objectives	In-depth knowledge of managed care, finance, business processes, and strategies and objectives
	Job-specific technical knowledge	Job-specific technical knowledge

Exhibit 2. Excerpts from the job descriptions of three types of medical directors.

(continued)

Exhibit 2.   *(continued)*

Other requirements	Board certification is highly desired; state license must be active and unencumbered	Board certification is optional
	Demonstrated commitment to professional development (e.g., CME, conferences)	Demonstrated commitment to professional development (e.g. seminars)

for the regional management team at his summer home at Lake Lanier, for example.

This meant considerable added workload due to supervision, performance review, objective setting, and process improvement. He typically worked from 7:00 A.M. to 6:00 P.M. 2 days per week, and 9:00 A.M. to 6:00 P.M. the other three and then usually had a couple of dinner meetings each week. Weekend activities such as a strategic planning retreat or a mock NCQA site visit exercise might tie up one weekend a month. Typically, he responded to about 60 internal e-mail messages a day and a large number of telephone calls. A 2-month review of his calendar showed that he spent on average 4 hours per day in meetings about 60% in the office and 40% outside. When he took the job, he was told to expect to be traveling 4 days per week. This market's business, however, was very heavily concentrated in Georgia, and in Atlanta in particular.

Management of Quality

In 1990, XM Data Driven, Inc. (XMDD) was established as an XMHC quality measurement subsidiary. With more than 280 employees, it had access to a data warehouse of claims information from hospitalization, outpatient visits, pharmacy claims and laboratory reports of 15 million enrollees. It was a pioneering and innovative unit with Xtra Mile Healthcare, developing clinical algorithms identifying and risk-stratifying seriously ill members for disease-management interventions, providing risk-adjusted performance reporting systems, maintaining a disease registry for members with any of more than 65 chronic illnesses, and working with participating academic medical centers to conduct applied research. A full description of XMDD is provided in Exhibit 3. An example of the type of report cards they provided to management and to providers is shown in Exhibit 4.

Vigilant-XMHC believed that ultimately the market would be defined by quality. This was so important to Vigilant-XMHC that the company had established a unique quality-driven compensation system for primary care physicians. The incentives in this system were balanced to attempt to avoid

The XMDD's health services research program is the dedicated research and development unit of Vigilant—Xtra Mile HealthCare. Physicians, Ph.D.-level researchers, methodologists, nurses, statisticians, programmers, medical coders, and other experienced professionals make up this unit. Staff members conduct applied research and develop methodologies that measure and improve the quality and efficiency of health care services for Vigilant—Xtra Mile HealthCare's membership. One of the main goals of the Health Services Research Program is to evaluate the outcomes and cost-effectiveness of managed care programs.

The XMDD Health Services Research Program has access to an abundance of health-related data on more than 14 million insured members throughout the United States, and routinely analyzes both primary and secondary data for hundreds of practical applications. Research conducted by this unit is designed to benefit four primary customers, which include: 1) individual members, 2) providers, 3) plan sponsors, and 4) the Vigilant—Xtra Mile HealthCare system.

When working with external organizations on collaborative research, XMDD staff members provide methodological, data acquisition and technical support, and assist with the grant application process as well.

Examples of XMDD Health Services Research

- Health profiling—Using a number of different data sets, clinical logic has been created to identify individuals with any of 65 chronic diseases. Each individual's disease-specific health status can be categorized and used in a number of applications. For instance, an individual's health profile is used as a predictor in risk-stratification models to determine who should be entered into disease management programs. Health status is also used as a risk adjuster in physician performance compensation models. Furthermore, these profiles are used to calculate employer group disease-specific prevalence rates, which help employers determine the best benefits package to purchase from Vigilant—Xtra Mile HealthCare.

- Risk Stratification Modeling—XMDD has created empirically driven risk-stratification models designed to identify individuals who are at high risk for certain types of disease-specific acute exacerbations. These multivariate predictive models use previous utilization patterns to assign chronically ill individuals into one of five risk strata. After extensive cross-validation, these models are used to determine appropriate disease management resources that are consistent with the health needs of each category of individuals.

- Clinical Outcomes Studies and Program Evaluation—Both pilot and long-standing managed care programs are evaluated to determine their impact on members' health status. A number of different econometric, epidemiological and statistical quasi-experimental models have been employed to evaluate these programs while controlling for important confounding variables.

- Severity-Adjusted Performance Measurement—Severity-adjusted performance measurement models have been developed for hospitals, specialists and primary care providers. These multivariate statistical models are used to provide feedback to providers and institutions about their performance relative to others in their field. Additionally, performance measurement information is used to determine a portion of each provider's reimbursement. By accounting for differences in patient mix by factoring in characteristics such as age, gender, and co-morbidities, the playing field is leveled between providers, and performance results are more valid.

- Health System Research—A number of research projects are under way to further investigate the health system overall. Cost-effectiveness and practice pattern variation studies, for example, have been undertaken to more fully understand costs and utilization of the country's health system. Additionally, the impact of different insurance arrangements on utilization and health status are being studied. Results from these studies will help Vigilant—Xtra Mile HealthCare better understand how to resource high-quality health services.

Exhibit 3. A comprehensive description of XMDD health services research.

both over- and underutilization. Each practice receives a capitation payment, which was adjusted for the age and gender of the covered population. This payment was further adjusted by a quality factor that was revised every six months. The example in Exhibit 5 illustrates how the quality factor is determined.

Practice Type:_Family Practice_____   Region: _XX_____   Office Number: _XX_____

Office Address: _1 Street Anytown, PA 19074_____   Reporting Period: _10/1/02–9/03/03____

Number of our current insured individuals identified with asthma: _232_____

	Office	XMHC Average
PREVALENCE MEASURES		
1 Estimated overall prevalence of asthma	4.5%	4.0%
2 Estimated overall prevalence of asthma age 0–9	9.0%	7.9%
3 Estimated overall prevalence of asthma age 10–19	7.2%	6.8%
4 Estimated overall prevalence of asthma age 20–39	5.7%	4.0%
5 Estimated overall prevalence of asthma age 40+	2.5%	2.8%
ASTHMA TREATMENT PATTERNS		
6 Asthmatics on prescription drugs for asthma	65.8%	66.4%
7 Asthmatics receiving sympathomimetics	58.3%	58.3%
8 Asthmatics receiving theophylline	6.4%	11.0%
9 Asthmatics receiving only theophylline	0.0%	0.7%
10 Asthmatics receiving cromolyn	8.0%	8.7%
11 Asthmatics receiving inhaled steroids	21.4%	18.8%
12 Average annual number of beta agonist prescriptions for asthmatics receiving beta agonist	4.29	3.72
13 Asthmatics on beta agonists receiving 2 or more prescriptions in one month	18.3%	17.9%
14 Asthmatics receiving one or more courses of oral steroids	17.1%	18.3%
ACCESS MEASURES		
15 Asthmatics seeing the PCP at least once	92.5%	86.9%
16 Average number of annual PCP visits per asthmatic	5.74	4.69
17 Asthmatics seeing a pulmonologist	8.8%	7.0%
18 Asthmatics seeing an allergist	14.5%	11.7%
PROCESS MEASURES		
19 Asthmatics with an outpatient chest X-ray	8.4%	8.9%
20 Asthmatics age 8+ receiving pulmonary function tests	8.3%	10.1%
21 Asthmatics receiving allergy testing	3.1%	4.8%
22 Asthmatics receiving allergy immunotherapy	7.5%	8.0%
23 Asthmatics using a home nebulizer	2.2%	2.4%
24 Asthmatics with at least one antibiotic prescription	63.1%	71.3%
25 Asthmatics on theophylline who have at least one theophylline level drawn	10.0%	18.9%
26 Average annual number of theophylline levels in asthmatics on theophylline	0.10	0.29
27 Asthmatics receiving at least one home care visit	3.5%	3.4%
OUTCOME MEASURES **ASTHMA-RELATED CONDITIONS**		
28 Emergency room visits specifically for asthma/1,000 asthmatics/year	57	86
29 Total admissions (acute) specifically for asthma/1,000 asthmatics/year	44	40
30 Total inpatient days (acute) specifically for asthma/1,000 asthmatics/year	273	177
ALL CONDITIONS FOR ASTHMATIC MEMBERS		
31 Total emergency room visits for all conditions/1,000 asthmatics/year	154	242
32 Total admissions (acute) for all conditions/1,000 asthmatics/year	128	149
33 Total inpatient days (acute) for all conditions/1,000 asthmatics/year	493	572
SATISFACTION MEASURES*		
34 Overall satisfaction with medical care at PCP office of asthmatic members	100.0%	95.9%
35 Satisfaction with the ability to make appointments for illnesses	95.4%	92.1%
36 Satisfaction with the response to an emergency call within 30 minutes	98.6%	93.0%

* Percent of respondents with Good, Very Good, or Excellent.

Exhibit 4. An example of the type of report cards that XMDD provided to management and providers.

Offices that failed to make a score of at least 2% received a 10% reduction in capitation payments during the subsequent 6 months. Those that maintained a score of at least 2% received an increase in their semi-monthly capitation payments equal to the percentage score. Thus the ABC Practice would have received a 14.55% increment in its capitation payments.

Each practice also received a 6-month quality-factored distribution based on its three utilization components (hospital, specialist, and ER) year-to-date, which was adjusted by the Quality Review and Comprehensive Care components (in Exhibit 5, 4.25% + 8.50% = 12.75%). If the practice had achieved a combined Quality Review and Utilization component score of at

---

Based on the quality of care, comprehensive service, and utilization, the ABC Practice earned the following quality factor, which is multiplied by their sex- and age-adjusted base capitation payment for the previous two weeks

Quality Review Components:

a.	Member Surveys (compared with others in HMO, range -0.75 to +3.0)	2.00%
b.	Focused Medical Chart Reviews (2/yr., comparative, -0.75 to +3.0)	0.75%
c.	Member Transfer Rates (comparative, -0.75 to +1.5)	0.50%
d.	Philosophy of Managed care (cooperation and participation with XMHC quality programs (subjective, -0.75 to +3.0)	<u>1.00%</u>
	Quality Review Subtotal	**4.25%**

Comprehensive Care Components:

a.	Membership Size (members/doctors or practice, e.g. range = 0, 1% at 100/doctor, 2% at 300/doctor)	1.00%
b.	Schedule Office Hours (range = 0, 0.5% for 50–59, 1.0% for 60–69, and 1.5% for >70 hours/week)	0.50%
c.	Available Office Procedures (e.g., flexible sigmoidoscopy = 1.0%, max. = 3%)	1.00%
d.	Program Education (completing XMHC educational courses [e.g., Current Concepts in Cancer = 0.5%] max. sum = 2%)	0.50%
e.	Internal Practice Coverage (1% if coverage is by practice for continuity)	1.00%
f.	Catastrophic Care (practice has greater than the HMO-type average total causes for catastrophic cases [e.g., >$20,000 = 1.5%])	1.50%
g.	Patient Management (1% if practice supports and participates in XMHC patient management and directs hospital care of own patients)	1.00%
h.	Practice Growth (XMHC membership growth [e.g., >10% = 1.0%])	1.00%
i.	Computer Links to XMHC (transmits encounter and referral data electronically = 1.0%)	<u>1.00%</u>
	Comprehensive Care Subtotal	**8.50%**

Utilization Components

a.	Hospital Utilization at the average bracket (range = -0.8 to +1.8%)	0.80%
b.	Specialist Utilization one bracket greater than average (-0.8 to +1.8)	0.40%
c.	Emergency Room Utilization one bracket less than average (-0.8 to +1.4%)	<u>0.60%</u>
	Utilization Subtotal	**<u>1.80%</u>**
	TOTAL QUALITY FACTOR =	**14.55%**

Exhibit 5. An illustration of how the quality factor is determined.

least 4% (4.25% + 1.80% = 6.05%), it was eligible for an office status payment of 5%, if it had remained open for XMHC enrollment throughout the period or if it had accepted current patients as XMHC members throughout that period.

The large employers that the company sought out tended to insist on NCQA certification. Therefore, one of Dr. Johnson's main performance objectives was to have the network meet the NCQA requirement of meeting its own written quality standards. He spent much time and effort making sure that the network conformed to NCQA requirements such as having a certain percentage of members within 15 minutes travel time of a primary care provider in the network and working with practices to help them achieve NCQA's HEDIS (Health Plan Employer Data and Information Set) standards for their patients. Another standard was that of keeping provider turnover below 5% per year.

The costs of achieving these standards can be substantial. In six months, the region had gone through a NCQA audit exercise, a Georgia exercise for Medicaid, and a federal exercise for Medicare. Then there were the operational costs of maintaining standards. NCQA standards, for example, required recredentialing each network physician every 2 years. With more than 7,000 physicians in their network in Georgia, that was a substantial workload, the cost of which made Dr. Johnson consider strategies for narrowing the network where possible. HMOs in Georgia were licensed county by county by the state. As geographic coverage was expanded, the number of physicians to be credentialed expanded. He found himself having to trade off greater choice for his patients with the costs of providing the larger provider network in the served areas as well as allocating scarce resources between served areas and new target market areas.

One decision that Dr. Johnson had to make was how much time to spend requesting and reviewing report cards on the physicians in the network. XMDD could generate an almost infinite number of reports like the one in Exhibit 4. They could also generate statistical reports identifying outlier individuals and practices. Much of the data on over- or underutilization were of more concern to the regional medical director responsible for patient management, but that medical loss ratio was part of his performance evaluation also.

DR. JOHNSON'S OBSERVATIONS ABOUT THE JOB

Dr. Johnson had been in the job only 6 months. So far, he was quite happy with the job and with its potential. He observed that the Dominion Northwest had been a useful transition for him to enable him to see the comparative advantages of various types of health care organizations and to get used to working in a large organization. He was no longer seeing patients, but he was comfortable with that fact. He had already "seen enough patients to fill Fulton County Stadium three times" and no longer found practice much of a challenge. He often compared the practice of medicine to flying an airplane: "When you need a skilled pilot, that individual is important and one's skills are critical during the unique takeoff and landing periods. However, in between take offs and landings, most of the system is on autopilot and that gets old over time. The same is true of medicine."

There were always the fires to fight and there were always special projects related to process improvement. The company had just gone through a major database cleanup of its provider records, for example. Many physicians had changed their affiliations due to mergers and acquisitions and thus their tax ID numbers, but had not informed their payers. A wrong provider ID number on a claim could hold up payment and distort the company's data on activities and costs. That had been a major effort for his group.

He observed that most physicians would not be comfortable with the length of time that it took to get things done in a large organization. They, like he, were used to dealing with and reaching closure on a presenting problem every 15 minutes. Recruiting a substantial group practice into the network might take as much as a year with a meeting every month to establish a trusting relationship and to work out the details of the contract.

Medical directors also had to be comfortable working as part of a management team, to influence others where possible, but take orders when necessary. They would have to know when to keep quiet and when to speak up. In the disease management arena, for example, the core management at Wheeling would often decide which disease management programs were "network impactable" and he would have to make them work. He noted that he still had more to learn about the politics of large organizations and about the insurance industry in general, about group selection, underwriting, claims management, contracting, and marketing. He certainly felt that he had a better idea of what groups such as independent practice associations (IPAs) could or could not do effectively. Having seen the information system investment that Vigilant-XMHC had to support membership enrollment, claims processing, disease management, and utilization review, he saw no way that much smaller, physician-led organizations could compete. Conversely, he felt that insurance organizations knew relatively little about managing practices or running hospitals and were better off not trying to integrate them.

Dr. Johnson was aware of the high turnover rate among medical directors in the industry. In his own words: "The health care environment is in turmoil and one needs a mentor, someone looking out for them, if one is to survive. One has to be careful to avoid the lose-lose situations that many medical directors had gotten into." By way of example, he cited medical directors of Medicaid managed care organizations when the Georgia State legislature decreed a 20% cut in funding, or those whose jobs were eliminated during mergers. He knew a local medical director working for MedPartners who was let go when the merger with Phycor was announced. Now that that merger did not go through, they were recruiting a replacement.

He noted that most physicians are not at all prepared for the practices of large organizations. He had heard them speak quite heatedly about the experience of a terminated medical director at another HMO who was given 20 minutes under observation to clean out her desk, escorted to the door with security person on each side, and asked to hand over her keys at the door. After a few months in a data-driven organization, he fully understood why. Why give anyone a chance to download proprietary information onto a computer disk or destroy a data set? No practicing physician, however, would ever expect to be mortified that way.

Dr. Johnson also felt that most physicians would have difficulty with having to clear so many decisions with the legal department or with public relations. Although there were policies and procedures governing most everything, he did not feel that they would constrain his team from setting aggressive goals, developing plans to compete in the markets that they chose, and implementing them quickly and efficiently. Most physicians, however, would have trouble at first being resource-constrained in what could be accomplished. When he was in practice, if he felt the practice would benefit from a piece of equipment, he bought it. It meant a loss in the profits distributed at the end of the month, but there was still enough. But when he wanted an additional employee to serve as a practice management coordinator, a highly skilled professional services consultant to go into network practices and help them solve billing or cost problems, he had to work hard to justify that position and show how it would contribute to meeting financial targets.

THE FUTURE

Dr. Johnson saw the provider community consolidating, which would give providers more power in the negotiations with the payer networks. He felt that the payers would have to learn how to do a better job of partnering with the providers so that, in sharing the risks, they would both succeed. Thus far, providers had had a very poor track record in profiting by taking on risk and he felt that one of his jobs in the future would be in helping them succeed.

He also saw many opportunities for expanding the network. There were many areas of Georgia, Mississippi, and Alabama that did not have rationalized provider networks. He recognized a need to tell the managed care story more effectively given the current hostility in the profession and in the media, which was being echoed politically in Georgia and Washington, D.C. He also saw the need to become more effective in negotiating good contracts, closely observing quality and utilization, and moving population to the good providers. There were many opportunities, many issues, and many unknowns to be faced.

13

Sibley Memorial Hospital

Kurt Darr
The George Washington University, Washington, D.C.

The Methodist Women's Home Missionary Society established the Lucy Webb Hayes National Training School for Deaconesses and Missionaries in 1891 for the purpose, in part, of providing health services to the poor of the Washington, D.C., area. The school was incorporated under the laws of the District of Columbia as a charitable, benevolent, and educational institution in 1894. The following year, the school built the Sibley Memorial Hospital, on North Capitol Street, to facilitate its charitable work. Over the years, operation of the hospital became the principal concern. As increasing demands were made on Sibley's facilities, it was renovated several times. In the mid-1950s, the hospital was relocated to Loughboro Road, in northwest Washington. This is an upper-class, affluent area of the city. The new 355-bed Sibley Memorial Hospital was dedicated on June 17, 1962. One half of the $8.8 million construction costs came from federal sources.

BOARD OF TRUSTEES[1]

In 1960, shortly after ground was broken for the new building, the board revised the corporate bylaws in preparation for an expected increase in the volume and complexity of hospital activities. The new bylaws required the board to meet at least twice a year and to consist of 25–35 members; the number varied from 27 to 33 during the 1960s and early 1970s. The board continued to be self-perpetuating (i.e., existing board members chose replacements to fill vacancies). Between meetings, an executive committee represented the board (see Appendix A). Several powers vested in this committee were financial: to open checking and savings accounts, to approve the hospital's budget, to renew mortgages, and to enter into contracts.

Most board members were prominent leaders in the community—a number were heavily involved in investment management and banking. The board chairman, Stacy M. Reed, was a Washington, D.C., attorney. Donald R. Ernst, former chairman of Steuart Investment Company, also in Washington, was the board treasurer. John M. Orem, M.D., was a board member and the administrator. All three were members of the executive committee. Others relevant to this case and their affiliations are listed in Table 1. As administrator, Orem was employed by the hospital. Although not an employee, Ernst was physically in the hospital on an almost-daily basis. All other trustees had principal vocations elsewhere, and service to the hospital was voluntary and incidental to their primary activities.

There were 11 members of the executive committee, and it was the real source of power on the board. Orem and Ernst were the most important members, as evidenced by the fact that their recommendations were routinely accepted and their actions ratified, usually without question. This relationship with the executive committee existed from the early 1950s until 1968, when Orem died after a brief illness. Ernst continued to be a dominant figure on the executive committee after Orem's death. Ernst died in 1972.

The 1960 changes in bylaws created a finance committee and an investment committee (see Appendix A). The former's primary functions were to review the budget and to report regularly the amount of cash available for investment. In turn, management of investments was to be supervised by the investment committee, which was to work closely with the finance committee.

Yet, from their creation in 1960 when the bylaws were modified until 1971—3 years after Orem's death—neither the finance nor the investment committee had ever met or conducted business. During this period—until 1968—Orem and Ernst made budgetary and investment decisions, like most other management decisions affecting the hospital's finances. The executive committee and the full board gave these decisions only cursory review.

Orem's death in 1968 obliged other board members to play a more active role in managing the hospital. The executive committee, and particularly Reed, who at that time was president of the hospital as well as chair-

Table 1.   Sibley trustees and their hospital and financial institution
responsibilities

Trustees responsibilities	Hospital responsibilities	Financial institution
Stacy M. Reed	Trustee (1956– Executive Committee (1961– Finance Committee (1961– Investment Committee (1961– Board Chairman (1960– President (1968–1972; 1973–	Security National Bank Director (1930– Executive Committee (1937– Minor stockholder
Lanier P. McLachlen	Trustee (1956– Investment Committee (1960–1973)	McLachlen National Bank Director (1974– Board Chairman (1953–1973) President (1922–1954) Principal stockholder (8.1%)
George M. Ferris	Trustee (1956– Finance Committee (1973– Investment Committee (1962–1970) Acting Treasurer (1972–1973)	Ferris & Co. Senior Partner (1971– Board Chairman (1971– Principal stockholder (42%)
Edward K. Jones	Trustee (1959– Executive Committee (1959– Finance Committee (1960–1973) Investment Committee (1971–1973)	Interstate Building Association Director (1932– Executive Committee (1932– Board Chairman (1969– President (1954–1969) Minor stockholder Riggs National Bank Director (1967– Executive Committee (1967–1974) Minor stockholder
Fred W. Smith	Trustee (1964– Executive Committee (1964– Investment Committee (1967–1973)	Riggs National Bank Advisory Director (1964– Minor stockholder Jefferson Federal Savings & Loan Director (1954– Executive Committee (1957– President (1959–

man of the board, became more deeply involved in day-to-day management
while efforts were made to find a new administrator. In 1970, he unsuccessfully pressed Ernst to activate the finance and investment committees.

It was some months after Orem's death until his replacement was
selected, and during this time there was a modest reorganization. The

position of executive director was created, and Garth L. Jarvis, M.D., was the first incumbent. Charles Blatchley was named administrator. Jarvis had little managerial experience, and Reed worked closely with him. It was generally agreed that Jarvis's performance was not entirely satisfactory. Ernst continued to make most of the financial and investment decisions for Sibley. His actions and failure to make prudent investment decisions, however, slowly came under increasing scrutiny by several other trustees, particularly after a series of disagreements between Ernst and the hospital comptroller led to the comptroller's discharge in 1971.

In 1971, Sibley Hospital applied for a $500,000 planning grant from the Department of Health, Education, and Welfare (HEW). It was denied. Major reasons cited by the reviewers were Jarvis's authority was substantially undercut by board involvement in the administrative operation of the hospital, and his function was undermined by the lack of an "effective" table of organization or "experienced and educated professional staff to support the chief executive officer." HEW also noted that the grant application had been developed without the knowledge of the hospital's medical staff and that the application was not of high quality, generally.

THE TREASURER

Ernst maintained almost exclusive control of the hospital's investments for more than a decade, until his death in 1972. As board treasurer, he shifted money among banks or accounts within banks and purchased or sold securities without consulting any other trustee. Because the investment and the finance committees never met, only Orem and a few other officers apparently were aware of Ernst's investment policies. Ernst did not consult with the hospital comptroller, although the comptroller did have some information about the accounts.

Ernst kept confidential the records of checking and savings accounts, the opening and closing of accounts, and the balance of various hospital accounts. Balances were never reported to other board members. Yearly audit reports were distributed to board members and other similar information was available for inspection, but the reports were treated as mere formalities. The executive committee did have to approve the opening of new accounts, however.

Board members approved Ernst's recommendations as a matter of course and rarely, if ever, read the relevant details of audits critically; investment decisions were left to the presumed expertise of Ernst. Some found that the treasurer regarded their suggestions as "interference" in these matters, and none forced the issue. A more vocal board member was Edward K. Jones. Over the years of Ernst's tenure, Jones repeatedly asked for information about the investment activities. He was more persistent after the hospital comptroller was forced out by Ernst. Jones did not, however, believe a move to oust Ernst would succeed, and no such effort was made. Jones's belief that, over the years, Ernst's investment activities had benefited the hospital also kept him from taking steps that otherwise might have been deemed necessary.

Under Ernst's direction, Sibley kept large amounts of money on deposit with certain banks and savings and loan associations. As shown in Table 2, the hospital maintained most of its liquid assets in savings and checking accounts rather than in U.S. treasuries or investment securities that would have yielded higher interest. Note in Table 2 the change from 1971 to 1972, which resulted from Reed's review of hospital investment policies. In 1971, for example, more than one fourth of the more than $4 million available for investment was deposited in checking accounts, compared to only $135,646 in securities and $310,436 in U.S. treasuries. Although substantial sums were used to purchase certificates of deposit, which produce at least a moderate amount of income, the hospital occasionally purchased from one financial institution a certificate yielding lower interest rates than were available elsewhere.

Most of these funds were deposited in financial institutions in which board members also served in ownership or managerial capacities. An example was a single checking account, drawing no interest and maintained alternately at Riggs National Bank and Security National

Table 2. Summary of Sibley financial assets, 1967–1972, as of December 31 (in dollars)[a]

Type of account	1972	1971	1970	1969	1968	1967
Sibley						
Checking	501,333	1,148,769	1,265,288	588,735	522,174	655,084
Savings	2,015,448	826,435	588,979	866,374	774,661	646,649
Certificates	2,043,435	2,029,211	1,325,000	900,000	900,000	900,000
U.S. treasuries	310,764	310,436	383,786	220,000	220,000	—
Securities (at cost)	135,749	135,646	140,446	71,621	71,621	70,052
All Hahnemann net financial assets[b]	413,152	588,464	538,755	505,046	687,909	427,638
Total	5,419,881	5,038,961	4,242,254	3,151,776	3,176,365	2,699,423

[a]Average liquidity equal to 6 weeks' operating expenses.

[b]Hahnemann Hospital, another Methodist charity, was merged with Sibley in 1956 in anticipation of the move to the new facility. Hahnemann had been retained as a separate corporate entity solely to receive certain charitable contributions under the terms of various wills and trusts, agreements that predated the merger. Sibley's board members also comprised the Hahnemann board, and Hahnemann funds had been maintained in most of the same banks as Sibley's.

Bank. It usually contained more than $250,000; once it grew to nearly $1 million.

Ernst's reasons for pursuing this conservative investment policy were not clear. It was suggested by some that his experience during the Depression (i.e., bank failures) was an important factor. That same experience probably helped explain his belief that Sibley should maintain close relationships with a few local banks and his apparent decision to favor those banks that held a mortgage on the hospital and that had interlocking directorships with the Sibley Hospital Board. Ernst had been chairman of Steuart Investment Co., whose majority owner was Curtis S. Steuart, a Riggs Bank director, executive committee member, and stockholder.

Ernst's decisions were reached without any apparent encouragement from the banks or board members who held directorships in interlocking fashion. These same persons, however, frequently approved transactions that benefited institutions with which they were affiliated, and occasionally they would even seek out such an arrangement, but there appears to have been no conspiracy or effort to obtain personal gain from such an arrangement. When the board's investigations in early 1971 showed the inadequacy of Ernst's policies, they moved toward a more realistic investment program in a manner that negated existence of a prior agreement.

Ernst's inability to work with the comptroller resulted in the comptroller's forced resignation in September 1971. He had joined the hospital as assistant director for finance and comptroller in 1969. Beginning in early 1971, Ernst refused to cooperate with him in any fashion. It was about this time that accounts shown in Table 2 exceeded the usual norm of 1 month's operating expenses. This factor may have caused the relationship to deteriorate. The animosity must have been significant because the minutes of a February, 1972, executive committee meeting show that, when Ernst was criticized by a board member about the extent of moneys being held in non–interest-bearing accounts, Ernst accused the already dismissed comptroller of misinforming the committee.

Prompted by these difficulties, Reed decided to activate the finance and investment committees in the fall of 1971. As chairman of the finance committee and member of the investment committee as well as board treasurer, however, Ernst continued to exercise dominant control over investment decisions and on several occasions discouraged and flatly refused to respond to inquiries into such matters. After Ernst's death in October 1972, other members of the board assumed a more identifiable supervisory role over investment policy and hospital fiscal management in general.

INTERLOCKING DIRECTORATES

Table 1 shows the extent to which board members who performed a variety of important hospital responsibilities also had significant positions in financial institutions with which Sibley had dealings.

One example of conflict of interest occurred when George M. Ferris advised and voted on the hospital's decision to contract for investment services. Jones raised the idea at a meeting of the reactivated investment committee in early 1971. It was decided that Ferris, a member of that committee, should present a proposal from Ferris & Co., of which Ferris was chairman of the board and principal stockholder, for the provision of continuing investment advisory services to Sibley. Ferris presented such a proposal on April 12, 1971, and the committee voted to recommend approval. Ferris urged acceptance and may have voted in favor of that recommendation at an informal session of the investment committee, but he then resigned from the investment committee to avoid further possible conflicts of interest. For a short time he served as acting treasurer following the death of Ernst, but several members of the board objected.

On formal approval by the hospital's legal counsel and the executive committee, of which Ferris was not a member, Sibley entered into the "investment advisory agreement" with Ferris & Co., and the written contract remained in effect for several years. Fees charged by Ferris & Co. were fair. There is ample evidence that Ferris & Co. did a good job, although shifts in market prices resulted in some loss in the account. This would not have occurred had the hospital kept the money in certificates of deposit.

A less clear example of conflict of interest occurred in the continuation of a mortgage dating from the late 1950s, when the board began negotiations with local banks to obtain a loan to finance construction of the new hospital building. When these negotiations broke off, the board obtained a commitment from a Texas bank. Although local banks had earlier refused to assist the hospital, several board members then organized a syndicate of Washington banks willing to provide the loan on terms equal to the Texas proposal and persuaded the board to accept the local offer. As a result, the syndicate agreed in 1959 to lend Sibley $3 million, secured by a mortgage on the hospital. The sum was increased to $3.5 million in 1961.

The loan was renewed in 1969 and repaid fully in 1972. Although Sibley had sufficient funds in 1969 to pay off the loan without totally impairing its ability to meet obligations as they came due, the executive committee voted instead for renewal. The committee reasoned that reduced cash flow would have put operations on a tight basis, and available funds might have been needed to renovate certain property owned by Sibley, or for new construction.

Terms of the loan were entirely fair to Sibley. There is no indication that the board could have received better terms elsewhere or that it had failed to diligently seek an optimal arrangement at the time of the original loan. The renewal in 1969 also appears to have been a reasonable, good-faith business decision. There is no indication that either decision was motivated by a desire to benefit the banks involved at the hospital's expense. Nonetheless, the hospital held significant amounts of funds in low– or non–interest-bearing accounts in many of the same banks to which it continued to pay interest on the mortgage.

It is unclear to what degree full disclosure preceded the frequent self-dealing that occurred during the 1960s. It is reasonable to assume that board members were generally aware of the various bank affiliations of their peers, but there is no indication that these conflicting interests were stressed in the executive committee or at meetings of the full board when it voted to approve particular transactions. At one time or another, all those on interlocking directorates approved self-dealing transactions, most of which were of relatively minor significance: one interested board member would join a dozen disinterested fellow members of the executive committee in unanimously approving a new bank account; two or three interested board members would support a similarly large group in voting to give or renew the hospital's mortgage.

There was no evidence that the financial institutions ever had any contact among themselves relating to handling Sibley's business, its apportionment, or even its existence. Board members as a group did not solicit business for any particular bank or savings and loan association, and, indeed, it appears that most of the Sibley business done with these interlocking institutions was initiated by hospital officers without advance knowledge or direction of the board. There was no recognizable pattern of dealing, no discussion, no complaint of deviation from a course of agreed conduct—in fact, nothing from which a conspiracy between board members and the banking institutions can be implied beyond the simple fact that the hospital did considerable business with financial institutions that had some interlocking ties to its board.

UNWELCOME PUBLICITY

In 1969 and 1970, Bradshaw Mintener, vice chairman of the board, began to raise questions about the quality of investment practices. Board minutes show that at various times he estimated losses as high as $50,000–$60,000 per year from failure of the board to have more aggressive investment policies. This amount was the estimated income that would have resulted from placing checking account funds in a savings account or similar investment rather than paying off the $7\frac{1}{8}\%$ mortgage. At one point in this controversy, Reed threatened Mintener with legal action.

In early 1973, information about the controversy over investment policy was leaked to the *Washington Post*, and a series of articles followed. The *Post* articles raised questions among various members of the public. The articles reported that as much as $1 million was being held in interest-free accounts, costing the hospital and its patients more than $100,000 per year in interest income. The articles estimated that the failure to pay off the mortgages added $1.11 to each patient day at Sibley. It was also reported, however, that the average *per diem* at Sibley of $111 was lower than that of most Washington, D.C., hospitals. More than a quarter of its $11.3 million annual revenue was received from the federal government, primarily through Medicare and Medicaid.

Reed was quoted in the article as saying that the hospital's attorneys did not believe board members were violating the law because, in Reed's view, they did not gain any personal benefit from transactions with the hospital. If there was any benefit, it was overshadowed by the benefit to the hospital of having the bankers' expert advice on financial matters. "Such advice," he said, "cannot be reckoned in terms of money." Reed went on to explain that large cash reserves were held in checking and savings accounts in order to pay for future remodeling or hospital expansion. This was done instead of retiring the mortgage.

The articles quoted a board member as saying that Reed and Ernst had periodically fought for control of Sibley since Reed had joined the board in 1956. As Reed got the better of these struggles, the balances in the account at his bank, Security, would rise. Likewise, as Ernst achieved more control, hospital balances at Riggs would go up. Reed became president of Sibley as well as chairman of the board in 1968. One year later, the hospital's primary checking account was switched from Riggs to Reed's bank, Security. When Ernst objected to the high balance at Security in September 1971, the primary account was transferred to Riggs and balances quickly rose to between $400,000 and $750,000.

On February 13, 1973, just over one week following disclosure of the alleged improprieties at Sibley Hospital, legal action was filed by David M. Stern and others as consumers of health services in a class action suit against the hospital and several board members and financial institutions. The plaintiffs contended that the five board members and five financial institutions were engaged in a conspiracy to enrich themselves at the expense of the hospital (and, ultimately, those who paid for services there). The interlocking relationships cited in the complaint are shown in Table 1. It was alleged that the defendants accomplished the conspiracy by arranging to have Sibley maintain unnecessarily large amounts of money on deposit with the defendant banks and savings and loan associations, drawing inadequate or no interest. Table 2 shows that the hospital did maintain its liquid assets in savings and checking accounts rather than in treasuries or securities, at least until the investment review instituted by Reed in late 1971. The plaintiffs also attempted to bolster the conspiracy theory by pointing to two other hospital transactions: continuation of a mortgage with the defendant financial institutions and the investment advisory agreement with Ferris & Co.

The plaintiffs also contended that the facts revealed serious dereliction of duty on the part of the defendants, who were alleged to have engaged in mismanagement, nonmanagement, and self-dealing; in other words, a breach of the fiduciary relationship that existed by reason of their service as board members.[2] Mismanagement was allegedly shown by the failure to use due diligence in investing and using hospital funds. Nonmanagement was alleged in the failure to supervise management of hospital investments or even to attend meetings of the committees charged with such supervision. The plaintiffs also alleged that self-dealing resulted from investing funds in financial institutions in which board members had director or officer status.

Prior to trial, but after suit was brought, the board adopted a new bylaw based on guidelines issued by the American Hospital Association (AHA). The AHA guidelines are shown in Appendix B. It uses the modified corporate rule, which relies on disclosure and abstaining from voting or any attempts to influence other members as means of eliminating or reducing potential conflicts of interest.

The fact that a lawsuit was filed against Sibley Hospital and against individual board members and their affiliated financial institutions shocked and angered virtually the entire board. They wondered what they had done to incur such an embarrassing reaction by members of the public, which they had labored to serve. It was a fine way to be thanked for their many hours of donated time and hard work on behalf of the community. They were, however, determined to fight the allegations and make every attempt to vindicate themselves.

ENDNOTES

1. The corporate board was called a board of trustees and its members were known as trustees even though no trust was involved and they actually functioned like corporate directors. This practice is common in health services organizations, especially hospitals.
2. To be a fiduciary means that one may not take selfish advantage of one's position or act in such a way as to benefit oneself. Fiduciaries must exercise good faith and serve the purposes of the organization. They must not utilize inside information or the power of office for personal benefit.

APPENDIX A

Administration of the Hospital's Finances

The bylaws of the hospital provided that business of the corporation should be transacted by a board of trustees (Article II), which should have regular meetings in October and May of each year (Art. III, Section 1):

> There shall be two regular meetings to be held in Washington, D.C., on dates to be fixed by the Executive Committee. One of said regular meetings shall be held in May of each year. The other regular meeting, to be known as the Semi-Annual Meeting, shall be held in October of each year.

Article V, Section 14, described the duties and responsibilities of the treasurer as follows:

> The Treasurer shall receive all funds and shall be the custodian of all securities belonging to the Corporation and shall perform the usual duties attendant upon this office, and the Treasurer may delegate such duties as are approved by the Board or Executive Committee of the Board.

Article VIII provided that the board shall elect from its members an executive committee. Section 2 of this article was as follows:

> The Executive Committee shall exercise general supervision and administration of the affairs of the corporation and during the interim of the meetings of the Board of Trustees shall be authorized to fully exercise the powers and duties of the Board, except that said committee shall have no power to amend the bylaws or to fill vacancies which may occur in the Board of Trustees.

Article IX, Section 1, provided for establishment of a finance committee consisting of the treasurer, the chairman of the investment committee, and three additional members. Section 2 was as follows:

> (A) It shall be the duty of the Finance Committee to administer all funds for the maintenance, operation, and development of the Hospital, including appropriations made by the Department of Work in Home Fields of the Woman's Division of the Board of Missions of the Methodist Church, and gifts, grants, bequests, and annuities from interested friends, patrons, and other sources.
>
> (B) The Finance Committee, with the President, shall prepare the annual budget and submit it to the annual meeting of the Board for its approval.
>
> (C) The Treasurer, under the direction of the Finance Committee, shall establish and maintain a separate fund, keeping the necessary

books and records thereof, to be known as the building fund, in which shall be kept all securities or cash which are intended to be set aside for use in the building expansion program of the Hospital.

Article X provided for an investment committee consisting of the treasurer and two members of the board. Its duties were set forth in Section 2 as follows:

(A)   It shall be the duty of the Investment Committee to invest all moneys belonging to the Corporation, which are available for investment purposes, under the direction of the Board of Trustees or the Executive Committee, and to see that all conditions, provisions, and specifications attached to any gifts, grants, and bequests to the corporation are complied with and carried out.

(B)   The Treasurer, under the direction of the Investment Committee, shall establish and maintain a separate fund, keeping the necessary books and records thereof, to be known as the endowment fund, in which shall be kept all securities and cash, which are to be retained as a permanent endowment. Only the income from said Endowment Fund shall be expended and such income shall be used solely for maintenance or current operating expenses of the Hospital, except that all or any of said fund may at any time be used for capital improvements or other expenditures as the Board may direct.

The following facts were established from hospital's bylaws, minutes of board meetings and various committees, and papers filed with the court during the legal proceedings:

1.   The finance committee was charged with the responsibility of and did review the budget of the hospital, approved it, and submitted it to the executive committee for approval. The finance committee determined what funds of the hospital were available for investment.

2.   The investment committee was charged with the responsibility of and did review the hospital's investments and submitted its recommendations to the executive committee.

3.   The treasurer, under the direction at times of the executive committee or the president and at other times on his own initiative, handled the funds of the hospital, opened checking and savings accounts, and purchased certificates of deposit from the various financial institutions as well as reviewed the balances in various accounts.

APPENDIX B

American Hospital Association—
Article XXVIII, Conflicts of Interest[1]

Section 1   Any duality of interest or possible conflict of interest on the part of any governing board member shall be disclosed to the other members of the board and made a matter of record through an annual procedure and also when the interest becomes a matter of board action.

Section 2   Any governing board member having a duality of interest or possible conflict of interest on a matter shall not vote or use his or her personal influence on the matter, and he or she shall not be counted in determining the quorum for the meeting, even where permitted by law. The minutes of the meeting shall reflect that disclosure was made, the abstention from voting, and the quorum situation.

Section 3   The foregoing requirements shall not be construed as preventing the governing board member from briefly stating his or her position in the matter, nor from answering pertinent questions of other board members since his or her knowledge may be of great assistance.

Section 4   Any new member of the board will be advised of this policy upon entering on the duties of office.

ENDNOTE

1.   Adopted by the board of trustees of Sibley Hospital in 1974.

Ethics Incidents

Kurt Darr
The George Washington University, Washington, D.C.

INCIDENT 1: THE ADMINISTRATIVE INSTITUTIONAL ETHICS COMMITTEE[1]

The CEO of Community Health Plan (CHP), a small not-for-profit HMO, has been approached by a group from "north of the river." This area of the city is economically depressed and has lost many of its health services organizations (HSOs) and physicians to the suburbs during the last decade. It seems to be in a downward vortex with no apparent bottom. An increasing number of uninsured patients means that HSOs are less and less able to continue serving the area. The city-owned hospital has made several ill-fated attempts to serve "north of the river" with a clinic system, but its efforts have been scandal-ridden. The system is a political football with little credibility in the community.

The representatives from "north of the river" are community leaders, none of whom appear to have any political ambitions. They seem genuinely willing to do whatever they can to assist in delivering high-quality health services in the community. They proposed that CHP establish and staff three store-front clinics in the area. The community leaders stated they would get volunteers to remodel the facilities and work in clerical capacities.

The CEO described the proposed activity to the administrative institutional ethics committee (IEC), which included members of governance, managers, and physicians and others from clinical areas. In making the presentation, the CEO stressed the plan's historical role in providing health services to those in need, its not-for-profit status, and its continuing modest surplus. The members listened patiently, but the minute the CEO finished all of them seemed to speak at once. Several were opposed and made the following points about the suggested venture:

1. "North of the river" is the city's responsibility. Providing care to the needy is not something a small, not-for-profit health plan should attempt.

2. They have a primary obligation to enhance benefits for their enrollees, rather than get involved in new schemes. Several of their physicians and many plan members have requested additional services.

3. The modest surplus that the plan has accumulated over several years could easily be consumed. The chief financial officer noted that they are expecting an increase in reinsurance premiums in the next quarter.

4. If the plan pulls the city's political chestnuts out of the fire by providing even stop-gap assistance, the city will never get its house in order and develop the system needed "north of the river."

Several spoke in favor of working "north of the river":

1. Helping the "north of the river" community is the right thing to do. The people there deserve health services. It was noted that CHP's own start had come about when several physicians in the community fought the prevailing attitude among their peers about prepaid practice.

2. Those opposed are putting dollars ahead of people's health. They must be willing to assist those less fortunate.

3. Plan members will support such an initiative if it is properly explained to them.

4. The positive publicity will further plan interests by increasing the number of enrollees.

It seems to the CEO that this is a no-win situation. The organizational philosophy is not well developed, and the proposal is a major step. Something should be done to assist the "north of the river" community. The IEC members are raising valid points that merit further discussion.

INCIDENT 2: MIRIAM HOSPITAL[2]

Before 1980, a six-channel analyzer performed routine blood tests at Miriam Hospital. In 1980, the hospital purchased and put into operation a 12-channel blood analyzer. Because of a computer programming error, patients continued to be charged for *both* sets of tests, even though only the 12-channel machine was used.

A year later, Blue Cross raised questions about the unusually high laboratory charges at Miriam compared with other hospitals. The explanation was that doctors at Miriam simply ordered more lab tests. In 1982, a professional standards review organization audit clerk uncovered the double billing. The manager of information systems was ordered by his immediate superior to eliminate the programming error. Shortly thereafter, however, he was told by "top officials" at Miriam to reinstate it.

Later in 1982, a Blue Cross auditor uncovered the same problem and asked for a copy of the program. The manager of data processing was told to erase any evidence in the program that showed the original error had been reintroduced. Blue Cross was provided the sanitized program.

Shortly thereafter, two data-processing personnel were accused of allowing an outside company to use Miriam's computer in contravention of hospital policy. Each was offered the opportunity to resign. Fearing he would be made a scapegoat, one of them went to Blue Cross with the information. Blue Cross took the case to the attorney general's office. Six months later, a grand jury handed up indictments against the hospital and several senior managers. The crimes charged included obtaining money under false pretenses, conspiracy, and filing false documents. The alleged overbilling amounted to almost $2.8 million.

The hospital's and managers' defense was based on their interpretation of the rules under which reimbursement was made. They argued that the rules required hospitals to continue with the same accounting methods for the entire fiscal year, even though there were errors of the sort found in this case. An end-of-fiscal year audit would then determine what financial adjustments were needed.

INCIDENT 3: MAILING LISTS[3]

University Hospital has a very active cardiac medicine service in its department of medicine. Over the years, it has treated thousands of persons with problems ranging from angina to congestive heart failure. A number of times, its patients have been included in special study programs, most often funded by either the National Institutes of Health or a national heart association.

As part of long-term patient follow-up, regular questionnaire surveys are conducted. In order to perform the surveys, an extensive mailing list is maintained by the cardiac medicine service. On one occasion, the development department of University Hospital used the mailing list to solicit general contributions. Once it had a special fund-raising effort to assist in converting and equipping a six-bed cardiac intensive care unit. Results of fund raising among the cardiac program's present and former patients have been excellent, primarily because of the superior rapport and reputation it has with them.

The physician director of the program and her administrative assistant have been approached by a prominent national life insurance company that has been impressed with results of the program. It wants to market life insurance among the program's participants. The proposal is attractive because the opportunity to obtain life insurance will benefit present and former patients, because many of them are otherwise uninsurable except at very high premiums, and because any data obtained by the insurance company will be available to the hospital at cost if the mailing list is provided to the insurance company.

The physician director and administrative assistant are very enthusiastic about the clinical possibilities (in addition to helping the patients), and the director of development sees the sale of mailing lists as an excellent means of raising money for the cardiac program's activities. They have just spent an hour making their arguments to try to convince the chief executive officer of the appropriateness of releasing the mailing list for such a worthy purpose.

INCIDENT 4: BITS AND PIECES[4]

John Henry Williams really liked his new job in the department of radiology at Affiliated Nursing Homes and Rehabilitation Center. He had recently been appointed acting head when his predecessor, Mary Beth Jacobson, went on maternity leave. As acting head of radiology, John Henry is responsible for two and a half full-time equivalent (FTE) technicians, an appointments clerk, and more than $250,000 worth of equipment. He has authority to purchase radiographic supplies, including certain types of film. The total value of these purchases is approximately $90,000 per year. Most are obtained from three vendors, companies with which the organization has done business for many years.

When Mary Beth oriented John Henry to the demands and responsibilities of the job, she told him that some of the best parts were the meetings with the sales representatives from the three vendors. She said that most of these meetings were held at nice restaurants in the suburban area around the center. Some were held in her office. When that was the case, she said, the sales representatives invariably brought along a "little something." When John Henry asked what that meant, Mary Beth gave examples: perfume, a bottle of French brandy, and a pen set in a nice case. John Henry remembered thinking that his wife might like the perfume.

He asked Mary Beth whether there was a policy concerning accepting gifts from vendors. Mary Beth was a little put out by the question, because it seemed to suggest something might be wrong with the practice. She responded somewhat curtly that the center's senior management trusted its managers and allowed them discretion in such matters.

Personally, John Henry was more interested in the lunches, because it seemed to be a chance for him to leave the facility occasionally and get away from the dreary cafeteria as well as his routine sack lunches. Mary Beth described the lunches as nothing especially fancy. She estimated their cost to the sales representative as about the same as small gifts—the $40–$50 range.

John Henry asked whether the action might not suggest to some members of the staff that her decisions were being influenced by the pecuniary relationship with the sales representatives. Mary Beth's anger flashed. She quickly gave four reasons in justification to John Henry:

1. Taking clients to lunch or providing small gifts was common in business relationships.

2. There was no cost to the center because the vendors paid for everything and they could charge it against their expense account, or get reimbursed by the company.

3. At least one of the sales representatives had become a friend over the years and she enjoyed his company on a social level as well.

4. There was absolutely no possibility her judgment could be influenced for the small amounts of money involved.

Somewhat heatedly, Mary Beth added, "I know you're thinking that somehow this whole thing doesn't look right. But that isn't fair at all. I work long hours as a manager and get paid very little extra. It also takes more effort and time to do the ordering and keep the inventory of supplies at a proper level. If anything goes wrong, it's my neck that's in a noose. These gratuities from vendors are a little something to help compensate me for those activities. My work for the center has been very effective. I'd be happy to talk to anyone who thinks otherwise!"

INCIDENT 5: PROTECTING THE COMMUNITY[5]

University Hospital has a unique role. It is not only a tertiary referral hospital for the region but also a major source of service to the community. In 1977, it experienced an outbreak of *Legionella* (the bacteria causing Legionnaire's disease). A number of patients were affected; several died.

Legionnella is a bacterial infection of the respiratory tract and lungs that may result in death if not diagnosed and treated early. It is especially dangerous for elderly people and those with medical problems that weaken their general resistance. A factor requiring even greater caution on the part of hospital management is that, at the time of the outbreak, the process for identifying the organism in the laboratory took several days. Thus, patients were at great risk until a confirmatory diagnosis was obtained. Epidemiological studies showed a relationship between air conditioning cooling towers and the fine mist they give off and spread of the disease through the aerosol. Workers exposed directly to the aerosol have contracted severe cases of *Legionnella*. Chlorinating the water in the cooling towers eliminates the organism.

Although a cooling tower was implicated in the 1977 outbreak at University Hospital, the relationship was never confirmed. The infection control committee of the hospital did not develop any standing orders or policies after the first outbreak. In May 1982, there was evidence of another outbreak of *Legionnella*. Chlorination was immediately undertaken and the number of new cases dropped dramatically. An undetected failure in the chlorination system, however, brought a second outbreak in early June.

When the first cases were detected in May 1982, the administrator was notified. He met with various staff members, including physicians on the attending staff. It was decided that information about the outbreak should be kept from the community, lest there be a panic and a sudden drop in census, as well as loss of public confidence. A confidential letter was sent to staff physicians advising them of the problem and asking that they keep in mind the *potential* for infection when making admissions decisions. Admissions were not limited to emergencies, however, and there was no prospective review of elective admissions to determine whether patients at risk for pulmonary infections such as *Legionnella* should be sent elsewhere. Nor was there any review of indications for, and necessity of, admission. The medical staff developed a protocol (standing order) stating that unexplained acute-onset pneumonias were to be treated immediately with a very potent antibiotic shown to be effective against *Legionnella*. No provision was made, however, for effective review to determine that the protocol was actually followed on a concurrent basis.

INCIDENT 6: DECISIONS[6]

Mrs. Nickleby is in her mid-forties and has severe multiple sclerosis, a chronic disease that impairs muscular control. She has been a resident of Hightower Nursing Home for almost 3 years. Her two teenage daughters live with her sister in a nearby subdivision and visit her often. Mr.

Nickleby, a middle-management executive with a local firm, divorced her 5 years ago.

Mrs. Nickleby has frequent acute attacks of asthma. To date they have been caught in time by the nursing staff; on a couple of occasions she has had to be rushed to the emergency room of the local community hospital. Her physician, who treats her at Hightower Nursing Home, has ordered "no code" if Nickleby has a cardiac arrest during an acute asthma episode at the nursing home—that is, she will not be resuscitated. (Skilled nursing facilities [and acute care hospitals] have different signals, or codes, that are used to call a resuscitation team over the loud-speaker system to respond to a cardiac arrest without alarming other patients and visitors.)

As far as the nurses know, Nickleby's physician made his decision without having discussed it with the patient or her family. One of the nurses is very upset because the decision conflicts with her professional values, although she admits in private that, if she were Nickleby, she would find the situation intolerable and that she would not want to continue living in those circumstances. None of the nurses has heard Nickleby express the same opinion about her condition, even though she has become increasingly depressed, especially after each episode. The nurses have asked the administrative director of the unit for advice.

INCIDENT 7: THE MISSING NEEDLE PROTECTOR[7]

E.L. Straight is director of clinical services at Hopewell Hospital. As in most hospitals, a few physicians deliver care that is acceptable but not of very high quality; they tend to make more mistakes than the others and have a higher incidence of patients going "sour." Since Straight took the position 2 years ago, new programs have been developed and things seem to be getting better.

Dr. Cutrite has practiced at Hopewell for longer than anyone can remember. Although once a brilliant surgeon, he has slipped physically and mentally over the years, and Straight is contemplating steps to recommend a reduction in his privileges. However, the process is not yet complete, and Cutrite continues to perform a full range of procedures.

The operating room supervisor appeared at Straight's office one Monday afternoon. "We've got a problem," she said, somewhat nonchalantly, but with a hint of disgust. "I'm almost sure we left a plastic needle protector from a disposable syringe in a patient's belly, a Mrs. Jameson. You know, the protectors with the red-pink color. They'd be almost impossible to see if they were in a wound."

"Where did it come from?" asked Straight.

"I'm not absolutely sure," answered the supervisor. "All I know is that the syringe was in a used surgical pack when we did the count." She went on to describe the safeguards of counts and records. The discrepancy was noted when the records were reconciled at the end of the week. A surgical pack was shown as having a syringe that was not supposed to be there. When the scrub nurse working with Cutrite was questioned, she remembered that he had used a syringe, but, when it was included in the count at the conclusion of surgery, she didn't think about the protective sheath, which must certainly have been on it.

"Let's get Mrs. Jameson back into surgery," said Straight. "We'll tell her it's necessary to check her incision and deep sutures. She'll never know that we're really looking for the needle cover."

"Too late," responded the supervisor, "she went home the day before yesterday."

Damn, thought Straight. Now what to do? "Have you talked to Dr. Cutrite?"

The supervisor nodded affirmatively. "He won't consider telling Mrs. Jameson that there might be a problem and calling her back to the hospital," she said. "And he warned us not to do anything, either," she added. "Dr. Cutrite claims it cannot possibly hurt her. Except for a little discomfort, she'll never know it's there."

Straight called the chief of surgery and asked a hypothetical question about the consequences of leaving a small plastic cap in a patient's belly. The chief knew something was up but didn't pursue it. He simply replied that there would likely be occasional discomfort, but probably no life-threatening consequences from leaving it in. "Although," he added, "one can never be sure."

Straight liked working at Hopewell Hospital and didn't relish crossing swords with Cutrite, who, although declining professionally, was politically very powerful. Straight had refrained from fingernail biting for years, but that old habit was suddenly overwhelming.

INCIDENT 8: DEMARKETING TO AVOID BANKRUPTCY[8]

Chris Hines had finally gotten down far enough in the stack of papers on her desk to get to last month's emergency department (ED) activity report. She had already digested the grim news about the continued financial hemorrhage affecting Community Hospital. The current deficit was $500,000— and it was only the fourth month of the fiscal year. Because Community served a largely inner-city population, many of whom were uninsured or whose care was paid by a chronically underfunded Medicaid program, there seemed to be little hope of the financial situation improving.

Hines knew that more than 40% of Community's admissions came through the ED, and that about half of those admissions arrived by taxi, by private automobile, or on foot. The other half was brought in by the ambulance service run by the city government. Hines had tried to implement a plan to increase the number of elective admissions (and thus improve the payer mix) by encouraging physicians to bring their private patients to Community. This effort failed, however, largely because of the difficulty physicians had in getting their patients admitted—ED admissions were taking too many beds. Hines then tried to work with city officials to implement a new ambulance routing system that would give Community a chance to improve its financial condition. This effort also failed because city officials were unsympathetic.

Hines knew that Community's endowment would carry the hospital about 3 years, but that it would be forced to close if it were not breaking even by then. Because there was nothing that could be done with the city, Hines concluded that the key to survival lay with reducing the number of uninsured and Medicaid admissions through the ED.

Hines spoke with several marketing consultants, one of whom offered to do *pro bono* work for Community. He seized on the idea of "demarketing" the ED. He reasoned that it was the fine reputation Community's ED had in its service area that was largely responsible for the 50% of ED patients who came in other than by city ambulance. He then set out to identify ways in which ED could be made less attractive to potential patients. The plan he developed included reducing ED staffing to the very minimum; closing the parking lot near the ED; reducing housekeeping services so that the physical plant would be dirty and unkempt; deferring indefinitely all non–safety-related maintenance; changing the triage policies, procedures, and staffing so as to increase waiting time for nonemergency patients; using staff who were most likely to be rude and inconsiderate; and encouraging rumors that the closure of the ED was imminent.

The consultant knew there might be repercussions beyond the ED, but Community Hospital was desperate, and he believed there was no choice but to take extreme action.

INCIDENT 9: SOMETHING MUST BE DONE, BUT WHAT?[9]

Stunned, Carolyn Aubrey, the CEO of Metropolitan Hospital, sank into her chair and stared out the window for a very long time. She realized when Dr. Midmore's wife had angrily insisted on seeing the CEO that something was afoot. Even in her worst nightmares, however, Aubrey could never have imagined that Mrs. Midmore would tell Aubrey that she was suing her husband, an orthopedic surgeon, for divorce because he had given her AIDS. As Mrs. Midmore left Aubrey's office, she had turned back and said, "I was sure you'd want to know—surely you'll want to do something."

Fleetingly, Aubrey thought Mrs. Midmore's remarks might be nothing more than the ravings of an angry, vindictive wife, but that was not likely. As she considered what she had just learned, she recalled an incident several years ago involving Dr. Midmore and a male orderly. In retrospect, it now suggested that he might be bisexual. Aubrey thought, too, about the department of surgery meeting last year when there had been a long discussion about the desirability of knowing the HIV status of all surgical patients. The special risks of torn gloves and cuts during orthopedic surgery had been described in detail.

Now it seemed that Dr. Midmore's patients were at special risk. Aubrey called operating room scheduling and learned that Dr. Midmore was maintaining a full surgical load. Aubrey asked her secretary to call the hospital attorney and the medical director and set up an emergency meeting for 7:00 A.M. the following morning. *Mrs. Midmore might have been telling the truth*, thought Aubrey. *We will have to do something, but what?*

INCIDENT 10: A POTENTIALLY SHOCKING REVELATION

Geraldene Jones had been a nurse before she earned her master of health services administration degree and began her trek to the top of the corporate ladder, a trek that sometimes seemed agonizingly slow. Her love of long-term care and improving the way it is provided fuels her goal to become the chief executive officer of a large nursing facility. Currently, Jones is the vice president for support services at a large nursing facility. It is part of a for-profit chain that owns more than 100 facilities; most of them are large and have more than 200 residents. The facility has an excellent reputation, and there is a waiting list for admission.

Jones's facility is undergoing a major expansion of its physical plant, one that will almost double the square feet. The new space will house rehabilitation services and will add a new respite care program and about 50 new private residents' rooms. Jones volunteered to be responsible for the building program, and some of her other duties were reassigned. She volunteered because she believed success in getting the building program completed on time and under budget would bring her to the attention of corporate headquarters and would make her more promotable.

One day as Jones walked through the half-completed structure, she overheard a heated conversation between the foreman for the electrical contractor and the county electrical inspector. The inspector was pointing out a long list of discrepancies, which ranged from the number of amperes of overall electrical service to the location and number of outlets. The contractor stated repeatedly that the inspector was being overly aggressive in applying the county electrical code. After the inspector left, Jones approached the electrical contractor and asked him whether there were any problems that she should know about. The electrical contractor rubbed two of his fingers and thumb together and said, "Nothing that a little 'grease' won't take care of." It was obvious that the contractor was talking about bribing the inspector. Jones expressed shock and was rebuked by the contractor. "Obviously, you're new to the construction game. Payoffs are common, and I've dealt with this kind of thing before. I know what to do and it's what we'll have to do if you want this building completed on time. I have an account for just such a contingency, but you may have to add to it if the electrical inspector isn't reasonable."

Jones was stunned. She had no idea what to say or what to do.

ENDNOTES

1. From Darr, K. (1997). *Ethics in health services management* (3rd ed., pp. 80–81). Baltimore: Health Professions Press; reprinted by permission.
2. From Darr, K. (1997). *Ethics in health services management* (3rd ed., pp. 110–111). Baltimore: Health Professions Press; reprinted by permission.
3. From Darr, K. (1997). *Ethics in health services management* (3rd ed., p. 136). Baltimore: Health Professions Press; reprinted by permission.
4. From Darr, K. (1997). *Ethics in health services management* (3rd ed., p. 107). Baltimore: Health Professions Press; reprinted by permission.
5. From Darr, K. (1997). *Ethics in health services management* (3rd ed., pp. 150). Baltimore: Health Professions Press; reprinted by permission.
6. Adapted from Aroskar, M. (1977, August). Case No. 461, Case studies in bioethics. *Hastings Center Report*, p. 17; used by permission.
7. From Longest, Jr., B.B., Rakich, J.S., & Darr, K. (2000). *Managing health services organizations and systems* (4th ed., pp. 725–726). Baltimore: Health Professions Press; reprinted by permission.
8. From Darr, K. (1997). *Ethics in health services management* (3rd ed., pp. 210–211). Baltimore: Health Professions Press; reprinted by permission.
9. From Darr, K. (1997). *Ethics in health services management* (3rd ed., p. 233). Baltimore: Health Professions Press; reprinted by permission.

PART III

Resource Utilization and Control

15

Endoscopes at Victoria Hospital

Elizabeth M.A. Grasby

Mark D. Applebaum
The University of Western Ontario, London, Ontario, Canada

Richard Ivey School of Business
The University of Western Ontario

Ivey

As manager of clinical engineering at Victoria Hospital in London,[1] Ontario, Canada, Mark Greig was part of a team responsible for managing the Hospital's medical technology. Greig knew something had to be done to improve the quality and cost of repairs being made to the Hospital's flexible endoscopes by outside firms. It was now early April 1994 and Greig was eager to prepare for the monthly team meeting, which was to take place on April 18.

VICTORIA HOSPITAL

Victoria Hospital (VH) was one of the larger hospitals in Canada with 667 beds, and an annual budget of $267 million in 1992. The majority of this budget (81%) came from the Ministry of Health. In addition to VH's budget, the Ontario Health Insurance Plan (OHIP) was a major source of funds which contributed on a per service basis. VH, St. Joseph's Hospital (SJH), and University Hospital (UH) were the three largest hospitals in London. There was significant coordination between these hospitals, which were linked through the University of Western Ontario as "teaching hospitals." Although VH specialized in Cardiology, Pediatrics, and Oncology, its services were extremely diverse with specialists in most areas.

THE BIOMEDICAL ENGINEERING DEPARTMENT

The Biomedical Engineering Department (BME) was a team of 17 people which focused on managing VH's medical technology. The BME team was directed by Steve Elder and was part of the Medical Operations Division of VH. Other members of the team included Paul Howarth, Dennis Pickersgill, Mark Greig, 12 special area technologists, and a secretary. Howarth, the equipment management coordinator, was responsible for the financial management of repair budgets and medical capital acquisitions. Pickersgill managed the technical concerns of the division as technical supervisor, and Greig was involved from an engineering perspective as manager of Clinical Engineering. Greig held a mechanical engineering degree and was a 1991 MBA graduate from the Western Business School,[2] London, Ontario.

Services provided by BME included the purchase, maintenance, repair, and disposal of hospital equipment, and assisting departments in bringing new technology on-line. BME had an operating budget of approximately $1.3 million in 1994 but was also responsible for managing VH's medical capital budget of approximately $4.0 million. Most equipment repair costs were covered by each department's budget.

ENDOSCOPY

VH used flexible and rigid "endoscopes" in gastroenterological and surgical procedures for both exploratory and corrective purposes. An endoscope was a device which could be inserted into the human body to view areas such as the lungs, stomach, digestive tract, or major joints. Under most circumstances, the patient was awake during the operation. Some endoscopes were flexible and could be manipulated using angulation knobs which controlled the vertical and horizontal movement of the device's head. Once inserted, a scope could perform various functions such as suction and fluid exchange, and was particularly useful because of high resolution video technology which allowed viewing of areas that would otherwise require major exploratory surgery. The Endoscopy department (Endoscopy) dealt with approximately 2,500 cases[3] in 1993.

Endoscopes were maintenance- and repair-intensive devices, which involved extremely sensitive technology. The scopes were tested before and after every case. This rigorous process included cleaning, leak testing, measuring of angulation ranges, and video picture testing. Despite this careful maintenance, the scopes frequently broke down during surgery, which required aborting the operation and rescheduling the patient for the next day. The scope requiring repair could be temporarily replaced by borrowing from SJH or UH (subject to availability). The quantity of each type of scope that VH owned varied but was as low as one or two scopes for some types.

Endoscopy purchased two or three new flexible scopes each year at a cost of approximately $20,000 each and spent an additional $20,000 to $30,000 per year on related equipment such as video processors. The operating room (OR) also used some flexible and rigid scopes. Rigid scopes cost approximately $5,000 to $10,000 and were often replaced if they required a significant amount of repair. Total spending by VH in 1993 on scope repairs, including Endoscopy and OR, was approximately $60,000.

ORIGINAL EQUIPMENT MANUFACTURERS

There were three original equipment manufacturers (OEMs) in Ontario that sold endoscopes. VH and UH bought and serviced most of their scopes at Barton Surgical Ltd. (Barton), while SJH dealt with Weber Inc. (Weber). The third OEM, Bowe Technical (Bowe), was not used by any of the three hospitals.

In choosing Barton as VH's scope supplier and servicer, VH's physicians were originally asked to decide which of the available scopes would be acceptable from a medical perspective. BME would then consider technical specifications and financial issues. VH had developed a long-lasting relationship with Barton and spent approximately $150,000 annually on Barton products and services such as flexible and rigid scopes, video equipment, and repairs.

Since, historically, OEMs were the only companies that could provide the highly technical parts, they had been the only option available for scope repairs, which usually took approximately two weeks. OEMs were extremely protective of their supply of parts. There was some concern among endoscope users that OEMs were charging unreasonable prices for repairs. There was also the suspicion that, occasionally, repairs were made that were unnecessary. Historically, there was no way to verify repair estimates since even the process of removing the sealed casing on an endoscope required technical tools and methods which were carefully guarded by the OEMs.

CHANGES TO THE ENDOSCOPE INDUSTRY

Recently, there had been other firms entering the endoscope repair industry in Canada and the United States. These firms offered free estimates, cheaper repairs, faster turnaround times, and written warranties.

In January 1994, a scope in need of repair was sent to an out-of-province repair firm as a test case. The work done took approximately three weeks and turned out to be unacceptable. The scope broke again after being used 25 times.

VH had intended to send the scope back to the out-of-province firm for further repairs. Inadvertently, the scope was sent to Barton, the OEM. A few days later, a representative from Barton brought the scope to the BME offices at VH. Greig was shocked at the repair work that had been done. The scope was severely damaged. The Barton representative explained that this was what could be expected when Barton scopes were repaired by third party servicers. Since Greig knew that the scope could not have been used 25 times in its current state, he concluded that Barton must have been responsible for the damage in an effort to discredit the out-of-province firm.

Greig was further disturbed when a scope which had previously been sent only to Barton for repairs was returned with an estimate for repairs which had resulted, Barton claimed, from a third party attempting to open the scope using improper tools.

Further attempts at having scopes repaired at firms other than Barton had resulted in unsatisfactory work and long delays—apparently due to difficulty in getting the necessary parts.

IN-HOUSE REPAIRS

VH repaired most of its equipment in-house. Due to the technical nature of the endoscopes and the difficulty of obtaining parts, all scope repairs were sent to outside firms. In November 1993, Steve Elder had attended a meeting of the Toronto Hospital's Consortium, which was a banded group of hospitals within Toronto similar to the three major London hospitals. The consortium had been successful in combining purchasing initiatives and had moved their scope repairs in-house resulting in significant savings.

The BME team had been discussing a similar coordination between VH, UH, and SJH. Combined, the three hospitals spent approximately $240,000 on scope repairs annually. There were four possible levels of service for an in-house repair operation including preventative maintenance, pre-repair screening (estimates), minor repairs, and major repairs. Historically, VH was only involved in the preventative maintenance level. Greig estimated that 80% of repair costs related to the first three levels of service. He also realized that the fourth level of repair would be impossible to move in-house due to the lack of technical knowledge. Recently, however, competitive pressure had made Barton more responsive to assisting with the second and third levels of service. If requested, the OEM would supply the parts and technical training for minor repair work and would give BME a list of necessary tools.

Paul Howarth, the equipment management coordinator, arrived at the following cost estimates for bringing the endoscope repairs in-house:

- The hospital would spend $25,000 annually on parts for VH or a total of $80,000 for all three hospitals.

- The same inventory of tools would be necessary regardless of whether the in-house operation was for VH only, or for all three hospitals. These tools would cost $20,000.

- A technician to perform the work could be hired at $25 per hour and would have to be in the hospital 40 hours per week, 50 weeks per year regardless of repair demand. Total repair time was projected to be 700 hours for VH and a total of 2,000 hours for all three hospitals.

- There was space available in the hospital which could be used for the operation. Renovations would cost $5,000.

- Training costs would be $2,000 initially, plus $1,000 each year in order to keep up with the rapidly changing technology.

- A parts inventory would have to be kept on hand at all times. This cost would be $35,000 for VH or a total of $100,000 for all three hospitals.

Each repair would take approximately three hours, which would significantly reduce the "downtime" that endoscopy would experience while the scope was out of service. Even at times when the technician might be overloaded with work, Howarth estimated that at least two days' turnaround time would be saved by doing the repairs in-house.

Greig knew he had many factors to consider. The monthly department meeting, which would focus on endoscopes, was less than three weeks away. Specifically, Greig wanted to report his findings and make the appropriate recommendations regarding the in-house scope repair possibility.

ENDNOTES

1. London's population was over 320,000, while Ontario's population of almost nine million accounted for one-third of Canada's citizenry.
2. Now known as The Richard Ivey School of Business.
3. Case: Term used to refer to an individual patient

16

Regional Health System

The Satellite Health Park Strategy

Jonathon S. Rakich
Indiana University Southeast, New Albany, Indiana

Michael F. Rolph
First Health of Carolina, Pinehurst, North Carolina

As he prepared for the December 1993 board meeting, Michael Reynolds, Senior Vice President and Chief Financial Officer of Regional Health System (RHS) felt exhilarated by the bold strategic initiatives that were implemented by RHS in July. The change to the organization had been breathtaking and the manner in which RHS delivered health services was fundamentally different from that of just a year ago. Reynolds was, however, still worried about the increasingly turbulent and threatening health services delivery environment. He knew that if "you rest you rust." He was still somewhat apprehensive about RHS's future and survival. The always-present prospect of marginal financial performance, or worse, the specter of acquisition by an aggressive for-profit hospital system remained in the deep reaches of his mind.

As the "money man" of the $140 million a year organization, Reynolds felt confident that the satellite health park strategy to be presented for consideration by the board at its December 1993 meeting was financially viable. Still, he had a sinking feeling that other considerations and external forces could affect the potential success of the strategy.

Reynolds, age 49, has always been comfortable with numbers. His MBA and CPA background, 5 years teaching experience as a professor of accounting at a major university, and 20 years experience in various financial positions at two nonprofit hospitals and a managed care insurance company provided him with an in-depth understanding of the financial dimensions of health services delivery. He had witnessed the industry evolve from rather simple reimbursement systems two decades ago to the exceedingly complex systems of today. He thought to himself:

> Can we keep up with the fast-paced changes? It seems that today's market place pressures, especially from government, managed care organizations, large third-party payers and competitors, including physicians, have turned traditional health services delivery upside down. I know what the numbers tell me. Robert Meek [President and CEO] and I should strongly recommend to the board that the satellite health park strategy be seriously considered for implementation. Yet, the numbers don't tell all. There are other considerations, some beyond control, that might affect them or cause them to unravel.

BACKGROUND

Prior to July of 1993, RHS was a stand alone 342-bed not-for-profit acute care hospital that served a predominantly elderly community in Florida. The hospital had been operationally profitable during the 1980s even after the implementation of the Medicare prospective payment reimbursement system (PPS) in 1983. Under PPS, the federal government reimbursed hospitals for Medicare acute care inpatient services based on diagnosis-related groups (DRGs). Each DRG represents an associated fixed reimbursement amount by case/discharge regardless of the hospital's cost in delivering the service. In the early 1990s, however, the hospital had begun to see its operating margin suffer as the federal government's efforts to reduce its deficit translated into reduced Medicare reimbursement.

Approximately 45% of the population of the hospital's primary and secondary markets are age 65+ compared to a national average of 13%. Due to the greater than proportionate utilization of health services by the elderly, the hospital's Medicare payer mix was and still is greater than that of 99% of hospitals nationally. The hospital's operating and capital costs of providing inpatient care per case/discharge for Medicare patients had been increasing at a rate in excess of 7% each year since 1983, while the Medicare program has provided less than a 3% reimbursement rate increase each year through the same period. Given the situation of declining margins, in July of 1992 Meek appointed Reynolds as chair of the strategic planning committee with the responsibility of exploring alternatives that would enhance revenues and the financial viability of the hospital. Meek said,

> Mike, we must respond to this deteriorating financial situation. We have to do something to increase revenues since inpatient dollars for Medicare patients will continue to be limited by the Feds. Remember, missions are nice, but no bottom line residual money means no long-term mission accomplishment. Put your pen to work, crunch the numbers, and give me the committee's recommendations by December.

With extensive analysis and review, Reynolds and the strategic planning committee conceived and evaluated numerous strategic alternatives that could meet Meek's charge of enhancing hospital revenues. All were framed within the planning premise of specifically choosing not to expand Medicare inpatient care but to expand other services to the senior and other market segments that would be eligible for alternate forms of reimbursement. The committee's report was submitted to Meek in December of 1992.

Reynolds's pen did indeed work wonders. Based on the committee report and with Reynolds at his side, Meek recommended to the board the following strategies that would transform the hospital into a vertically integrated health system. They were:

1. *Convert 36 general acute care medical/surgical beds to a Medicare certified hospital-based skilled nursing unit.* Meek told the board that "this unit would provide an alternative setting within which patients and others would receive rehabilitation, transfusion, and other skilled care. With treatment in such a unit, revenue would be enhanced beyond the Medicare inpatient acute care DRG fixed amount and would be based upon the actual cost of providing the services."

2. *Acquire a Medicare certified hospital-based home health agency.* Meek explained to the board that a home health agency "presents an opportunity to provide health services traditionally performed in a hospital acute care setting in a less costly setting, thereby increasing reimbursement and reducing costs while maintaining quality. We have a unique opportunity to acquire an existing agency which is the dominant home health provider in our service area."

3. *Acquire a 120-bed free-standing nursing home.* Meek was particularly excited as he presented this strategy to the board. He indicated that at this time there was not a critical shortage of nursing home beds in the service area. Based on future growth projections, however, "we can seize a rare opportunity to acquire an upscale nursing home from private investors who want to sell." He added that state certificate-of-need regulations prohibit the building of more nursing home beds in our area. "If we do not purchase this facility now there is little likelihood that another opportunity would present itself for many years. There will be barriers to entry."

Since all three strategies met the criteria of being financially viable and enhancing revenues, the board approved them at its January 1993 meeting. The three strategies were implemented by July 1993. Furthermore, to facilitate implementation, the board approved a restructuring of the hospital and changed its name (effective July 1993) to RHS in order to reflect the fact that it had now become an integrated health system offering a range of services beyond just that of acute inpatient care.

REGIONAL HEALTH SYSTEM 1993

Throughout his twenty-three year career as a hospital manager, Meek has always been an idea and big picture person. Having earned his MHA degree from a leading university in 1970, he gained substantial experience at three different hospitals before joining what is now RHS as President and Chief Executive Officer (CEO) in 1990. His success was largely due to his aggressiveness. One of the most telling events in his career was the fact that the 400 bed not-for-profit hospital where he was previously the Chief Operating Officer (COO) was sold to a for-profit hospital chain. When informed that his services were no longer needed he vowed to himself that he would never let the for-profits "zap" him again. Meek's proclivity to initiate programs and strategies without clearly assessing all factors and environmental forces beyond the financials or how they could affect the financials was known to Reynolds. In their meetings Meek would often say to Reynolds, "Just show me the numbers."

In late August of 1993 Reynolds returned from a well-earned vacation. The task of implementing the skilled nursing unit, home health agency, and nursing home acquisition strategies by July 1993 had been delegated to him by Meek. Drained, he looked forward to a few months of peace and calm. This was not to be. During the monthly meeting of senior managers, Meek told those assembled that he thought that RHS should embark on another strategy that he called the Satellite Health Park. Turning to Reynolds, Meek said, "Reconvene and chair the strategic planning committee, run the numbers, and make a recommendation to me by November. I want to make a presentation to the board at its December meeting and, if the health park strategy is approved, implementation would begin in 1994."

THE SATELLITE HEALTH PARK STRATEGY— BACKGROUND DATA

Meek visualized the satellite health park strategy as a means to expand RHS's outpatient services to a nonhospital site. The satellite health park would include the following: (a) an ophthalmology surgery center, (b) a diagnostic facility, and (c) a rehabilitation facility, in addition to the building and sale of physician office condominiums. Meek told Reynolds,

> Progressive advances in technology have significantly increased the ability of health care providers to deliver traditionally inpatient care in settings such as the health park. The setting offers the opportunity of enhanced reimbursement while also providing economies that result in reduced overhead and other costs. Also, because of the need for a critical mass, I believed that all components of the health park must be included. It is an all or nothing proposition.

In terms of resources, Reynolds knew that RHS had approximately $6,000,000 of proceeds remaining from a recent bond issue that had an effective interest cost of 7%. An additional $10,000,000 of capital was available from a board-designated fund for plant replacement and expansion. That fund has been professionally managed in recent years and was expected to continue yielding 9% per annum. Accordingly, incremental cost of capital is a weighted average of 8.25%. The health park strategy would require approval from the State Agency for Health Administration in the form of a certificate of need (CON). It was anticipated that such approval would be forthcoming.

At the committee's request, the Planning Department conducted a demographic study of the RHS market and provided Reynolds and the committee with information and several exhibits that were of assistance in evaluating the financial viability and long range strategic value of the health park. The population age distribution, for example, indicated the significant contrast in age of this community from the national average. Nearly 45% of the RHS service area is age 65+ as compared to the national average of only 13%.

Exhibit 1 (Service Area Population and Market Share Capture) provides 1990 census data for the primary and secondary service area as well as estimates of annual growth rate, projected 1995 census and RHS's market share of outpatient services to be offered at the health park before and after the health park would open. Exhibit 2 (Payer Mix) is the Planning

Service Area	Census 1990	Growth Rate 1991-2000	Projected Census 1995
Primary:			
North	15,099	3.2%	17,674
South	9,262	4.5%	11,542
Center	12,219	2.1%	13,557
East	26,484	5.5%	34,614
Total	63,064	4.1%	77,387
Secondary:			
North	3,695	3.5%	4,389
East	16,353	7.1%	23,043
South	32,407	6.1%	43,573
Total	52,455	6.2%	71,005
Total Service Area	115,519	5.1%	148,392

Outpatient Market Share Capture

Before Addition of Health Park			After Addition of Health Park		
Surgical	Diagnostic	Rehab	Surgical	Diagnostic	Rehab
25.00%	40.000%	50.000%	34.000%	60.000%	64.000%
18.103%	14.921%	19.906%	54.051%	47.204%	69.281%
21.700%	28.000%	35.600%	43.594%	53.877%	66.527%

Exhibit 1.   Service area population and market share capture.

	Health Park	
Payer	Surgery	Other
Medicare	90	65
Medicaid	2	3
Commercial/Other	6	28
Bad Debt/Charity	2	4
Total	100	100

Exhibit 2. Payer mix.

Department's best estimate of the payer mix to be experienced for each of the initiatives contemplated. Again the dominant payer is the Medicare program.

Planning developed estimates of service area use rates per thousand population as a means of computing total market demand for the services contemplated. A summary is provided in Exhibit 3 (Service Area Use Rates). As may be inferred from the Exhibit, advent of the Medicare prospective payment system, managed care, and technology advances in surgery and medicine, all contributed to a national and regional shift from inpatient to outpatient utilization. Planning analyzed population growth, use rate trends, and other factors in projecting the volume of services for each health park component and they are presented in Exhibit 4 (Projected Service Volume).

Cost data specific to each health park component were compiled by the Fiscal Services Department, Management Engineering, key operating personnel, and others. The Operations Standards presented in Table 1 provide a summary of their effort to identify relevant variable and fixed operating costs. The cost/volume relationships may be assumed to be valid in later years. All costs with the exception of initial outlay and depreciation are assumed to inflate at an average rate of 4% per annum. Depreciation of building and equipment is based upon the useful life of the assets.

	Year	
Healthcare Encounters	1990	1995
Inpatient Discharges	211.1	172.0
Outpatient:		
Surgeries	36.1	37.1
Diagnostic Tests	1,922.40	1,999.30
Rehab. Therapy Visits	289.7	298.4

Exhibit 3. Service area use rates.

Description	Service		
	Surgery	Diagnostic	Rehab
A. Use Rate per 1,000 (Exhibit 3)	37.1	1,999.30	298.4
B. Projected Population (1,000's) (Exhibit 1)	148.392	148.392	148.392
C. Projected Total Market (A x B) (Rounded) *	5,505	296,680	44,280
D. Market Share (%) After Addition of Health Park (Exhibit 1)	43.594%	53.877%	66.527%
E. Market Share After Addition of Health Park (Rounded)	2,400	159,843	29,458
F. Market Share (%) Before Addition of Health Park (Exhibit 1)	21.700%	28.000%	35.600%
G. Market Share Before Addition of Health Park (Rounded)	1,195	83,071	15,764
H. Market Share Increase (E-G)	1,205	76,772	13,694
I. Percent of Hospital Volume to Shift to the Health Park	100.000%	40.000%	40.000%
J. Hospital Volume Shift to Health Park (G x I)	1,195	33,228	6,306
K. Total 1995 Volume at Health Park (H + J)	2,400	110,000	20,000
L. Total 1994 Volume at Health Park (K x 50%)	1,200	55,000	10,000

*Projected market is assumed to remain constant through 1998 to simplify the case. A more exact solution would require total market to change with projected use rate and population each year.

Exhibit 4. Projected service volume.

THE HEALTH PARK STRATEGY— FINANCIAL ANALYSIS

As Exhibit 1 illustrates, RHS's service area growth rate (1991–2000) was projected to be the greatest in the secondary market, particularly in the east and south. Growth, as well as the industry trend toward greater out-patient utilization per capita, appears to assure an adequate demand for services proposed for the health park.

The Planning Department's estimates of the cumulative shift in market from competitors and from the RHS Hospital itself to the health park are provided in Exhibit 1 (Market Share Capture). The capture rate in conjunction with use rates and service area population provide the basis upon which the projected service volumes given in Exhibit 4 (Projected Service Volume) were developed.

In order to obtain additional information on the economic viability of the health park strategy, Reynolds and his committee engaged a project management firm to evaluate the proposed site to determine construction cost, adequate access, environmental impact, and other development issues. The site has two parcels with 39 combined acres. The acquisition cost is $110,000

Table 1. Operations standards

Description of Cost	Surgery	Diagnostics	Rehab
Variable cost/unit	$500	$40	$50
Fixed Expenses:			
Staff and supplies	$175,000	$150,000	$180,000
Allocated overhead	0	0	0
Depreciation	$80,000	$250,000	$110,000

per acre. Site development cost will approximate $2,450,000. The project management firm recommended that the infrastructure be developed for the total acreage even though only 25 acres will be required to accommodate the health park. A number of *bona fide* buyers were known to exist for the remaining 14 acres. After site development, the per acre market value would increase to $250,000. For purposes of this analysis it is assumed that 6 acres will be sold in 1994 with the remaining 8 acres sold in 1995. Table 2 shows the capital investment costs that will be required for each health park service.

The physician offices that will be built will be divided into office condominiums and sold during 1994 at a total net sales price of $2,330,000. Title to the land will remain with RHS and a land lease executed with each physician purchasing an office. The lease payments will aggregate $145,000 per year and will run a term of 99 years. At the completion of the term, all leasehold improvements will revert to RHS. Working capital requirements will approximate $1,100,000.

Medicare reimbursement for free-standing ophthalmology surgery and diagnostic services is based upon a fee schedule. The surgical procedures will be primarily cataract, which will be reimbursed at $795 per procedure in 1994. Diagnostics are expected to have a Medicare reimbursement rate of $85 per procedure in 1994. The Medicare reimbursement rate is expected to increase 3% per annum.

Medicare reimburses certified outpatient rehabilitation facilities (CORF) based on actual cost. Cost is computed as the direct cost of oper-

Table 2. Capital investment costs for surgery, diagnostic, and rehabilitation

	Building	Equipment
Ophthalmic Surgery	$1,050,000	$270,000
Diagnostics	1,680,000	850,000
Rehabilitation	2,090,000	195,000
Physician Offices	2,025,000	0
Total	$6,845,000	$1,315,000

ating the facility (operating expenses and depreciation) plus allocated over-head from support departments such as RHS administration using a complex cost finding process. For purpose of this case it is assumed that the reimbursement rate will be $80 per therapy in 1994 and increase at 4% per annum.

Medicaid reimburses free-standing centers for surgery, diagnostic, and rehabilitation services in a manner similar to Medicare. Thus, the Medicare and Medicaid payer mix may be combined in analyzing total reimbursement received from those programs.

Patient charges per procedure in 1994 will be $1,200 for cataract surgery, $120 for diagnostic tests, and $100 per rehabilitation visit. Rate increases are projected to approximate 7% per annum. Commercial/other payers receive a 10% discount from charges during the entire forecast period.

Procedures captured from the RHS Hospital will reduce contribution margin there. The revenue and variable expense relationships at the RHS Hospital are similar to those projected for the health park. Thus, it may be assumed that the contribution margin lost at the RHS Hospital due to the shift in services to the health park will equal the contribution margin per unit generated at the health park multiplied times the health park volume captured from the RHS Hospital. All of the ophthalmology but only 40% of the diagnostic and rehabilitation volume will shift to the health park.

Determining the Cost–Benefit of the Health Park Strategy

Knowing that Meek and the board required a complete financial analysis of the health park strategy, Reynolds worked on a cost–benefit analysis for the 5 year period, 1994–1998. His analysis of cash flow from operations covering the years 1994–1998 for the a) surgery, b) diagnostic, and c) rehabilitation services is provided in Exhibits 5–7. Exhibit 8 provides the contribution margin lost by the hospital for each service. Exhibit 9 presents the cost–benefit analysis for the years 1994–1998 for all three services, as well as the sale of physician offices.

Reynolds provided this information to you, his assistant. His instructions to you to were to use the Operational Standards information and that provided in Exhibits 5–8, and interest rate of 8.25%, do the following:

1. Calculate the payback in years (the number of years for the net cash flow to equal the initial investment outlay).

2. Calculate the net present value (present value of benefits less initial outlay).

3. Calculate the profitability index (present value of benefits divided by initial outlay).

4. Based on your analysis, make a recommendation to me whether the health park strategy should be recommended to Meek and the board.

	1994	1995	1996	1997	1998
Patient Volume by Payer:					
Medicare/Medicaid (95%)	1,140	2,280	2,280	2,280	2,280
Commercial/Other (3%)	36	72	72	72	72
Bad Debt/Charity (2%)	24	48	48	48	48
Total Patient Volume (100%)	1,200	2,400	2,400	2,400	2,400
Reimbursement Rate Per Case ($):					
Medicare/Medicaid	795.0000	818.8500	843.4155	868.7180	894.7765
Commercial/Other	1,080.0000	1,155.6000	1,236.4920	1,323.0464	1,415.6597
Bad Debt/Charity	0.0000	0.0000	0.0000	0.0000	0.0000
Operating Revenue ($):					
Medicare/Medicaid	906,300	1,866,978	1,922,987	1,980,677	2,040,097
Commercial/Other	38,880	83,203	89,027	95,259	101,927
Bad Debt/Charity	0	0	0	0	0
Total Operating Revenue ($)	945,180	1,950,181	2,012,015	2,075,936	2,142,025
Variable Expenses ($)	660,000	1,372,800	1,427,712	1,484,820	1,544,213
Contribution Margin ($)	285,180	577,381	548,303	591,116	597,811
Fixed Expenses ($):					
Staff and Supplies	175,000	182,000	189,280	196,851	204,725
Depreciation	80,000	80,000	80,000	80,000	80,000
Total Fixed Expenses ($)	255,000	262,000	269,280	276,851	284,725
Income (Loss) from Operations ($)	30,180	315,381	315,023	314,265	313,086
Expenses Not Requiring Cash ($):					
Depreciation	80,000	80,000	80,000	80,000	80,000
Cash Flow from Operations ($)	110,180	395,381	395,023	394,265	393,086

Exhibit 5. Cash flow from surgery.

	1994	1995	1996	1997	1998
Patient Volume by Payer:					
Medicare/Medicaid (74%)	40,700	81,400	81,400	81,400	81,400
Commercial/Other (21%)	11,500	23,100	23,100	23,100	23,100
Bad Debt/Charity (5%)	2,750	5,500	5,500	5,500	5,500
Total Patient Volume (100%)	55,000	110,000	110,000	110,000	110,000
Reimbursement Rate Per Case ($):					
Medicare/Medicaid	85.0000	87.5500	90.1765	92.8818	95.6682
Commercial/Other	108.0000	115.5600	123.6492	132.3046	141.5660
Bad Debt/Charity	0.0000	0.0000	0.0000	0.0000	0.0000
Operating Revenue ($):					
Medicare/Medicaid	3,459,500	7,126,570	7,340,367	7,560,578	7,787,395
Commercial/Other	1,247,400	2,669,436	2,856,297	3,056,237	3,270,174
Bad Debt/Charity	0	0	0	0	0
Total Operating Revenue ($)	4,706,900	9,796,006	10,196,664	10,616,815	11,057,569
Variable Expenses ($)	2,200,000	4,576,000	4,759,040	4,949,402	5,147,378
Contribution Margin ($)	2,506,900	5,220,006	5,437,624	5,667,414	5,910,192
Fixed Expenses ($):					
Staff and Supplies	150,000	156,000	162,240	168,730	175,479
Depreciation	250,000	250,000	250,000	250,000	250,000
Total Fixed Expenses ($)	400,000	406,000	412,240	418,730	425,479
Income (Loss) from Oper. ($)	2,106,900	4,814,006	5,025,384	5,248,684	5,484,713
Expenses Not Requiring Cash ($):					
Depreciation	250,000	250,000	250,000	250,000	250,000
Cash Flow from Operations ($)	2,356,900	5,064,006	5,275,384	5,498,684	5,734,713

Exhibit 6.   Cash flow from diagnostic.

	1994	1995	1996	1997	1998
Patient Volume by Payer:					
Medicare/Medicaid (74%)	7,400	14,800	14,800	14,800	14,800
Commercial/Other (21%)	2,100	4,200	4,200	4,200	4,200
Bad Debt/Charity (5%)	500	1,000	1,000	1,000	1,000
Total Patient Volume (100%)	10,000	20,000	20,000	20,000	20,000
Reimbursement Rate Per Case ($):					
Medicare/Medicaid	80.0000	83.2000	86.5280	89.9891	93.5887
Commercial/Other	90.0000	96.3000	103.0410	110.2539	117.9716
Bad Debt/Charity	0.0000	0.0000	0.0000	0.0000	0.0000
Operating Revenue ($):					
Medicare/Medicaid	592,000	1,231,360	1,280,614	1,331,839	1,385,113
Commercial/Other	189,000	404,460	432,772	463,066	495,481
Bad Debt/Charity	0	0	0	0	0
Total Operating Revenue ($)	781,000	1,635,820	1,713,387	1,794,905	1,880,593
Variable Expenses ($)	500,000	1,040,000	1,081,000	1,124,864	1,169,000
Contribution Margin ($)	281,000	595,000	631,787	670,041	710,735
Fixed Expenses ($):					
Staff and Supplies	180,000	187,000	194,688	202,476	210,575
Depreciation	110,000	110,000	110,000	110,000	110,000
Total Fixed Expenses ($)	290,000	297,200	304,688	312,476	320,575
Income (Loss) from Operations ($)	(9,000)	298,620	327,099	357,566	390,160
Expenses Not Requiring Cash ($):					
Depreciation	110,000	110,000	110,000	110,000	110,000
Cash Flow from Operations ($)	101,000	408,620	437,099	467,566	500,160

Exhibit 7. Cash flow from rehabilitation.

	1994	1995	1996	1997	1998
Surgery:					
Health Park Contribution Margin ($)	285,180	577,381	584,303	591,116	597,811
Health Park Volume	1,200	2,400	2,400	2,400	2,400
Contribution Margin per Unit Volume ($)	237.6500	240.5755	243.4595	246.2983	249.0881
Volume Shift from Hospital to Health Park	1,195	1,195	1,195	1,195	1,195
Contribution Margin Lost by Hospital ($)	283,992	287,488	290,934	294,326	297,660
Diagnostic:					
Health Park Contribution Margin ($)	2,506,900	5,220,006	5,437,624	5,667,414	5,910,192
Health Park Volume	55,000	110,000	110,000	110,000	110,000
Contribution Margin per Unit Volume ($)	45.5800	47.4546	49.4239	51.5219	53.7290
Volume Shift from Hospital to Health Park	33,228	33,228	33,228	33,228	33,228
Contribution Margin Lost by Hospital ($)	1,514,532	1,576,821	1,642,558	1,711,971	1,785,307
Rehabilitation:					
Health Park Contribution Margin ($)	281,000	595,820	631,787	670,041	710,735
Health Park Volume	10,000	20,000	20,000	20,000	20,000
Contribution Margin per Unit Volume ($)	28.1000	29.7910	31.5893	33.5021	35.5367
Volume Shift from Hospital to Health Park	6,306	6,306	6,306	6,306	6,306
Contribution Margin Lost by Hospital ($)	177,199	187,862	199,202	211,264	224,094

*The change in the contribution margin per unit each year is based upon the net effect of a combination of reimbursement rate changes by payer and unit variable expense increases.

Exhibit 8. The contribution margin lost by the hospital to the health park for surgery, diagnostic, and rehabilitation.

	Outlay	1994	1995	1996	1997	1998
Cost ($):						
Land	4,290,000					
Site Development	2,450,000					
Construction	6,845,000					
Equipment	1,315,000					
Working Capital	1,100,000					
Contribution Margin Lost by Hospital						
Surgery		283,992	287,488	290,934	294,326	297,660
Diagnostics		1,514,532	1,576,821	1,642,558	1,711,971	1,785,307
Rehabilitation		177,199	187,862	199,202	211,264	224,094
Total Cost ($)	16,000,000	1,975,723	2,052,171	2,132,694	2,217,562	2,307,062
Benefit ($):						
Cash Flow from Operations						
Surgery		110,180	395,381	395,023	394,265	393,086
Diagnostics		2,356,900	5,064,006	5,275,384	5,498,684	5,734,713
Rehabilitation		101,000	408,620	437,099	467,566	500,160
Land Sales		1,500,000	2,000,000			
Physician Office Sales		2,330,000				
Land Lease		145,000	145,000	145,000	145,000	145,000
Total Benefit ($)		6,543,080	8,013,007	6,252,505	6,505,515	6,772,959
Net Cost/Benefit ($)	(16,000,000)	4,567,357	5,960,836	4,119,811	4,287,953	4,465,898

Additional Financial Analysis:

Payback Period (years)	
Present Value of Net Benefits ($)	
Outlay ($)	(16,000,00)
Net Present Value ($)	
Profitability Index	

Exhibit 9. The cost–benefit analysis for the years 1994–1998 for surgery, diagnostic, and rehabilitation.

17

The ER that Became the Emergency

Managing the Double Bind

Earl Simendinger

Mary Anne Watson

Mike Jasperson

Bryan Boliard
University of Tampa, Florida

FRIDAY SENIOR STAFF MEETING

"I finally have some good news concerning our marketing activities," Bill Coffman said with a smile at the weekly senior staff meeting. "Our radio advertising and other marketing efforts over the past 5 months seem to be paying off. In the last $2\frac{1}{2}$ months, we've seen a dramatic increase in our emergency room visits, and I feel quite positive about the increase in demand." It was easy to see that Bill, the Chief Financial Officer of Community Memorial Hospital (CMH) was quite pleased about his monthly report.

From Simendinger, E., Watson, M.A., Jasperson, M., and Boliard, B. (1998). "The ER that became the emergency: Managing the double bind." *Business Case Journal*, 6(2). Used by permission.

Ralph Peterson, Chief Executive Officer of the hospital, returned Bill's grin and responded, "That's great, Bill, especially since 30% of all of our admissions come through our emergency room."

Bill went on to note that admission increases were directly related to the growth in the amount of emergency room visits. He estimated that ER visits were expected to rise 15%–20% next month.

"Do we have enough staff, or should we start looking at hiring more physicians and nurses?" Ralph asked.

Bill promised he would look into the staffing matter before next week's meeting. As Bill continued with his report, Ralph's attention kept drifting back to the new ER figures on the income statement and balance sheet. For some unexplained reason, an uneasy feeling settled in his gut. He couldn't help but think something didn't fit—it seemed too good, too quick, and too lucky that the increase in admissions had occurred almost solely through CMH's marketing efforts. He wondered if the 15%–20% increase in ER visits in such a short time was realistic. The advertising seemed a bit too effective. One of his friend's favorite sayings popped into his head: "If it seems too good to be true, it probably is!"

In an attempt to gain more information from Bill about the emergency room activity, Ralph interrupted Bill's report and asked whether he had analyzed the ER visit numbers, tracking what types of new patients are using the emergency room. He also wanted to know when and from where they had come and what the payer mix was. "I don't have that information right here," Bill answered, "but we assumed that the payer mix was the same as it had been for the past 2 or 3 years. Why would it be any different?" (Payer mix is a term in health care that refers to the fact that different insurers, such as Medicare, Medicaid, HMOs, and PPOs, reimburse the hospital at different rates for the same service to patients.)

"Let's get the numbers. I have an uneasy feeling about this one," Ralph replied with an irritated shake of his head.

After a few minutes, the burn intensified, and Bill, visibly frustrated replied, "Do you realize how much time that analysis would take, and I'm up to my ears right now just trying to get the financials, capital, and operating budgets out on schedule!"

Ralph sat there thinking for a moment, wondering if there was something he was missing. As the senior staff at the meeting paused, Ralph finally answered. "Bill, do the analysis please."

As the Friday senior staff meeting concluded and everybody got ready to go home for the weekend, Ralph caught up with Bill on the way out. "Could you get me that ER information as soon as possible?" he asked.

BACKGROUND

CMH, a 400-bed medical/surgical hospital, is located in Middleville, Ohio, a mid-sized city of about 650,000 residents. It is a private, not-for-profit facility that has been located in the downtown area for 75 years. There has always been strong community support for the hospital. Its medical staff consists of 350 physicians and the hospital employs 1,700 people. The payer mix is typical of many hospitals with 25% private pay, 50% Medicare, 10% Medicaid, and the rest composed of HMO, medically indigent, and self-pay patients. The Medicaid program provides medical aid by the federal government although administered at the state level to provide benefits according to established criteria for the poor, aged, blind, disabled, and dependent children. The hospital's clinical reputation has been positive but community members, the board, and the medical staff have raised some concerns regarding its declining financial situation over the past 5 years.

City Hospital, a very well respected, 600-bed health care facility, is located about a quarter mile from CMH. City Hospital has two primary missions: 1) It is a teaching hospital and trains large numbers of residents in conjunction with the local medical school; 2) given its location in the poorest part of the city and its distinction as the city's only publicly funded hospital, it takes care of the city's Medicaid patients as well as other categories of medically indigent patients. A medically indigent patient is one who has insufficient income or savings to pay for medical care without having to sacrifice other essentials for living (i.e., food, clothing, shelter). Treating high numbers of these patients, coupled with the physician training programs, is extremely costly and produces very high operating costs for the City Hospital facility. The Emergency Medical Treatment and Active Labor Act (EMTALA) requires that hospitals receiving federal reimbursement treat, stabilize, and admit (as needed) all patients (regardless of payment) who present at their emergency departments. Patients whose conditions require capability that the hospital lacks may be sent elsewhere after the hospital stabilizes them. City tax funds make up any loss sustained each year by City Hospital for the cost of taking care of this population. The funds transferred to City Hospital have increased to $10 million over the past few months. Jim Harding, who has been the administrator at the City Hospital for the last five years, has worked with the mayor and other city commissioners to try to reduce City Hospital's high operating expenses. Despite several cost-cutting initiatives and two rounds of layoffs, City Hospital still is predicted to have a loss of $12 million for the coming year. The city can't cover this loss with its tax funding, and Mr. Harding is feeling a lot of pressure to, as the mayor says, "find a way."

In addition, there are five other hospitals throughout the city that provide medical care to the residents of the area. St. Marks, a 350-bed, religious-based hospital, is located on the north side of town, approximately 12 miles from CMH. OhioCare, a for-profit, 300-bed, medical/surgical hospital, is situated on the south side of the city about eight miles away from CMH. A third facility, Health Associates, is a specialty hospital, concentrating on serving cancer victims. The Ohio Women's Center Hospital, which is located on the east side of town, is a 200-bed facility that provides services primarily to women and children. Finally, Doctor's Hospital, another medical/surgical facility that has been in town for 20 years, is located on the west side of the town and is an osteopathic hospital.

CMH has competed aggressively with the other hospitals in the city through an expensive, active marketing campaign to get its occupancy rate up from 56%. With the recent increase in emergency room visits, CMH's efforts seemed to be paying off. Then, Bill Coffman did the analysis and found some alarming data on the new ER patients.

FOLLOW-UP MEETING (RALPH, I HAVE THE INFORMATION YOU ASKED FOR)

Over the weekend, Bill Coffman went into the office because he couldn't stop thinking about the strained interaction he had with Ralph, his concerns regarding the ER payer mix, and from where the new patients were coming. Sitting at his computer, feeling like Sherlock Holmes, he pored through the ER data with a fine-toothed comb. "From where are they coming? Let's look at the zip codes. When are they coming? How are they paying (type of insurance coverage)—or are they?" The printer was buzzing, pumping out the information. Sipping on his cold coffee and munching a sandwich from the vending machine, Bill began to analyze the stack of computer printouts on his desk. After looking at several sets of data, Bill began to shake his head in amazement and tried to avoid the sinking feeling in the pit of his stomach. "I'm seeing, but I don't believe it!" he said to himself. There was a clear pattern emerging as he looked at the information. Not only were the majority of new ER patients medically indigent patients, but also the zip code analysis showed that they were coming primarily from a high demand area not seen before. They were primarily coming in on the weekends during the busiest times for ERs and the most likely time to draw medically indigent patients. Bill sat back in his chair and thought, "Ralph isn't gonna believe this!" Looking more closely at the figures, he was shocked to learn that the medically indigent patient increases were going to be responsible for CMH losing $70,000 to $80,000 this coming month. He groaned and reached for the phone to call Ralph but changed his mind when he looked at his watch and saw it was 1:30 A.M. He realized that waking Ralph in the middle of the night, combined with delivering the bad news would be an unwise move, especially considering the interaction they had had in the staff meeting.

The following morning, Ralph received a message from Bill Coffman asking if they could get together to discuss the findings that he had come up with concerning the jump in patient activity. At 10 A.M., Ralph popped his head into Bill's office. "So what did you find out, Sherlock?"

"I don't think you're gonna like it—you're not going to believe what's happening and it makes no sense to me. I can't figure it out," Bill said, grimacing. "That jump in emergency room activity was all made up of medically indigent patients coming from one zip code area, and it'll cause a huge ER loss this month."

Ralph sat back in his seat abruptly, and said, "I knew it," and asked for the zip code map. "They're from 00010," Bill stated abruptly. "Get a zip code map, Bill," Ralph commanded.

As soon as Ralph's eyes hit the location on the map, he knew. "These patients are coming from City Hospital's area!" Ralph asked Bill, "What times were the peaks occurring?"

"Peak ER times—the weekends," was the glum reply.

"I think it's time to have a little chat with Jim Harding at City Hospital," Ralph said emphatically, "I'll set up a meeting with him and get to the bottom of this."

TUESDAY MEETING WITH MR. HARDING

Jim Harding, City Hospital's CEO, appeared as scheduled at Ralph's office at 10 A.M. sharp on Tuesday and remarked, "I knew it was just a matter of time before we would be sitting down and discussing this particular issue." He went on to discuss the problems that City Hospital was having with the lack of staffing in its emergency room. Even with the additional government funding, it was unable to afford the number of physicians, residents, and nurses needed to meet the demands of patients coming through its facility. City Hospital's concern for patient's quality of care and lack of staffing, Jim explained to Ralph, was the reason that City Hospital's diversion process had commenced. Diversion is the tactic used by hospital ER administrators to reroute patients to other facilities' emergency rooms when they have reached their capacities. Sometimes this tactic can be used deceptively: A hospital ER may go on diversion to avoid the high costs associated with taking certain types of ER patients, specifically those who provide low reimbursement to the hospital. Jim also admitted that

CMH would be the logical choice for patients diverted from City Hospital based on proximity and patient safety/liability issues. Ralph broke in and said, "I understand your circumstances and why you're going on diversion, but is there any way we can form some kind of financial relationship when you send us your patients? When you go on diversion, can we at least have some kind of a cost-based reimbursement arrangement for the medically indigent patients we take from you?" As the meeting came to a close, Jim agreed that a relationship between the two hospitals would be a good idea and that he would put together a cost-based reimbursement proposal in the next few days for Ralph to consider.

A week later, Ralph received a proposal on his desk from Jim and quickly sent it to Bill Coffman to analyze. Bill quickly ran the numbers and stopped into Ralph's office with the report. After giving Ralph a minute for an initial glance he summed it up, "So. . . the reimbursement of $100 per visit to CMH that City Hospital is offering us to reduce the expenses isn't even close to covering the losses from the influx of its medically indigent patients. At best they would only reduce our average losses by 20%. In 6 months we will be in serious financial trouble."

Ralph thanked Bill for the fast turnaround on the information as he left the office. Frustrated, he thought to himself, "Okay, I've got an ER that's bleeding us to death. What's my next move?"

Ralph immediately called Jim and told him the proposal was unacceptable based on CMH's financial situation. Jim responded by saying, "I'm not surprised, but that's the best I can do." In the conversation that followed, Jim inadvertently shared the fact that City Hospital received $550 a visit for medically indigent patients from city funds. Ralph immediately challenged him, "OK, Jim, let me get this straight. If a medically indigent patient in our city walks through your ER doors, the city gives you a visit rate of $550 as an all-inclusive amount, but if the same patient comes through my doors we will only receive $100 a visit? How is that fair?!" Jim reiterated, "Like I said, that's the best I can do given our financial situation. Sorry."

A WEEK LATER (MEETING WITH COMMISSIONERS)

Finding no acceptable alternatives in his conversation with Jim, Ralph decided his next step was to call a couple of the city commissioners he knew and ask their advice on the situation. Inasmuch as it had to do with city funds, they suggested that Ralph needed to speak with the mayor. After getting off the phone with the last city commissioner, feeling somewhat like a basketball being tossed around in warm-ups, Ralph finally realized he needed to go to the top. He phoned the mayor's office and was able to get an appointment for the following Friday morning.

FRIDAY MEETING WITH THE MAYOR

Ralph made his way promptly to his first ever meeting with the mayor. To his surprise, the mayor, Bill Cane, walked in on time despite his very busy schedule and escorted Ralph into his office. Feeling very impressed and a little intimidated by being in the mayor's office, Ralph brought the mayor up to date on the situation. He proposed that the city increase funding to City Hospital to deal with its financial situation. He also suggested that CMH would be willing to help with the diversion problem but it would need reasonable funding from the city for the care of the city's medically indigent patients.

The mayor expressed understanding, "I see your predicament, but right now the city is battling its own health care financial crisis. We're significantly lacking in funding for health care. You may not know that currently the tax funds can only be spent on medically indigent patients that receive care in a city facility. Any changes will take some time to get passed. We could try to change the city code that was passed with the health tax referendum but, as you are well aware, it is a very long, complex process. As you know it typically takes 3 years to complete all the procedural and legal steps, even before it could be put to the voters."

With the meeting coming to an end, it was clear to Ralph that the city's financial problems and the politics behind trying to get something done was digging a financial grave for CMH.

As Ralph drove back to CMH, he started realizing the lack of options and began to contemplate the extent of the double bind he was facing. First, he thought the hospital would reach a serious financial problem within 6 months if the problem weren't resolved quickly. On the other hand, if the hospital took a stance of refusing to accept the city patients coming through the ER doors, CMH could experience severe bad press that would bring a negative image on the facility and him. All Ralph could picture was the front page of the city's newspaper with a cartoon picture of himself holding the ER doors closed, preventing a bleeding, medically indigent patient, on his knees, from getting needed medical care. Ralph trembled to think of the board reaction to that picture.

Observing the traffic jam growing in front of him, Ralph turned to take an alternate route home. As he drove past Doctor's Hospital, it suddenly occurred to him that this issue went beyond CMH. Other hospitals might feel threatened as well, even though they were not currently affected by an influx of medically indigent patients. He thought a brainstorming session with other hospital administrators might be in order. As Ralph passed by City Hospital en route to his facility, he felt a slow burn across his back thinking about the fact that City Hospital could divert patients with no flack but he shuddered to think what would happen if CMH diverted just one patient. Over time, diversion of medically indigent patients had become an accepted practice from City Hospital. Although infrequent, City Hospital's ER was sometimes understaffed and unable to deal with the incoming patient volume. As a result, the facility went on diversion without notice or criticism. In the past, however, the duration of the diversion was typically short and involved only a few patients. Never had so many patients been diverted for so long!

SUGGESTED MEETING WITH OTHER CEOs

As soon as Ralph returned to the office, he made phone calls to each of the local hospital CEOs asking them to attend a meeting to discuss the situation. He was sure that he would be able to convince the other hospital's administrators, his friends, to take their fair share of medically indigent patients for the city.

As a week passed, Ralph was very frustrated at the lack of response from any of the other hospitals' administrators concerning the proposed meeting. In an attempt to get answers, Ralph called his good friend, Dick Rusk, CEO of Health Associates, to find out why he hadn't heard from him. Dick remarked, "I know what you're going through over at CMH and understand why you called the meeting, but we at Health Associates wouldn't want to change a system that would increase our costs." Dick also added he, as most of the other hospital CEOs, felt that they were already taking their fair share of medically indigent patients! Dick concluded by saying, "City Hospital has the funding support through the local referendum to take responsibility for a larger percentage of the area's medically indigent patients. Let them deal with the problem." As Ralph got off the phone, he realized that if he were one of the other CEOs he would probably do the same thing.

MEETING WITH HIMSELF

Later that afternoon, Ralph sat staring through his window at work. The image of getting doors slammed in his face—first Jim Harding's, the mayor's, the city commissioners', then all those hospital CEOs' who were his supposed friends—kept running through his head. Although Ralph realized the problem was complex and had financial, political, and public relations implications, he was humbled by the fact that he had no clear idea what to do next. As he sat perplexed at his desk, the wail of an ambulance siren grew louder, and then passed directly below his window. "Oh great," he thought, "there goes another 550 bucks out the window!"

18

Attica Memorial Hospital

The Ingelson Burn Center

Bonnie Eng-Suess
Central Health MSO, Inc., Covina, California

Robert C. Myrtle
University of Southern California, Los Angeles, California

INTRODUCTION

In late 2001, Attica Memorial Hospital purchased and absorbed its nearest competitor, Delphi Hospital, in what was termed an alliance. Attica Memorial's plans were to consolidate duplicate services and to realign all remaining units. Services unique to the acquired hospital were thoroughly evaluated in order to determine if they would survive the alliance. Services that were not essential to the community or added minimum value to Attica Memorial would not be supported. The Ingelson Burn Center was one of those unique lines of service that Attica Memorial thoroughly evaluated in order to determine its fate.

Used by permission of the authors. Copyright © 2004 by Bonnie Eng-Suess and Robert C. Myrtle.

Note: All names and identifiable characteristics of the organization have been modified to ensure anonymity.

BACKGROUND

Attica Memorial and Delphi Hospitals competed for more than 40 years for patients, physicians, and favorable insurance reimbursement rates. The two hospitals were nonprofit, acute care facilities located in Norton County, less than a half mile from each other and both offered similar types of services, creating a fiercely competitive environment. Many Attica Memorial physicians also had privileges at Delphi Hospital and could refer patients to either hospital. Physicians took their patients to the hospital that offered greater pay and benefits. In addition, both hospitals competed for limited resources such as staff, health plans, and medical group contracts. Before Attica Memorial acquired Delphi Hospital, health plans and medical groups pitted the hospitals against each other in order to obtain favorable reimbursement rates. Attica Memorial CEO Richard Ponti was left with the dim view that "Any contract rate is a good rate," even if the health plan reimbursed the hospital $4,000.00 for an open-heart procedure. When Delphi's parent organization placed the hospital for sale, Attica Memorial saw a strategic opportunity to purchase its long-time competitor and strengthen its position in the marketplace.

The initial plan of the alliance was to have both hospitals as recognizable "Center of Excellence" facilities by completely realigning the services between the two structures. Attica Memorial transitioned into an acute care inpatient facility while Delphi Hospital became an ambulatory care outpatient pavilion. The original Attica Memorial facility became Attica Memorial East Campus (AMH East Campus) and Delphi Hospital was renamed Attica Memorial West Campus (AMH West Campus). By combining resources with Delphi Hospital, the new Attica Memorial became a stronger and more vital community presence. The hospital would be able to expand its spectrum of patient care by offering new services, more outreach, improved access to care, and an increased focus on quality. Achieving the efficiencies promised by the consolidation of redundant services, however, required careful evaluation of each department and service line, transfers of personnel, and, inevitably, layoffs.

MACRO ENVIRONMENT

Before the 1980s, hospitals did not worry much about charges since they were reimbursed at fee-for-service rates (i.e., their charges were paid at full-price rates). The 1980s, however, brought dramatic changes to the health care environment. The trend was toward continual increases in the cost of health care due to increased costs of pharmaceuticals, aging of the general population, advancements in medical technology, shortage of nurses, and increases in the number of higher-acuity patients. Managed care organizations (MCOs) started to monitor hospital services closely in order to control health care costs. Health maintenance organizations (HMOs) began dictating the length of stay and reimbursement rates for hospitals, making competition for market share extremely difficult in Norton County, which contained a dense concentration of hospitals. In response, the demand for health care services shifted dramatically from the inpatient to the outpatient setting, leaving too many hospital beds for the shrinking number of inpatients. At the same time, the federal government attempted to contain and reduce costs by reimbursing hospitals' Medicare patients on diagnosis-related group (DRG) rates. Reimbursement for services from health plans and Medicare declined substantially. Hospitals started to see their revenue streams shrink on lower reimbursement and discounted fee-for-service rates, making it very difficult to cover costs.

COMPETITIVE ENVIRONMENT

Not only was Attica Memorial affected by trends in the macro-environment brought on by the evolution of managed care, but also pressures were even greater in the competitive environment. In Norton County, competition was fierce for market share because there were too many hospitals within a small geographic area. Within a 5-mile radius, Attica Memorial was surrounded by seven other hospitals, all competing for patients, physicians, and health plan contracts. Within a 10-mile radius, Attica Memorial's competition increased to more than 16 hospitals. The managed care penetration in Norton County was approximately 46%— almost double the national average of 24.3%—thereby creating concerns for managed risk and contract liability.

Excess capacity in hospitals was an increasingly steady trend; in 2000, the hospital room occupancy rate in the state was 45.6%, while Norton County's hospital room occupancy rate was slightly lower at 42.6%. A further external threat pressuring hospitals was California State Bill 1953 (SB 1953). This legislation mandated retrofitting of existing hospitals to current building seismic safety codes by the year 2008 and required significant capital expenditures and interruption of services of many hospitals. In addition, the health care market was experiencing a nursing shortage, thereby increasing costs and competition for quality staff.

ANALYSIS OF THE INGELSON BURN CENTER

Nature of Burn Injuries

Burn injuries are unique occurrences. Burn is a service line unlike obstetrics, in which OB physicians can estimate how many deliveries they will perform within a given time based upon patient base. Burns can be the result of fire, the sun, chemicals, heated objects, heated fluids, and electricity. The injury resulting from burn can be diagnosed as minor burn, needing non-emergent care, or major burn, needing life saving emergent care. The degree of burn is determined by the damage to the tissue of the body.

Burn Statistics

In the United States, approximately 2.4 million burn injuries are reported per year. Medical professionals treat approximately 650,000 of the injuries; 75,000 are hospitalized. Of those hospitalized, 20,000 have major burns involving at least 25% of their total body surface. Between 8,000 and 12,000 patients with burns die, and approximately 1 million sustain substantial or permanent disabilities resulting from their burn injury.

The Bureau of Labor Statistics published the following burn statistics for 1992:

- 41,000 heat burns resulted in an average of 4 lost days of work each. Breakdowns of industrial burns were as follows: 16,500 retail trade; 9,500 manufacturing; 8,600 service industry (e.g., restaurants).

- 15,700 chemical burns resulted in an average of 2 lost days of work each. Breakdowns were: 5,800 manufacturing (e.g., chemical manufacturers); 3,200 service industry; 2,600 retail industry.

Children age newborn to 2 years old are the most frequently admitted patients for emergency burn treatment. The kitchen is the most common area in the home where burn injuries occur for children of these ages. The next most frequent area is in the bathroom, where scalding hot water burns children. Scalds are the leading cause of accidental death in the home for children from birth to age 4 and are 40% of the burn injuries for children up to age 14.

Burn Center Background

In 1993, Dr. Craig Ingelson felt that there was a need to provide his unique standard and continuum of care to burn victims in three large counties by establishing a burn center in Norton County. The center would serve as a regional center of excellence by utilizing the same coordinated approach to the acute, surgical, and rehabilitative continuum of burn services for which he first established Ingelson Burn Center, 50 miles from Delphi Hospital, was noted. In 1997, Dr. Ingelson helped Delphi Hospital establish the Ingelson Burn Center as a state-of-the-art, six-licensed inpatient bed facility coupled with a dedicated outpatient burn center adjacent to the hospital, with himself as the Medical Director. The Ingelson Burn Center of Norton County had earned a reputation for excellent care delivery and superior outcomes by a highly motivated and trained team. The burn center received referrals from other hospitals, employers, insurance companies, and fire departments for both acute inpatient care and continuing outpatient reconstructive and therapy treatments.

Patient Care

Once a patient arrived at the emergency department, the team, consisting of emergency medical physicians, nurses, and emergency medical technicians, all of whom were fully trained in specialized burn care, conducted a preliminary assessment and performed emergency treatment of the patient's injuries based upon the category of burn. The emergency team was in contact with the team of burn surgeons, headed by Dr. Ingelson, relaying all information regarding the status of the patient's injuries. The patient was admitted to the inpatient burn unit where the progress of the patient's injuries was monitored for 48–72 hours postinjury. Burn care specialists coordinated patient care.

Staff

The staff of a burn team was comprised of a variety of members. It consisted of plastic surgeons; neurologists; psychologists; infectious disease physicians; neonatologists; pulmonologists; ophthalmologists; nurses; occupational, physical, recreational, respiratory, and speech therapists; and case managers.

All staff were trained in the most current treatment protocols for burn care, receiving continuous education throughout the year. In addition, all staff was ACLS (advanced cardiac life support) certified and ABLS (advanced burn life support) trained.

Nurse staffing in the inpatient burn center was based on the ratio recommended for any critical/intensive care patient. All specialists utilized were trained in the emergent, acute, immediate, and progressive treatment of burn injuries and were called upon on an as-needed basis after a full evaluation was made of the patient's needs. The burn center had four full-time scheduled personnel, one part-time, and one *per diem* nurse. Normally, the burn center patient staff ratio was 1:1, 2:1, and 3:1, respectively, which was based on patient classification and patient care needs.

Staffing needs were continuously assessed and adjusted based on patient census and condition fluctuations, the staff's experience and training, technological equipment used, and degree of supervision needed. Policy required not less than two nursing personnel physically present in the unit when a patient was present, with at least one of the nursing personnel an RN.

On average, approximately 20% of the Ingelson Burn Center's patients were children. To serve this special population, the burn center provided a bilingual licensed clinical social worker on staff who was paneled by State children's services. The social worker provided recreational therapy and worked with the children and their families to address concerns and fears in dealing with their burn injury.

Communication among the burn team and a patient's employer, insurer, and medical management representative was critical to delivering quality patient care. In order to maintain continuous flow of communication among all members of the team, the burn center coordinated weekly patient care conferences moderated by the case manager. The purpose of the conferences was to discuss and evaluate all inpatient and outpatient burn cases in order to ensure a complete continuum of patient care.

Quality/Image

Dr. Ingelson was a nationally recognized plastic surgeon, a graduate of Emory University and The University of Tennessee Medical School. He was board certified in general surgery as well as plastic surgery. Dr. Ingelson had a unique method of treating burns, characterized by his high utilization of surgery when he debrided and grafted burn patients, which was less painful than the traditional method of debridement and grafting. He was able to combine an extensive burn and reconstruction surgical practice with an aesthetic surgical practice.

The Ingelson Burn Center of Norton County had earned a reputation in the community for excellent care delivery and superior outcomes by a highly skilled and patient-focused team. Patients of the burn center were referred from local and regional hospitals, employers, insurance companies, and fire departments for both acute patient care and continuing outpatient reconstructive and therapy treatments.

License Requirements

In order to have a burn unit; the hospital had to comply with the California State Code of Regulations for both state operations codes and state building codes.

State Operations Codes   According to the Department of Licensing, regulations dictate that a burn center must be a dedicated, closed unit.

In order to treat severe burns, the burn center beds must be licensed for the treatment of burn patients only. In addition, due to the lowered immune response of the burn patient, the unit must be isolated from traffic.

- A burn unit is defined as an intensive care unit (ICU) with services and staff specializing in burn treatment, used solely to treat burns or similar/ related conditions.

- A burn unit must be located to prevent through traffic.

- A burn unit must have a minimum of four beds and no more than twelve.

- A burn unit must treat at least 50 burn patients per year.

State Building Code   According to the architecture firm contracted by Attica Memorial, a burn center, as defined in the state building codes, described a unit that must meet requirements for the operation of an intensive care unit, a rehabilitation space, and a respiratory care service space.

The code did not state or imply that any of these referenced areas may be shared, but only that the design guidelines for a burn center needed to comply with requirements needed for an intensive care unit, rehab unit, and a respiratory care service space. Given the unique nature of the treatment and potential for airborne contamination in a burn center, the architects believed it was the intention of the code to designate this department to function as a stand-alone department or unit. In the past, the office of state health and licensing had categorized the Ingelson Burn Center as a separate unit used for the purpose for the treatment of burn patients.

Burn center regulations closely paralleled the state building codes for the operation of an intensive care unit. The following summarize the key requirements:

- At least one negative pressure isolation room shall be provided for patients with an airborne communicable disease (state building code)

- Nursing station with control desk, charting space, lockable medicine cabinet, refrigerator, and hand wash fixture (state building code)

- At least 132 square feet of floor space per bed with no dimension of less than 11 feet, at least 4 feet of clearance around the bed, and at least 8 feet between beds (state building code)

- 24-hour coordination and physical space requirements for Respiratory and Rehabilitation (state building code)

Physician and Nursing Supervision

There were very specific California State Operation Codes regulations related to supervision of a burn center. Based on these requirements, Attica Memorial would be required to provide medical and nursing staff with significant burn care experience and training as follows.

- Two accredited physicians experienced in burn therapy shall be responsible for supervision and performance of burn care (state operation code).

- Continuous in-house physician coverage is required (state operation code).

- A registered nurse with at least 6 months of experience in treating burn patients and with evidence of burn care continuing education shall be responsible for nursing care and management in the burn center (state operation code).

- A registered nurse with at least 3 months experience in treating burn patients shall be on duty each shift (state operation code).

Members of the medical and nursing staff at Attica Memorial and Delphi Hospital were interviewed to determine the level of experience and interest in the treatment of burn patients. Based on those interviews, it was determined that many of the RNs who had already trained in burn care had resigned from Delphi Hospital. It was the opinion of the Attica Memorial intensive care unit (ICU) and critical care unit (CCU) leadership that the staff of Attica Memorial did not have the necessary competencies in burn treatment to continue the required level of care.

STATE CHILDREN SERVICES (SCS) IMPACT

California State Children Services (SCS) is the body that regulates the treatment of Medicaid children aged birth to 21 years who experience disabilities resulting from congenital anomalies or severe debilitating injury. SCS certification was vital to the operation of the burn center. According to the director of business development for the Ingelson Burn Center, SCS patients represented 74% of the pediatric inpatient burn volume and 26% of all pediatric outpatient visits in 2000. For the first and second quarters of calendar year 2001, 59% of inpatients and 31% of outpatients were SCS.

SCS Certification Requirements

State children services (SCS) guidelines provided for specialized care of pediatric patients and for adults with delayed mental development in an acute care environment. These guidelines consisted largely of policies and procedures designed to support the psycho-social and emotional well-being of the pediatric patients. Meeting SCS certification requirements had very little impact on the normal operations of a burn unit. The following applied to SCS requirements:

- Pediatric play room and age-appropriate toys
- Increased security provisions for pediatric patients
- Specialized pediatric burn intake and admission nursing protocols
- Cribs and crib nets functional 24 hours
- Pediatric CRASH carts, thermometers, scales, BP cuffs, and so forth
- Pediatric PT available 24 hours
- Child life therapist available 24 hours

SCS Current State

The Ingelson Burn Center applied for SCS certification 3 years ago but was granted only provisional status because the burn center had not fulfilled all the requirements dictated by the Department of Health Services. The provisional status was to expire on October 31, 2001. If this status were allowed to expire without immediate written notification to SCS regarding the future of the center, the burn center would no longer be reimbursed for treating the largest percentage of its pediatric burn patients. Recertification was unlikely if provisional status was allowed to lapse.

Even if the provisional status was renewed after October 31, 2001, SCS could not be applied to the burn center at Attica Memorial East Campus since SCS status was not transferable from one facility to another. Applying for SCS accreditation was an extensive process that could take more than two years. Without SCS, the burn center would not be able to treat pediatric patients and would have to transfer them to University Hospital, 5 miles to the south. University Hospital was able to treat pediatric burn patients under its SCS medical center umbrella policy; however, the medical center was applying for SCS specifically to treat pediatric burn patients, which would be a threat to Attica Memorial's ability to capture this important burn population.

FACILITY CONSTRAINTS

Based on the findings regarding the licensing and regulatory requirements of operating a burn center, the burn unit was required to be located near critical/intensive care because of the severity of burn injuries and the complications that could arise. Because infection was so threatening to a burn victim, both positive and negative pressure rooms were required to handle the most critical patients. Children typically comprise 50% of all burn patients. In order to treat pediatric burn inpatients, SCS required a playroom within the burn unit. The playroom was for parents to visit with their children, adolescents to visit with their friends, and for staff or social workers to perform play and recreational therapy with children. According to the business director for the burn center, the existing playroom was too small (190 square feet) and needed to be expanded by 5%.

A Hydrotherapy room was a critical element in the treatment of a severe burn. Hydrotherapy cleaned the burn area, allowed the removal of dressings, and performed gentle skin debridement.

Hyperbaric oxygen therapy (HBO) was the second critical element in treating burn. HBO was the process of placing a patient in an environment that allowed them to breathe and be surrounded by oxygen at two to three times atmospheric pressure. HBO had proven to be significant in promoting rapid healing.

Equally important was the third element of the Ingelson Burn Center, the Outpatient Burn Center, located close to Delphi Hospital. At the Outpatient Burn Center, the patient's progress was continually monitored and modified when appropriate, not only by the physicians, psychologist, and nurses, but also by the therapists and the burn case manager.

CAPACITY ANALYSIS

Based on the findings regarding the licensing and regulatory requirements of operating a burn center, a capacity analysis was conducted to locate space for the integration of a dedicated burn unit into the existing Attica Memorial East Campus physical plant. The current East Campus ICU/CCU space was identified as a potential location for the burn center. Two capital build-out scenarios were considered: 1) Integration of a burn unit into current ICU/CCU configuration, and 2) Expansion of inpatient space through a full unit build out. Based on ICU/CCU post-campus integration capacity constraints and the state operation code and state building code regulations, it was determined that it was not feasible to integrate the burn unit into the existing ICU/CCU unit. Therefore, a new unit would have to be built to accommodate the program. The architecture firm determined the cost for a full build out of a dedicated six-bed burn unit would be approximately $1,604,958; a dedicated four-bed burn unit full build-out would cost approximately $1,505,525. There would, however, be potential cost savings if the burn unit moved to the Attica Memorial rehabilitation space. Moving the burn unit to the rehabilitation space would cost approximately $820,147 for a six-bed burn unit, or approximately $735,618 for a four-bed burn unit (see Exhibit 1, p. 252).

PHYSICIAN RELATIONS

Dr. Ingelson was the medical director of the Ingelson Burn Center. He was not, however, an on-site physician at Delphi Hospital. Dr. Ingelson and his team of burn surgeons were only on site for difficult and acute burn patients; otherwise, Dr. Fred Peace was the local burn physician who managed all the burn cases that came through the Ingelson Burn Center. Dr. Peace then reviewed all the burn cases with Dr. Ingelson for a confirmed patient treatment plan. All phases of inpatient care were coordinated on the same unit and were supervised by Dr. Ingelson and his team of specially trained burn physicians. Nurses, therapists, and other allied health professionals had all been trained to treat and deal with burn injuries and issues associated with burn. The continuity of care continued to the outpatient burn center with familiar physicians and staff working with the patients and their families on a daily basis toward full physical and emotional recovery.

Edward Totino, former CEO of Delphi Hospital, stated that Dr. Ingelson was an extraordinary physician and commanded special treatment from clinical and administrative staff. Whenever Dr. Ingelson was needed at Delphi, the hospital provided limousine service for his trip to the burn center. Totino gave a firm warning that if Attica Memorial did not treat Dr. Ingelson correctly, Dr. Ingelson would leave and set up his burn service elsewhere. A burn center without Dr. Ingelson would no longer be regarded as a center of excellence in Norton County. Therefore, burn patients would have to use other burn centers that might not be well known for their burn treatment. In addition, the hospital would lose a vital source of revenue generated from the Ingelson Burn Center.

PHYSICIAN POLITICS

When Attica Memorial CEO Rick Ponti surveyed the physicians with practicing privileges at both Attica Memorial East and West Campuses and who knew of Dr. Ingelson and his burn practice, all the physicians had negative comments about Dr. Ingelson. The physicians categorized Dr. Ingelson as a "Diva Physician." They did not like the fact that the administration gave special treatment to Dr. Ingelson and did not treat all physician staff the same. Attica Memorial East Campus physicians had mixed feelings about the Ingelson Burn Center joining their facility. Some of the physicians were indifferent to the burn program; however, there was a lack of support from all of the general surgeons and plastic surgeons interviewed. The surgeons did not like Dr. Ingelson's customary practice of reserving large blocks of OR time each week since that blocked OR time was typically underutilized (see Exhibit 3, p. 254).

When Dr. Ingelson met with Ponti and his executive team for a tour of the East Campus, it was noted that Dr. Ingelson's requested location of the burn unit would be extremely expensive. If the hospital determined to transition the Ingelson Burn Center to East Campus, a dedicated unit just for burn would have to be built out, requiring tearing down existing structures and shifting around services. Dr. Ingelson's request to convert the RN's rest area into the burn pediatrics playroom was not well received by Debra Walker, the VP of Patient Care. Converting the physician work-out room into the HBO facility was also not well received by the physicians.

COMMUNITY IMPACT

Through Dr. Ingelson's dedication to superior patient care, continuing education, and community outreach, the burn center had earned the respect and support of local fire departments. In interviews regarding the Ingelson Burn Center, all local firefighters contacted supported the burn center. One interviewee had been treated at the Ingelson Burn Center and was extremely satisfied with his outcome. According to a local fire department spokesperson, they preferred the Ingelson Burn Center treatment to the University Hospital burn treatment. The firefighters stated in their memorandum of understanding (MOU) that if they were ever victims of burn, they preferred to be treated at the Ingelson Burn Center over other burn centers.

The Progressive Group health care consultants claimed that burn units should admit 100 patients annually for 3 consecutive years in order to maintain the appropriate level of proficiency with burn care. Based on Norton County statistics, University Hospital admitted approximately 384 burn patients from 1998 to 2000 and its burn center was meeting NCOS standards. The Ingelson Burn Center had approximately 279 admissions for the same period. In addition, 85% of the burns treated in Norton County were 0%–20% burns, not considered "severe" burn. Lower severity burns could be treated in nondedicated inpatient units and through the emergency department. These statistics indicated that there might not have been a need for two burn centers serving Norton County.

Dr. Matthew Suess, Medical Director of Norton County, stated that a preliminary study of burn treatment in Norton County indicated that University Hospital provided more than adequate coverage for the county. Dr. Suess did not support the continuation of the Ingelson Burn Center and did not support Dr. Ingelson's methodology of treating burn with extensive plastic surgery that was not within the norm of burn treatment. Dr. Suess felt that there was no need for two programs in Norton County based on the low volume of critical burn cases and he claimed Norton County would not be affected by having the University Hospital as the sole provider for burn treatment.

OPPORTUNITY FOR MARKET GROWTH

With the Ingelson Burn Center as a Center of Excellence, there was potential for branding Attica Memorial and driving up volume with Dr. Ingelson's treatment for burn care. As part of the center's continuum of service, the Ingelson Burn Center provided outreach and educational services to pre-hospital personnel, emergency department personnel, schools, employers, and insurance carriers. The center hosted educational seminars, participated in community and employer health fairs, and provided in-service training, utilizing materials on burn safety, first aid for burn injuries, and breakthrough treatments of burn injuries and other pertinent information. In addition to hosting burn educational seminars, the Ingelson Burn Center held an annual Burn Survivors Reunion for all former and current patients, their families, and friends. Attica Memorial could establish relationships with local medical centers and community physicians in order to secure transfers post-stabilization and pre-admission.

Opportunities for market growth could be dimmed, however, by significant competition with University Hospital's burn center nearby. This leading burn center reported greater volume due to a Level 1 trauma emergency department, and had 123 inpatient cases reported in 1999. Without Level 1 trauma, the Ingelson Burn Center was limited to receiving only burn patients and was not able to treat patients with combinations of burn and other non-burn emergency injuries. According to Norton County's Emergency Medical Services, in the past 3 years, burn volume had been trending down from 23% to 15% of all emergencies.

Obtaining worker's compensation, patients could be limited because patients must either predesignate a program or wait 30 days postadmission to transfer to a different burn center. In an interview, Dr. David Carpenter, owner of a large medical group contracted with Attica Memorial, stated that his medical group would not use the Ingelson Burn Center for his occupational patients because of Dr. Ingelson's high cost of treating burn patients. Although Dr. Ingelson's plastic surgery approach to treating burn had impressive outcomes, his treatment costs were more than the norm. Dr. Carpenter referred all of his occupational patients to University Hospital because it was known to have positive outcomes and the burn treatment costs were within the norm.

PROFITABILITY

Based on the financial data provided by Delphi Hospital's decision support system and factoring in the impact on inpatient surgery, the Ingelson Burn Center's net margin in FY 2000 was $309,939, while FY 2001 decreased to $232,745 (see Exhibit 1).

If the Ingelson Burn Center were moved to Attica Memorial East Campus, the capital expense for a full build out expansion of six beds was $1,604,958, based on either FY 2000 or FY 2001 financials. The payback of this capital investment was 5.18 years based on FY 2000 patient volume and revenue, or 6.9 years based on FY 2001.

If the burn program were moved into the present rehabilitation space at Attica Memorial East Campus, the capital expense could be lowered to $820,147 for six beds, with payback of the full build-out expansion in 2.65 years based on FY 2000, or 3.52 years based on FY 2001 (see Exhibit 1).

	FY 2000	FY 2001	FY 2000	FY 2001
Contribution Margin				
Net Revenues	$1,901,953	$1,904,538	$1,901,953	$1,904,538
Variable Expenses	967,066	1,047,561	967,066	1,047,561
Fixed Expenses	433,068	432,352	433,068	432,352
	$501,819	$424,625	$501,819	$424,625
Impact to Inpatient Surgery	191,880	191,880	191,880	191,880
Burn Center Net Margin	$309,939	$232,745	$309,939	$232,745

	Moved to present rehabilitation space at Attica Memorial East		Moved to Attica Memorial East (full build out expansion)	
Capital Expense - 6 Beds	$820,147	$820,147	$1,604,958	$1,604,958
Capital Expense - 4 Beds	$735,618	$735,618	$1,505,525	$1,515,525
Analysis				
Payback (in years) - (6 Beds)	2.65	3.52	5.18	6.90
Payback (in years) - (4 Beds)	2.37	3.16	4.86	6.51

Exhibit 1. Ingelson Burn Center summary (without loss of SCS).

Moving Ingelson Burn Center to the East Campus, whether into a new building or into the existing rehabilitation space, however, meant that the loss of SCS certification had to be considered. Because SCS status would not transfer to the AMH East Campus, the financial health of the program quickly worsened. According to the financial analysis for FY 2001, lost SCS contribution margin was $114,885. The lost savings for surgery call coverage was ($70,080), and the lost cost savings for a blood bank technician was ($32,120), therefore the total net margin was $12,685. Without SCS certification, the payback of the capital investment in the burn program for a full build out expansion for six beds was 126.52 years; if the program moved to the AMH East Campus rehabilitation space, the payback for six beds was 64.65 years. The dramatic financial impact of the loss of SCS status could make it financially untenable for the hospital to support such a unique program (see Exhibit 2).

The practice of reserving large blocks of OR time by the Ingelson Burn Center Physician Medical Group would dramatically affect the Attica Memorial Surgical Services if the burn center moved to AMH Campus. The burn physician group currently scheduled two $4\frac{1}{2}$-hour OR time blocks per week at the West Campus in anticipation of as-needed surgical services. According to Attica Memorial's Surgical Services Coordinator, it was standard practice at East Campus to release OR time 72 hours in advance. The burn physician group, however, released blocked OR time for rescheduling only 14 hours in advance, at 5:00 P.M. on the day prior to blocked time that had no scheduled sur-

	FY 2001	FY 2001
Loss of State Children Services		
Lost Contribution Margin	$114,885	$114,885
Lost Savings	102,200	102,200
Burn Center Net Margin	$12,685	$12,685
	Present rehab space at AME	Moved to AME (full build out)
Capital Expense - 6 Beds	$820,147	$1,604,958
Capital Expense - 4 Beds	$735,618	$1,505,525
Analysis		
Payback (in years) - (6 Beds)	64.65	126.52
Payback (in years) - (4 Beds)	57.99	118.69

Exhibit 2. Ingelson Burn Center summary (with loss of SCS).

geries. The surgical services coordinator claimed that the late cancellation practice of Dr. Ingelson would result in idle OR time and affect scheduling and hospital revenues.

Attica Memorial East Campus OR suites were operating at or near capacity and constraints on OR scheduling were anticipated when services from the West Campus were integrated. In addition, interviews with Attica Memorial West Campus Surgical Services personnel revealed that the Ingelson Burn Center Physician Medical Group was currently underutilizing its block schedule by 3 hours each week, which impacted inpatient surgery at the Attica Memorial East Campus facility. The practice of reserving large blocks of OR time might affect Attica Memorial East Campus Surgical Services by $191,880 (see Exhibit 3). When the capital expenditure for a new, six-bed, dedicated burn unit at the East Campus of $820,147, when using rehab space, or $1,604,958 for the full build out, was coupled with a decrease in the overall inpatient surgery contribution margins, the burn program would have a negative impact on the financial health of AMH East Campus.

EASE TO IMPLEMENT

Intentions to close the Ingelson Burn Center were met with great resentment by the former Delphi Hospital's staff and administration. Delphi's

Total Inpatient Cases	1,420
Avg. Gross Revenue Per Inpatient Case	$35,920
Avg. Deduction Inpatient Case	24,406
Net Revenue per Inpatient Case	$11,514
Avg. Variable Costs Per Inpatient Case	6,773
Avg. Direct Fixed Costs Per Inpatient Case	1,051
Avg. Contribution Margin Per Inpatient Case	$3,690
Number of Inpatient Procedures Impacted Each Week by Underutilization of Blocked Operation Room Time	1
Impact Per Week	$3,690
Number of Weeks Per year	52
Impact Per Year	$191,880

Note:
(1) According to Jamie Patel in Surgical Services Department at AMH West Campus, Dr. Ingelson on average underutilizes his Operating Room time by 3 hours each week. Assuming that average inpatient surgery takes 3 hours and Operating Room time is near or at capacity, the underutilization of OR time will impact 1 surgery per week.

Exhibit 3.   Impact on inpatient surgery contribution margins.

former CEO believed that Dr. Ingelson's reputation for his burn treatment and outcomes were far superior to nearby competitors that had medical residents treating burn patients. In addition, with provisional SCS status, Attica Memorial West Campus would be able to drive up volume and surpass University Hospital, its nearest competitor. Following the alliance's plan for an East Campus acute/inpatient care facility and a West Campus ambulatory care facility would, however, require moving the program to the East Campus and building a new critical/intensive burn unit and hyperbaric facilities.

Implementing the burn center at the East Campus would require investment to train all emergency clinical and critical/intensive care staff in emergency burn care. In addition, during the interim transition, essential burn staff would be required to train the East Campus clinical staff that will be administering burn treatment. In addition, some of the current burn nurses had expressed discontentment working with Dr. Ingelson and with burn patients, and had stated they want to transition out of the burn unit. The burn center had a trend of high nursing staff turnover because, as one burn nurse stated, working with Dr. Ingelson could be challenging, and hiring and training burn nurses was costly.

THE INGELSON BURN CENTER DECISION

After Ponti reviewed the Burn Center analysis, he knew that a decision had to be made on the fate of the program. In order to clearly delineate the implications and ramifications of whichever course was to be taken with the Burn Center, there were a number of issues that Ponti need take into consideration. In deciding, Ponti knew that the community impacts and emotional issues could not be overlooked, but that the financials were vital to the decision about whether to continue the Burn Center. Three alternatives emerged from the analysis: 1) Status Quo—The Ingelson Burn Center remains at Attica Memorial West Campus, the former Delphi Hospital; 2) Relocation—The Ingelson Burn Center transitions to Attica Memorial East Campus; 3) Termination—Attica Memorial closes the Ingelson Burn Center.

19

Brunswick Community Hospital Cash Flow Crisis

Michael Wiltfong

Gary R. Wells

William E. Stratton
Idaho State University, Pocatello, Idaho

Peter Butler recently assumed the position of chief financial officer (CFO) at Brunswick Community Hospital (BCH), which was organized under state law as a county institution. As such it is not subject to income, sales, or property taxes. The hospital is managed under contract by a large national hospital management corporation that hires and pays the hospital administrator and provides management oversight. With the exception of the hospital administrator, all individuals working for the hospital are county employees.

Prior to assuming his duties, Peter discussed the situation faced by the hospital with the regional financial vice president and the chief executive officer (CEO) of the hospital services firm. The financial vice president told him, "There is a lot of work to do at Brunswick. Internal reporting is inadequate and no one seems to know about the computer. Most of the problems can be addressed long term, but there won't be a long term unless we can get the cash situation under control."

The CEO was concerned about the cash situation, too, but he had additional concerns for BCH as well. "We can't get anywhere if we don't build revenue," he stated. "To build revenue we must attract new physicians. If we can't free up money for equipment, these doctors won't come. I have just recruited a urologist, and he will need equipment. I know that we are short of cash, but we must buy what these doctors need. We need money for capital expenditure and we need it quickly."

Peter had accepted the job offer at BCH partly because of the challenge it afforded him. After spending a week becoming familiar with the hospital and meeting the other key employees, Peter thought further about the situation. With the words of the regional financial vice president and the CEO still ringing in his mind, Peter wondered what options were available to the hospital, in both the long and short term, to resolve the cash problem. He felt considerable pressure as the CFO to come up with a viable solution and to come up with it soon.

BACKGROUND

Brunswick Community Hospital is a 54-bed acute care hospital with an attached 58-bed long-term nursing care and 16-bed residential care facility providing health care services to residents of its county. The hospital service area covers approximately 35,000 people. Three larger hospitals are within 25 miles of Brunswick. Two are located in a city of 60,000 people and one is in another city of approximately 50,000. One smaller hospital also operates within the county. Brunswick often refers its more specialized cases to the other three larger hospitals. The area hospitals have been discussing the collective purchasing of mobile equipment such as a machine for MRI, CT scanners, and a mammography unit as a way to provide additional services at reasonable cost.

Subsequent to changes in the Medicare program, BCH experienced trends common among hospitals throughout the healthcare industry in the United States. The Medicare program funds a majority of health care costs for patients covered by Social Security. Historically, the payments provided by the Medicare program were changed from a cost-based system to a fixed payment system. In place of billing for the actual costs of treating a patient, under the fixed payment system hospitals received a set fee for a given diagnosis, regardless of the expense incurred in treating any specific patient. In conjunction with this change, Medicare, as well as other insurance payers, began to challenge the appropriateness of care provided to their covered beneficiaries. The processes implemented to control alleged inappropriate delivery of care resulted in an initial decline in activity at BCH. Recently, extended care and residential care suffered additional declines (see Table 1).

During the same time, the percent of patient days devoted to Medicare/Medicaid increased from 43.0% to 49.7% (see bottom of Table 1). These changes led to significant decreases in cash inflows, which were covered by bank loans during the past two years.

An additional possible impact on the hospital cash flows was the conversion of the hospital computer system in October of year 4 (see the Appendix for a description of the computerized charging system). The conversion was blamed by some for all the problems the hospital was currently experiencing. The business office manager represented the opinion of many of the employees involved in the collection of the patient accounts when he stated, "We never had these problems in the past. We were always current in paying our bills until we decided to change that blasted computer."

The conversion included all data processing systems. In November of Year 4, shortly after the conversion, receivables climbed to an average of 140 days outstanding. Industry averages were approximately 80 days. The effect was to decrease the hospital's operating cash by $36,000 over a period of just 30 days. This result led to the forecast of a critical cash crisis for Year 5 (see Table 2). The cash flows from operations are expected to accrue evenly throughout the year. The capital expenditures are sched-

Table 1. Brunswick Community Hospital patient days and occupancy rates (for the year ended June 30)

	Patient Days			
	Year 1	Year 2	Year 3	Year 4
Hospital				
Adults & Children	5,649	5,525	5,148	5,576
Newborn	861	834	800	804
Extended Care	19,922	19,839	20,602	19,907
Residential Care	5,905	6,391	5,871	5,329
	Occupancy Rate			
	Year 1	Year 2	Year 3	Year 4
Hospital				
Adults & Children	28.7%	28.0%	26.1%	28.3%
Newborn	19.7%	19.0%	18.3%	18.4%
Extended Care	97.5%	96.8%	97.0%	94.0%
Residential Care	77.0%	83.2%	96.6%	91.3%
Medicaid/Medicare Inpatient Utilization of Hospital (Inpatient Days)	43.0%	46.9%	44.0%	49.7%

Table 2. Brunswick Community Hospital cash forecast (for the year ending June 30)

	Year 5
Cash Flow from Operations	$450,000
Capital Expenditures	(200,000)
Deposits designated for capital improvements	(100,000)
Increase of funds on hand	(100,000)
Decrease in A/P held in excess of term	(150,000)
Increase in Due to Third-party Payers	75,000
Decrease in Unsecured Debt	(100,000)
Cash Deficit	−$125,000

uled for the first 6 months of the year. Peter's immediate challenge is to develop a plan to meet the predicted cash deficit.

ALTERNATIVE APPROACHES TO A SOLUTION

Long-Term Financing Options

Hospital policy regarding long-term financing limited the courses of action open to Peter. The board of trustees, as a matter of principle, wanted to avoid all unsecured debt and to liquidate all debt currently outstanding.

Revenue Bonds Long-term financing, such as a revenue bond, was a possibility. Two weeks after arriving at BCH, Peter met for the first time with the finance committee of the board of trustees, whose membership included county commissioners and other community leaders. Peter presented an overview of the cash situation at BCH to the committee and recommended they consider increasing long-term borrowing by issuing revenue bonds for the hospital. His proposal received little support and one committee member, the treasurer of the board of trustees, stated, "If the hospital tries to borrow money, people in this community will string us up." Such financing would require a vote of the citizens of the county, with a positive outcome in no way assured. The school district had recently made several attempts to obtain voter approval for long-term debt, and all of them were unsuccessful. Peter's meeting with the finance committee ended with no progress made toward resolving the cash crisis of the hospital. The finance committee, and by extension the board of trustees, was reluctant to consider long-term borrowing to provide the needed infusion of cash, although it had not been ruled out categorically.

Deferred Compensation Plan Funds Other possible sources of financing are two alternative off-balance-sheet sources of financing available to the hospital. The first involves the deferred compensation plan sponsored by the hospital, which is structured and operated under the provisions of the Internal Revenue Code Section 457 (457 Plan). Under this plan, salary is withheld tax-free from an employee's current pay and deposited with a third-party administrator. The funds are invested in fixed interest contracts with a highly-rated insurance company.

Brunswick Community Hospital operates as a governmental entity under the Internal Revenue Code, which is more liberal for governmental entities than for nongovernmental entities. In governmental units, the 457 Plan funds are legally general assets of the entity. Under other types of deferred compensation plans, the funds are assets of the individual participant. Governmental entities are allowed to use deferred compensation funds to meet current obligations. In a bankruptcy proceeding, the participants in the deferred compensation plan would be treated as general creditors of BCH instead of preferential creditors. Withdrawal of funds from the plan is available at any time to governmental entities without paying a penalty assessed under other types of deferred compensation plans. In addition, pension plans for nongovernmental entities require minimum funding by the entity based on an actuarial evaluation. A governmental entity is not required to fund its plan.

For a 457 Plan of this type, generally accepted accounting principles require that the deferred compensation be shown as an asset and a liability on the hospital's balance sheet. The amount of the hospital's Plan 457 funds held by the third party administrator on June 30 of Year 4 was $967,763.

Pension Plan Funds Another source for increasing the availability of cash funds is the hospital sponsored pension plan. The hospital maintains a defined benefit plan. As a governmental pension plan, contributions can be delayed until pay-outs are made to the beneficiaries. In fact, the hospital had historically deferred funding of the plan during previous cash crises. The available pension assets as a percentage of the present value of projected pension benefits was close to 95% in Year 4. Discontinuing scheduled contributions to the pension plan would increase available cash by $120,000.

Working Capital Options

Another alternative available to Peter is to generate cash through managing components of working capital. The following is a discussion of the components of working capital on June 30 of Year 4.

Cash   The primary cash account is the operating account held in a local bank. Deposits are made to this account daily, and general expenses of the hospital are paid out of it daily as well. The hospital tries to keep just enough money in this account to cover the expenses being paid, with excess funds being invested in short-term, interest-bearing accounts.

Accounts Receivable   Patient receivables/third party payer receivables represent more than 80% of current assets. The length of time in days that receivables have been outstanding (unpaid) on June 30 of Year 4 is shown in Table 3. Of a total of $2,600,297 owed the hospital, $1,212,786 has been owed for more than 120 days.

The patient receivables by type of payer are shown in Table 4. Accounts are classified by payer based on which source will pay the majority of the bill. Private pay accounts, for example, will be paid by the patient, and insurance accounts will be paid by an insurance company such as Blue Cross or Blue Shield. This table indicates that the largest group of accounts is the private pay category accounting for 38.4% of receivables. This account is followed by the insurance account at 27.5%.

Contracts that the primary payers (insurance companies, Medicare, and Medicaid) have with the hospital dictate the terms of payment. These payers dictate the timing and the amount of payment for a given diagno-

Table 3.   Brunswick Community Hospital aging of patient receivables (at June 30)

Days Outstanding	Year 4 Amount of Receivables
0–30	$768,660
31–60	240,448
61–90	231,592
91–120	146,811
121–360	746,032
Over 360	466,754
	$2,600,297

Table 4. Brunswick Community Hospital patient
receivables by type of payer

Type of Account	Year 4
Private Pay	38.40%
Insurance	27.50%
Medicaid	17.30%
Medicare	16.80%
	100.00%

sis or procedure. Potentially more flexiblity exists for balances due from
private payers. These are amounts due from the patient after payment has
been made by the primary payer and include coinsurance and deductible
payments and amounts due from patients without primary coverage. Two
factors, however, restrict this flexibility. The hospital's largest commercial
insurance carrier, accounting for approximately 20% of total revenues, had
a favored nation clause in its contracts with all health care providers. The
crux of this clause was to guarantee the commercial insurance carrier the
best pricing available. The original intent of such a clause was to promote
competitiveness in health care pricing. This state's insurance commissioners, however, have concluded that this type of clause has the opposite
effect. But as long as the clause exists, offering discounts to private payers
to accelerate payment of their bills may result in the commercial insurance
carriers requesting the same discount.

The historical terms-of-sale offered to private pay patients also constituted a complicating factor in attempting to lower the level of patient
receivables. As a matter of policy, the hospital provided care regardless of
the ability of the patient to pay. The hospital had no formal charity policy.
Therefore, all write-offs were treated as bad debt. To maximize the cash
received from patients, the hospital allowed them to make payments over
time without interest. Formal records of the commitments patients had
made to the hospital to pay their bills did not exist. Over the years, the
number of these accounts had grown to the point that more than 1,200
accounts owing a total of $300,000 fell into this category.

Collection Efforts Along with the favorable terms-of-sale provided to private pay patients, other factors hampered collection efforts.
One factor was the previous hospital write-off policy, which dictated an
account be charged directly to expense at the time of write-off. To control
this expense, write-offs were limited to a maximum of $10,000 per month.
This amount included any defaults due to bankruptcy. To avoid exceeding

the $10,000 limit, some accounts that the hospital did not consider collectible were maintained in the system as accounts receivable. The lack of formal records of commitments made by private payers combined with personnel turnover resulted in collection efforts on old patient accounts coming to a standstill. One accounts receivable collector summed up her frustration by saying, "I am afraid to come in to work on Monday. I don't know which account will blow up this week. Which account should I make a collection effort on? Which account needs to be billed after six months? There is just no way of knowing." Personnel could no longer determine whether to bill, dun, or write off an account with no activity. In addition, the hospital's billing system complicated the collection of this type of account.

The hospital billing system was designed to facilitate the collection of an account within 120 days of the service date. Three to five days after a patient is discharged, for example, a final bill is generated by hospital staff. This bill is submitted to the patient's insurance carrier or the applicable governmental agency. The employee in accounts receivable then flags the account for follow up at a future date. The follow-up date may be different for each account and requires some judgment on the part of the billing clerk. Typically, 30–60 days later the clerk reviews the account to determine if action has been taken by the insurance carrier or governmental agency. If the appropriate action has been taken, then the clerk bills the patient for the residual amount due on the account. At this same time, the account is flagged again for subsequent follow up. If appropriate action has not been taken by that later time, the clerk ascertains the problem with the account and takes appropriate action and again flags the account for subsequent collection. Due to this billing process, at any one time the billing clerk is only working a small number of the total number of accounts for which he or she is responsible. This process does not readily accommodate accounts making irregular payments for up to 12 years after the patient's discharge. Consequently, the monitoring of this type of account was haphazard.

Supplies Inventory   Inventories consist of two categories—supplies related directly to patient care and those related to general services (see Table 5 for the components of the supplies inventory). Medical, intravenous, pharmacy, central supply, lab, and surgery constitute the inventory of items required for the care of patients. The need for any particular item may be very sporadic. Not having an item in stock when needed, however, may be potentially life threatening. The operating room supervisor stated her opinion concerning inventory management as follows: "I'm not going to jeopardize my patient because of some wild thing called carrying cost." Control is vested with patient caregivers for

Table 5. Brunswick Community Hospital supplies inventory (at June 30)

	Year 4	
Medical Supplies	$29,016	19%
Office Supplies	22,559	15%
Housekeeping Supplies	1,190	1%
Intravenous	4,251	3%
Linens	9,587	6%
Maintenance	187	0%
Pharmacy Drugs	31,149	20%
Central Supply	14,011	9%
Lab Supplies	21,507	14%
Surgery	20,905	14%
Total	$154,362	100%

these inventories. Their primary motivation is to stock inventory at such a level as to provide generous safety stock. General service departments maintain the remaining inventories. The use of these items is more predictable and out-of-stock situations less critical. Physical inventory counts are scheduled once a year. Base safety levels are used to maintain medical supplies inventories. Central supply was in the process of establishing these base safety levels. There was very little interest or understanding by other managers of the idea of efficient inventory levels. Day-to-day management of inventories was largely each department manager's concern. No formal control system was in place to establish or maintain inventory levels.

Prepaid Expenses/Other Current Assets Prepaid expenses comprise annual organization dues and annual maintenance contracts that provide for discounts of 5%–10% for annual up-front payment. Other current assets consist of the quarterly subsidy paid by the county government. By July 31 of Year 6, this balance will be paid in full. A long-term goal of the hospital board of trustees is for the hospital to be self-supporting.

Current Liabilities The cash forecast (see Table 2) outlines the hospital's goals for levels of unsecured debt, accounts payable, and amounts due to third-party payers. These goals could be changed; this would, however, require the approval of the board of trustees of the hospital.

Accounts payable are amounts owed to physicians who are members of the hospital medical staff and to national medical supply companies. The hospital also owes a small amount to local vendors for supply purchases. The local vendor and physician payments are current. National vendors do not emphasize credit worthiness to the extent common in other industries. Generally, community hospitals are good credit risks and some slowness in payment is not a source of concern to these vendors.

The amount due for accrued expenses is mainly attributable to payroll functions. As a practical matter, extending the payment of these accounts is impossible. Historical balance sheets and income statements are presented in Tables 6 and 7.

PETER BUTLER'S DECISION DILEMMA

Peter Butler realized the officers of the national company overseeing the hospital, the hospital administrator to whom he directly reported, and the members of the board of trustees all expected him to come up with a solution to the cash crisis at BCH. Peter knew he had considerable information about the hospital's operations that should be useful in designing a recommended solution. He felt his first job should be to determine exactly how the cash crisis had developed. He wondered what had changed recently compared to prior years when there had been no such problem. He thought this knowledge might then give him some clues as to where solutions may lie.

In general, Peter knew that there were many possible approaches to resolving a cash crisis in any organization. He realized there were several long-term financing options open to the hospital, including issuing revenue bonds, borrowing from deferred compensation funds, or deferring payments to the pension plan. Another set of possibilities included some kind of management intervention in managing the several different working capital accounts—accounts receivable, supplies inventories, prepaid expenses and other current assets, and current liabilities. Peter wondered what he could recommend that would result in the most effective, timely, and permanent solution to the cash crisis being experienced by the hospital.

Table 6. Brunswick Community Hospital balance sheets (at June 30)

ASSETS	Year 1	Year 2	Year 3	Year 4
Current Assets				
Cash & cash equivalents	$53,354	$110,070	$67,698	$43,125
Patient receivables	2,109,146	2,316,550	2,557,518	2,600,297
Less: uncol. & allowances	−380,000	−420,000	−480,000	−1,228,000
Taxes receivable from county	34,950	34,189	35,000	40,700
Due from 3rd-party payers			91,445	
Supplies & inventory	169,084	182,958	192,802	154,363
Prepaid expenses	13,268	18,208	15,797	26,032
Total Current Assets	$1,999,802	$2,241,975	$2,480,260	$1,636,517
Investment & Other Assets				
Interest-bearing deposits designated by board for capital improvements	185,978	236,238	135,565	30,486
Investment in medical office bldg.	227,039	213,759	200,479	187,199
Deferred financing costs	12,554	8,295	4,036	
Deferred compensation plan			822,424	967,763
	$425,571	$458,292	$1,162,504	$1,185,448
Property & equipment at cost	$8,197,389	$8,293,573	$8,442,491	$8,613,363
less accum. depreciation	3,094,171	3,464,918	3,858,022	4,269,538
	$5,103,218	$4,828,655	$4,584,469	$4,343,825
Total Assets	$7,528,591	$7,528,922	$8,227,233	$7,165,790
Current Liabilities				
Unsecured notes payable to bank			$85,101	$136,334
Current maturities of long-term debt	$129,524	$160,437	117,165	22,589
Accounts payable	260,700	221,372	266,534	348,013
Due to third-party payers	31,960	15,588	75,000	
Accrued expenses	226,895	226,309	258,008	301,394
Total Current Liabilities	$649,079	$623,706	$726,808	$883,330
Long-term debt less current maturities	$267,357	$156,947	$41,909	$6,078
Deferred compensation payable			822,424	967,763
Fund balance	6,612,155	6,748,269	6,636,092	5,308,619
Total Liabilities and Fund Balance	$7,528,591	$7,528,922	$8,227,233	$7,165,790

Table 7.   Brunswick Community Hospital statement of revenues and expenses and changes in fund balance (year ended June 30)

REVENUE AND EXPENSES	Year 1	Year 2	Year 3	Year 4
Net Patient Service Revenue	$5,879,092	$6,181,456	$6,660,092	$6,033,569
Other Operating Revenue	26,895	31,268	4,000	11,563
Total Operating Revenue	$5,905,987	$6,212,724	$6,664,092	$6,045,132
Operating Expenses				
Professional care of patients	$3,815,929	$3,718,098	$4,291,207	$4,753,848
General services	804,724	764,489	820,010	869,964
Fiscal and admin. services	1,259,970	1,225,901	1,270,212	1,453,754
Depreciation	469,128	484,200	512,503	492,287
Total Operating Expenses	$6,349,751	$6,192,688	$6,893,932	$7,569,853
Income from operations	−$443,764	$20,036	−$229,840	−$1,524,721
Nonoperating Gains (Losses)				
Property taxes	$69,900	$69,189	$70,000	$149,700
Income on interest-bearing deposit for capital improvements	22,227	4,296	13,545	6,591
Operating funds	3,872	5,066	25,569	12,175
Gain (Loss) on disposal of equip.	200	−2,038	−1,081	
Unrestricted gifts and requests	1,638	1,380	14,670	7,508
Other	1,030	−7,322	−7,204	−6,876
Net nonoperating gains	$98,867	$70,571	$115,499	$169,098
Rev. & Gains in excess of exp.	−$344,897	$90,607	−$114,341	−$1,355,623
CHANGES IN FUND BALANCE				
Balance, Beginning	$6,950,052	$6,612,155	$6,748,269	$6,636,092
Rev. & gains in excess of exp.	−344,897	90,337	−114,341	−1,355,623
Funds restricted for equipment purchases	7,000	45,777	2,164	28,150
Balance Ending	$6,612,155	$6,748,269	$6,636,092	$5,308,619

APPENDIX

Billing and Collection Processes

Hospital billing and collection processes are unique to the industry. The objective of the BCH computer conversion was to make these processes more efficient. The following is an overview of the BCH computerized billing and collection system.

Charges

Generally the three origins of hospital charges are rooms, procedures, and supplies. Processing each type of charge varies somewhat from the others. Under the previous computer system all charging had been done on a batch basis rather than a continuous online basis. A batch system is more labor intensive, more prone to error, and results in more delays in the billing and collection process than is the case with an online system. The new computer system was designed to process more charges on an online basis.

Room Charges   The charge for a room covers nursing care, food, utilities, depreciation, housekeeping, and linen. The patient is charged a standard rate for each day spent in the facility, except for the day of discharge. If a patient was admitted at 11:00 P.M. on Friday and discharged at 11:00 P.M. on Sunday, for example, the patient would be charged for 2 days.

Under the previous computer system, the room charges were batched daily and entered into the accounts receivable system through a remote terminal. The remote processing center would then run an update. The update would then be reviewed and corrected if necessary.

This system was streamlined by the new computer system. At midnight, the computer checks the room census database. Every account that exists in this database is charged with a room charge.

Procedure Charges   A procedure charge is for the cost of performing a treatment procedure. Most patients admitted for surgery need a chest X ray, for example. These patients are charged a fee for this procedure.

Procedure charges were charged on a batch basis under the previous system. This system required a charge sheet for each procedure. In addition, each charge was entered through the remote terminal. The remote location processed these entries and the input was balanced.

The charging system with the new computer system is more efficient. When a procedure is ordered, the order is entered into the computer. After the procedure has been performed, the results are entered into the computer. The benefit of this system is that the status of the procedure can be checked by referring to the computer. In addition, charging to the patient's account is done automatically at the end of the day.

Supply Charges Supplies are charged as used. All consumable supplies are affixed with a sticker when received. As a supply item is used, the sticker is removed from the item and affixed to a charge card bearing the patient name and account number. These cards are used to enter the charge into the patient's account. This system remains unchanged under the new computer conversion.

Billing

Before a bill can be submitted, all of the above charges must be charged to the patient's account. Submitting charges to a payer after the initial billing significantly increases the time to receive payments. In some cases, late submissions are not paid. Noncharge information also must be submitted with the bill. This information concerns the patient's medical condition and treatment. This subsystem interfaces with the new computer system.

To start the billing process, which determines cash flow, a number of pieces of information must be available. Initially, not all of the new systems to generate this information functioned during the conversion. Some of the breakdowns were attributable to the computer system. Other breakdowns were due to employee misunderstanding of the requirements of the new system.

20

Cardinal Health Care Systems

Some Behavioral Issues in Corporate Cost Allocation

Joseph F. Castellano
Wright State University, Dayton, Ohio

Harper A. Roehm
University of Dayton, Dayton, Ohio

Several months ago, Cardinal Health Care Systems (CHCS) hired Fred Bird as its chief financial officer. CHCS is a for-profit corporation that operates a number of health care subsidiaries in the greater St. Louis area:

1. Smith Valley Hospital—a full-service acute care hospital

2. Herr Care Services—outpatient clinics capable of providing both medical and surgical care

3. Coleman Long Term Care—a full-service, long-term care nursing home complex

---

From Castellano, J.F., & Roehm, H.A. (1988). Cardinal Health Care Systems: Some behavioral issues in corporate cost allocation. In C.C. Ling (Ed.) (1987), *Annual advances in business cases* (pp. 1–5). Nacogdoches, TX: Society for Case Research. Copyright © 1988 by Joseph F. Castellano and Harper A. Roehm; reprinted by permission.

Fred Bird was one of a dozen candidates interviewed for the CFO job. Bird was hired on the basis of his extensive experience with a large firm that specialized in consulting services for health care facilities.

At the time Bird was hired, CHCS, like other health care corporations, was under increasing pressure to control costs. The board of directors was especially concerned with CHCS's inability to control corporate overhead costs.

In addition, the presidents of the three subsidiaries had been complaining vigorously about CHCS's policy of allocating all corporate overhead costs on the basis of the revenue generated by each of their units. All three presidents were in agreement that the current policy of cost allocation provided no incentive to the staff service departments for controlling costs and, in addition, was putting the subsidiaries under extreme pressure to reduce their direct costs (i.e., costs under their control) in order to meet corporatewide profit targets. Tom Herzog, president of Smith Valley Hospital, was particularly upset because his unit generated the largest share of total revenue and, hence, received the largest allocation of corporate overhead costs even though in a number of cases his subsidiary used very little of a particular service.

Shortly after Bird joined CHCS, he and Dale Maxvill, CHCS's chief executive officer, met to review the corporate overhead cost problem. Maxvill communicated the board's concern about the need to control these costs. He also pointed out his reluctance to order across-the-board cuts in these staff services because this would be treating the symptom and not the problem. He instructed Bird to make a study of the overhead cost area, including the methods of allocating these costs, and report his preliminary recommendations within 30 days.

Bird soon learned that there were six principal service departments supporting CHCS's three subsidiaries.

- Information Systems and Databases

- Personnel and Employee Relations

- Communications/Advertising

- Controller

- Central Purchasing

- General Counsel

Although other service functions could be identified (i.e., CEO and staff, Tax Department, CHCS Foundation), their costs represented only 2% of total overhead costs. Because these costs were not allocated in the existing system, Bird decided to focus his efforts on the six principal service departments, which accounted for $10 million in overhead costs. Bird was quick to note that last year CHCS's earnings after expenses were $7 million. It was obvious that the need to control overhead costs was not just a mere accounting exercise.

Bird was acutely aware of some of the classic pitfalls associated with allocating corporate overhead on the basis of total revenues, as CHCS had been doing: 1) It was too easy for service departments to pass along inefficiencies to line departments, and 2) these types of allocations provided little direct linkage between the amount of resources needed to provide particular services and the demand for such services. Therefore, he decided to develop a charge-back procedure for CHCS's six principal corporate service departments.

Under the new system, all of the six service departments' costs would be charged back to the subsidiaries based on their use of services. The new system would have a number of significant advantages over the current system. First, service departments would have to identify their costs associated with providing the activities they are responsible for. Second, the subsidiaries (users or consumers of service department activities) would have to develop a better understanding of their demand for services and the costs associated with these services. In addition, the subsidiaries would no longer have to worry about being charged for services they did not want or use, and the corporation could more easily target service areas for cuts based on low demand for services.

Although anxious to report back to Maxvill, Bird decided to meet with the presidents of the three subsidiaries and the directors of each of the service departments. The meetings went as Bird had expected. The presidents seemed pleased with the prospect of being charged only for services they used. In addition, they all expressed the general feeling that, "This will force these support services to get a handle on their costs because we won't be forced to subsidize their inefficiencies."

The reaction from the service departments was neutral at best. They were fully aware of the opposition to the current allocation method and the concern about rising costs. They uniformly believed, however, that they were being singled out as the scapegoats. Several asked Bird why it was even necessary to allocate these costs at all. Others expressed strong reservations about the problem of getting agreement on the costs to be used in the charge-back plan. Bird listened attentively, but remained convinced that in time his plan would achieve positive results.

Bird's report to Maxvill received an enthusiastic reception. Maxvill saw positive results for all concerned; the subsidiaries would no longer be saddled with arbitrary allocations and the service departments would be spared across-the-board budget cuts, which were inevitable if the current cost trends continued. Maxvill sent a memo to all who would be directly involved in the project, urging their full cooperation with Bird in developing the specific details of the charge-back plan.

Several weeks into the process of developing the specific details of the plan, across-the-board resistance was increasingly apparent. In a series of joint meetings Bird was holding with subsidiary personnel and service department staff, both groups expressed serious opposition. Users (the subsidiaries) were anxious about trying to forecast demand for certain services (e.g., legal) and wanted to know the implications if they under- or overestimated their needs. In addition, they wanted the right to seek outside quotes for services and, if these charges were lower, to seek the services in the external market if the lower prices were not met internally.

The service departments were concerned about "being put under the microscope" in the process of detailing the services they would provide and the corresponding charges for these services. A number of department managers indicated that their employees were wondering if this entire process was a ruse to identify areas for elimination and budget cuts.

Bird, sensing that support for his plan was quickly eroding, decided to meet with the CEO to fully apprise him of the situation. After exchanging pleasantries, they had the following conversation:

Maxvill: I've been expecting your call. I understand you've been getting it from both sides. I know I've been getting an earful.

Bird: And how! But it's nothing unusual. I've seen this reaction many times in these kinds of situations. Everyone is initially afraid of change even though they are unhappy with the present system.

Maxvill: Did you anticipate this kind of reaction after your preliminary meeting with each group? I know I didn't.

Bird: Not really. The subsidiaries seemed anxious to try anything that would replace the existing system. The service departments seemed neutral. I tried to sell them on the idea that the proposed system could go a long way toward eliminating the need for across-the-board cuts. But I really didn't get into specifics with each group.

Maxvill: I understand that the subs are primarily concerned about having the right to get outside quotes.

Bird: That's true. But they want to go farther and have the right to acquire the services from outside vendors.

Maxvill: Is that realistic? Can they readily find these services cheaper outside the corporation?

Bird: In many cases, yes. But I think they are rushing things. They are trying to read too much into the plan.

Maxvill: What do you mean?

Bird: The proposal I've made is essentially an alternative to our current cost allocation policy. At the heart of the proposal is an attempt to control overhead costs. They seem to be reading more into it than what I have proposed.

Maxvill: What about the service departments? I know what they have been saying, but what is their real problem?

Bird: They feel like they're out on a limb. They have to identify the services they can provide and attach a cost to each. They are used to thinking of their department costs on a macro, not micro, basis.

Maxvill: But they think we are playing a game with them and that we really want them to make these identifications so we can cut their budgets.

Bird: I think that kind of talk is just a smoke screen. My system will force them to become cost managers. Naturally, their initial reaction will be to resist this change.

Maxvill: Do you think we should try to get some additional dialogue started before we proceed?

Bird: Absolutely not! I think it will just harden positions. Each group will just lobby for their vested interests and concerns. I think we should go ahead with the plan as I envisioned it—a straight charge-back cost allocation. However, for the time being, let's rule out outside quotes. This should relieve the service department manager's concerns. The subs get the relief from the present system they want so that should make them happy. Later on, we can look at other alternatives. That's my input. But it's your decision.

Maxvill: The buck stops here. Right?

Bird: Right.

Maxvill: I'll get back to you in a few days. I want to think about this.

As Maxvill pondered his conversation with Bird, he was struck by Bird's confident assurance in the plan he had proposed. From his standpoint, the charge-back plan had engendered the most resistance to any proposal during his 10 years as CEO. Yet, he knew something had to be done. The board was insisting that overhead costs be brought under control. Given his personal abhorrence to across-the-board cuts, Bird's plan had seemed the ideal solution. The resistance and suspicion of so many people, however, was equally troubling. Only one thing was clear: he would have to decide on some course of action soon.

21

West Florida Regional Medical Center (A)

Curtis P. McLaughlin
University of North Carolina at Chapel Hill

Now that West Florida Regional Medical Center (WFRMC) had successfully completed the Joint Commission on Accreditation of Healthcare Organizations (JCAHO) survey, John Kausch, its administrator/CEO, felt that he and his management team should start 1992 by focusing on their continuous quality improvement (CQI) process. There were a number of issues that he and the quality improvement council could address, including 1) performance reviews under CQI, 2) speeding up the work of the task forces, 3) focusing the process more on key competitive issues, and 4) deciding how much money to spend on it.

WEST FLORIDA REGIONAL MEDICAL CENTER

The WFRMC is a Hospital Corporation of America (HCA) owned and operated, for-profit hospital complex on the north side of Pensacola, Florida. Licensed for 547 beds, West Florida Regional operated approximately 325 beds in December 1991, plus the 89-bed psychiatric pavilion, and the 58-bed Rehabilitation Institute of West Florida. The 11-story office building of the Medical Center Clinic, P.A., is attached to the hospital facility, and a new cancer center is under construction.

The 130 doctors practicing at the Medical Center Clinic and its satellite clinics admitted mostly to WFRMC, whereas most of the other doctors in this city of 150,000 practiced at both Sacred Heart and Baptist hospitals downtown. Competition for patients was intense, and in 1992 as much as 90%–95% of patients in the hospital were admitted subject to discounted prices, mostly Medicare for the elderly, CHAMPUS for military dependents, and Blue Cross/Blue Shield of Florida for the employed and their dependents.

The CQI program had had some real successes during the past 4 years, especially in the areas where package prices for services were required. All of the management team had been trained in quality improvement techniques according to HCA's Deming-based approach and some 25 task forces were operating. The experiment with departmental self-assessments, using the Baldridge award criteria and an instrument developed by HCA headquarters, had spurred department heads to become further involved and begin to apply quality improvement techniques within their own work units. Yet Kausch and his senior leadership sensed some loss of interest among some managers, while others who had not bought into the idea at first were now enthusiasts.

THE HCA CQI PROCESS

Kausch had been in the first group of HCA CEOs trained in CQI techniques in 1987 by Paul Batalden, M.D., corporate Vice-President for Medical Care. Kausch had become a member of the steering committee for HCA's overall quality effort. The HCA approach is dependent on the active and continued participation of top local management and on the Plan-Do-Check-Act (PDCA) cycle of Deming. Exhibit 1 shows that process as presented to company employees. Dr. Batalden does not work with a hospital administrator until he is convinced that that individual is fully committed to the concept and is ready to lead the process at his own institution, which includes being the one to teach the Quality 101 course on site to his own managers. Kausch also took members of his management team to visit other quality exemplars, such as Florida Power and Light and local plants of Westinghouse and Monsanto.

In 1991, Kausch became actively involved in the total quality council of the Pensacola Area Chamber of Commerce (PATQC), when a group of Pensacola area leaders in business, government, military, education, and health care began meeting informally to share ideas in productivity and

FOCUS-PDCA

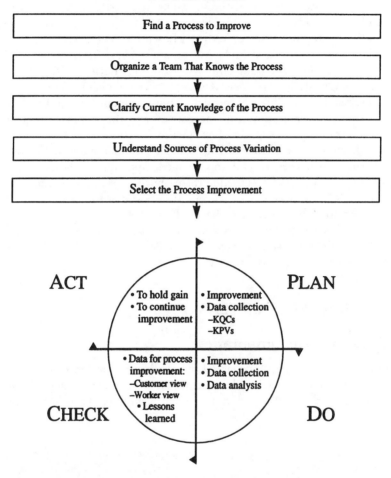

Exhibit 1.   The FOCUS-PDCA problem-solving approach.

quality improvement. Celanese Corporation (a Monsanto division), the largest nongovernmental employer in the area, also supported PATQC. From this informal group emerged the PATQC under the sponsorship of the chamber. The vision of PATQC was "helping the Pensacola area develop into a total quality community by promoting productivity and quality in all area organizations, public and private, and by promoting economic development through aiding existing business and attracting new business development." The primary employer in Pensacola, the U.S. Navy, was using TQM (total quality management) extensively and was quite satisfied with the results and supported the chamber program. In fact, the first 1992 1-day, community-wide seminar presented by Mr. George F. Butts, consultant and retired Chrysler Vice President for Quality and Productivity, was to be held at the Naval Air Station's Mustin Beach Officers' Club.

The CQI staffing at WFRMC was quite small, in keeping with HCA practice. The only program employee was Ms. Bette Gulsby, M.Ed., Director of Quality Improvement Resources, who serves as staff and "coach" to Kausch and as a member of the quality improvement council. Exhibits 2 and 3 show the organization of the council and the staffing for quality improvement program support. The "mentor" was provided by headquarters staff, and in the case of WFRMC was Dr. Batalden himself. The planning process had been careful and detailed. Appendix A shows excerpts from the planning processes used in the early years of the program.

WFRMC has been one of several HCA hospitals to work with a self-assessment tool for department heads. Exhibit 4 shows the cover letter sent to all department heads. Exhibit 5 shows the scoring matrix for self-assessment. Exhibit 6 shows the scoring guidelines, and Exhibit 7 displays the five assessment categories used.

FOUR EXAMPLES OF TEAMS

Intravenous Documentation

The nursing department originated the IV documentation team in September 1990 after receiving documentation from the pharmacy department that, over a 58-day period, there had been $16,800 in lost charges

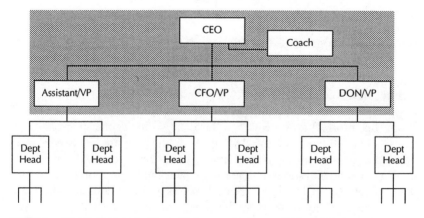

Exhibit 2. Organization chart with quality improvement council (shaded box).

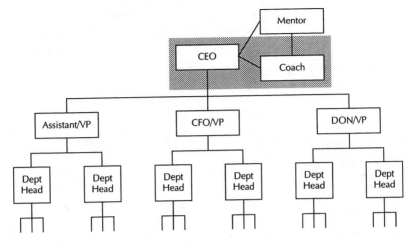

Exhibit 3. Organization chart with CEO QIP support (shaded box).

related to the administration of intravenous (IV) solutions. The pharmacy attributed the loss to the nursing staff's record keeping. This was the first time that the nursing department was aware of a problem or that the pharmacy department had been tracking this variable. There were other lost

In an effort to continue to monitor and implement elements of improvement and innovation within our organization, it will become more and more necessary to find methods that will describe our level of QI implementation.

The assessment or review of a quality initiative is only as good as the thought processes that have been triggered during the actual assessment. Last year (1990), the quality improvement council prepared for and participated in a quality review. This exercise was extremely beneficial to the overall understanding of what was being done and the results that have been accomplished utilizing various quality techniques and tools.

The departmental implementation of QI has been somewhat varied throughout the organization and, although the variation is certainly within the range of acceptability, it is the intent of the QIC to understand better each department's implementation road map and, furthermore, to provide advice/coaching on the next steps for each department.

Attached please find a scoring matrix for self-assessment. This matrix is followed by five category ratings (to be completed by each department head). The use of this type of tool reinforces the self-evaluation that is consistent with continuous improvement and meeting the vision of West Florida Regional Medical Center.

Please read and review the attachment describing the scoring instructions and then score your department category standings relative to the approach, deployment, and effects. This information will be forwarded to Bette Gulsby by April 19,1991, and, following a preliminary assessment by the QIC, an appointment will be scheduled for your departmental review.

The review will be conducted by John Kausch and Bette Gulsby, along with your administrative director. Please take the time to review the attachments and begin your self-assessment scoring. You will be notified of the date and time of your review.

This information will be utilized for preparing for the next department head retreat, scheduled for May 29 and 30, 1991, at the Perdido Beach Hilton.

Exhibit 4. QI assessment cover letter sent to department heads.

APPROACH	DEPLOYMENT (Implementation)	EFFECTS (Results)
* HQIP design includes all eight dimensions[a] * Integration across dimensions of HQIP & areas of operation	* Breadth of implementation (areas or functions) * Depth of implementation (Awareness, knowledge, understanding and application)	* Quality of measurable results

100% ───

* World-class approach: sound; systematic; effective; HQIP based; continuously evaluated, refined, and improved * Total integration across all functions * Repeated cycles of innovation/improvement	* Fully in all areas and functions * Ingrained in the culture	* Exceptional, world-class, superior to all competition; in all areas * Sustained (3–5 years), clearly caused by the approach

80% ───

* Well-developed and tested, HQIP based * Excellent integration	* In almost all areas and functions * Evident in the culture of all groups	* Excellent, sustained in all areas with improving competitive advantage * Much evidence that they are caused by the approach

60% ───

* Well-planned, documented, sound, systematic, HQIP based: all aspects addressed * Good integration	* In most areas and functions * Evident in the culture of most groups	* Solid, with positive trends in most areas * Some evidence that they are caused by the approach

40% ───

* Beginning of sound, systematic, HQIP based; not all aspects addressed * Fair integration	* Begun in many areas and functions * Evident in the culture of some groups	* Some success in major areas * Not much evidence that they are caused by the approach

20% ───

* Beginning of HQIP awareness * No integration across functions	* Beginning in some areas and functions * Not part of the culture	* Few or no results * Little or no evidence that any results are caused by the approach

0% ───

[a]The eight dimensions of HQIP are: leadership constancy, employee-mindedness, customer-mindedness, process focused, statistical thinking, PDCA-driven, innovativeness, and regulatory proactiveness.

Exhibit 5.   QI scoring matrix for self-assessment.

charges not yet quantified, resulting from recording errors in the oral administration of pharmaceuticals as well.

The team formed to look at this problem found that there were some 15 possible reasons why the errors occurred, but that the primary one was

In order to determine your department's score in each of the five categories, please review the scoring matrix for self-assessment. The operational definitions for Approach, Deployment, and Effects are listed in the small boxes on the top of the scoring matrix. Each criterion is divided into percent of progress/implementation (i.e., 0%-100%). For example, you may determine that your departmental score on category 3.0 (QI Practice) is:

APPROACH	DEPLOYMENT	EFFECTS
20%	20%	20%

This means that your departmental approach has fair integration of QIP practice, your departmental deployment is evident in the culture of some of your groups, and it is not actually evident that your departmental effects are caused by the approach.

Please remember that this is a *self-assessment* and only *you* know your departmental progress. This assessment is not a tool to generate documentation. However, if you would like to bring any particular document(s) to your review, please do so. This is only meant to provide a forum for you to showcase your progress and receive recognition and feedback on such.

Remember, review each of the self-assessment criteria of approach, deployment, and effects and become familiar with the levels or percentages described. You have three scores for each Departmental QI Assessment Category (categories 1.0–5.0).

Exhibit 6. The QI scoring guidelines used.

that documentation of the administration of the IV solution was not entered into the medication administration record (MAR). The MAR was kept at the patient's bedside and, each time that a medication was administered, the nurse was to enter documentation into this record.

The team had to come to understand some terms as they went along. The way that the pharmacy kept its books, anything that was sent to the floors but not billed within 48–72 hours was considered a "lost charge." If an inquiry was sent to the floor about the material and what happened and a correction is made, the entry was classified as "revenue recovered." Thus the core issue was not so much one of lost revenue as one of unnecessary rework in the pharmacy and on the nursing floors.

The team developed Pareto charts showing the reasons for the documentation errors. The most common ones were procedural (e.g., patient moved to the operating room, patient already discharged). Following the HCA model, these procedural problems were dealt with one at a time to correct the accounting for the unused materials. The next step in the usual procedures was to get a run chart developed to show what was happening over time to the lost charges on IVs. Here the team determined that the best quality indicator would be the ratio of "lost" charges to total charges issued. The pharmacy management realized, at this point, that it lacked the denominator figure and that its lack of computerization led to the lack of that information. Therefore, the task force had been inactive for 3 months, while the pharmacy implemented a computer system that could provide the denominator.

Ms. Debbie Koenig, Assistant Director of Nursing, responsible for the team, said the next step would be to look at situations where the MAR was not at the patient bedside, but perhaps up at the nursing station, so that a nurse could not make the entry at the appropriate time. This was an especially bothersome rework problem, because of nurses working various shifts or occasionally an agency nurse who had been on duty and was not

---

1.0   DEPARTMENTAL QI FRAMEWORK DEVELOPMENT

The QI Framework Development category examines how the departmental quality values have been developed, and how they are projected in a consistent manner, and how adoption of the values throughout the department is assessed and reinforced.

Examples of areas to address:

- Department mission
- Departmental quality definition
- Departmental employee performance feedback review
- Department QI plan
- QI methods

APPROACH	DEPLOYMENT	EFFECTS
_____ %	_____ %	_____ %

2.0   CUSTOMER KNOWLEDGE DEVELOPMENT

The Customer Knowledge Development category examines how the departmental leadership has involved and utilized various facets of customer-mindedness to guide the quality effort.

Examples of areas to address:

- HQT family of measures (patient, employee, etc.)
- Departmental customer identification
- Identification of customer needs and expectations
- Customer feedback/data review

APPROACH	DEPLOYMENT	EFFECTS
_____ %	_____ %	_____ %

3.0   QUALITY IMPROVEMENT PRACTICE

The Quality Improvement Practice category examines the effectiveness of the department's efforts to develop and realize the full potential of the work force, including management, and the methods to maintain an environment conducive to full participation, quality leadership, and personal and organizational growth.

Examples of areas to address:

- Process improvement practice
- Meeting skills
- QI storyboards
- QI in daily work life (individual use of QI tools, i.e., flowchart, run chart, Pareto chart)
- Practice quality management guidelines
- Departmental data review
- Plans to incorporate QI in daily clinical operations
- Identification of key physician leaders

APPROACH	DEPLOYMENT	EFFECTS
_____ %	_____ %	_____ %

Exhibit 7.   The five QI assessment categories used.

4.0 QUALITY AWARENESS BUILDING

The Quality Awareness Building category examines how the department decides what quality education and training is needed by employees and how it utilizes the knowledge and skills acquired. It also examines what has been done to communicate QI to the department and how QI is addressed in departmental staff meetings.

Examples of areas to address:

- JIT training
- Employee orientation
- Creating employee awareness
- Communication of QI results

APPROACH	DEPLOYMENT	EFFECTS
_____ %	_____ %	_____ %

5.0 QA/QI LINKAGE

The QA/QI Linkage category examines how the department has connected QA data and information to the QI process improvement strategy. Also examined is the utilization of QI data-gathering and decision-making tools to document and analyze data (how the department relates the ongoing QA activities to QI process improvement activities).

Examples of areas to address:

- QA process indentification
- FOCUS-PDCA process improvement
- Regulatory/accreditation connection (JCAHO)

APPROACH	DEPLOYMENT	EFFECTS
_____ %	_____ %	_____ %

---

available to consult when the pharmacy asked why documentation was not present for an IV dose of medication.

Universal Charting

There was evidence that a number of ancillary services results, or "loose reports," were not getting into the patients' medical records in a timely fashion. This was irritating to physicians and could result in delays in the patient's discharge, which under diagnosis-related groups (DRGs), essentially fixed payment per case, meant higher costs without higher reimbursement. One employee filed a suggestion that a single system be developed to avoid running over other people on the floor doing the "charting." A CQI team under Ms. Debbie Wroten, Medical Records Director, was authorized. The 12-member team included supervisors and directors from the laboratory, the pulmonary lab, the EKG lab, medical records, radiology, and nursing. They developed the following "opportunity statement":

> At present, six departments are utilizing nine full-time equivalents 92 hours per week for charting separate ancillary reports. Rework is created in the form of re-pulling in-house patient records, creating an ever-increasing demand for chart accessibility. All parties affected by this

process are frustrated because the current process increases the opportunity for lost documentation, chart unavailability, increased traffic on units creating congestion, and prolonged charting times, and provides for untimely availability of clinical reports for patient care. Therefore, an opportunity exists to improve the current charting practice for all departments involved to allow for the efficiency, timeliness, and accuracy of charting loose reports.

The team met, assessed, and flow charted the current charting processes of the five departments involved. Key variables were defined as follows:

Charting timeliness—number of charting times per day, consistency of charting, and reports not charted per charting round

Report availability—indicated by the number of telephone calls per department asking for reports not yet charted

Chart availability—chart is accessible at the nurses' station for charting without interruption

Resource utilization—staff hours and number of hours per day of charting

Each department was asked to use a common "charting log" for several weeks to track the number of records charted, who did the charting, when it was done, the preparation time, the number of reports charted, the number of reports not charted (missed), and the personnel hours consumed in charting. The results are shown in Exhibit 8. These data gave the team considerable insight into the nature of the problem. Not every department was picking up the materials every day. Two people could cover the whole hospital in .75 hour each or one person in 1.5 hours. The clinical chemistry laboratory, medical records, and radiology were making two trips per day, while other departments were only able to chart every other day and failed to chart over the weekends.

The processes used by all the groups were similar. The printed or typed response had to be sorted by floors and room numbers added if missing, then taken to the floors and inserted into patient charts. If the chart was not available, they had to be held until the next round. A further problem was identified in that, when the clerical person assigned to these rounds was not available, a technical person who was paid considerably more and was often in short supply had to be sent to do the job.

A smaller team of supervisors who actually knew and owned the charting efforts in the larger departments (medical records, radiology, and clinical chemistry) was set up to design and assess the pilot experiment. The overall team meetings were only used to brief the department heads to gain their feedback and support. A pilot experiment was run in which these three departments took turns doing the runs for each other. The results were favorable. The pilot increased timeliness and chart availability by charting four times per day on weekdays and three on weekends. Report availability was improved and there were fewer phone calls.

Department	Mean records per day	range	Mean hours per day	range	Comments
Medical Records	77.3	20–140	1.6	0.6–2.5	Daily
Pulmonary Lab	50.3	37–55	1.0	0.7–1.5	MWF
Clinical Lab	244.7	163–305	3.2	1.9–5.4	Daily
EKG Lab	40.2	35–48	0.8	0.1–1.0	Weekdays
Microbiology	106.9	3–197	1.4	0.1–2.2	Daily
Radiology	87.1	6–163	1.5	0.1–2.9	Daily

Exhibit 8. Results of each department tracking the number of records charted, who did the charting, when it was done, the preparation time, the number of reports charted, the number of reports not charted (missed), and the personnel hours consumed in charting.

Nursing staff, physicians, and participating departments specifically asked for the process to be continued. The hours of labor dropped from 92 weekly to less than 45, using less highly paid labor.

The Team decided, therefore, that the issues were important enough that they should consider setting up a separate universal charting team (UCT) to meet the needs of the entire hospital. "However, an unanticipated hospital census decline made impractical the possibility of requesting additional staffing. Consequently, the group reevaluated the possibility of continuing the arrangement developed for the pilot using the charting hours of the smaller departments on a volume basis. It was discovered that this had the effect of freeing the professional staff of the smaller departments from charting activities and a very minimal allocation of hours floated to the larger departments. It also increased the availability of charters in the larger departments for other activities." The payroll department was then asked to develop a system for allocating the hours that floated from one department to another. That proved cumbersome, so the group decided to allocate charting hours on the basis of each department's volume. "In the event that one or more departments experience a significant increase/decrease in charting needs, the group will reconvene and the hourly allocation will be adjusted."

The resulting schedule had the lab making rounds at 6 A.M. and 9 A.M. and radiology at 4 P.M. and 9:30 P.M. Monday–Friday, while medical records did it at 6 A.M., 1 P.M., and 8 P.M. on Saturdays and Sundays. Continuing statistics were kept on the process, which is shown in Appendix B. The system continues to work effectively.

Labor, Delivery, Recovery, Postpartum (LDRP) Nursing

Competition for young families needing maternity services had become quite intense in Pensacola. WFRMC obstetrical (OB) services offered very traditional services in 1989 in three separate units—labor and delivery, nursery, and postpartum—and operated considerably below capacity.

A consultant was hired to evaluate the potential growth of obstetrical services, the value of current services offered by WFRMC, customers' desires, competitors' services, and opportunities for improvement. Focus group interviews with young couples (past and potential customers) indicated that they wanted safe medical care in a warm, homelike setting with the lowest possible number of rules. More mothers were in their thirties, planning small families with the possibility of only one child. Fathers wanted to be "actively involved" in the birth process. The consultant challenged the staff to come up with their own vision for the department based on the focus group responses, customer feedback, and national trends.

It became clear that there was a demand for a system in which a family-centered birth experience could occur. The system needed to revolve around the customers, rather than the customers following a rigid traditional routine. Customers wanted all aspects of a normal delivery to happen in the same room. The new service would allow the mother, father, and baby to remain together throughout the hospital stay, now as short as 24 hours. Friends and families would be allowed and encouraged to visit and participate as much as the new parents desired. The main goals were to be responsive to the customer's needs and provide safe, quality medical care.

The hospital administration and the six obstetricians practicing there were eager to see obstetrical services grow. They were open to trying and supporting the new concept. The pediatricians accepted the changes, but without great enthusiasm. The anesthesiologists were opposed to the change. The OB supervisor and two of the three head nurses were dead set against it. They wanted to continue operations in the traditional manner.

When the hospital decided to adopt the new LDRP concept, it was clear that patients and families liked it, but the nursing staff, especially nursing management, did not. The OB nursing supervisor retired; one head nurse resigned, one was terminated, and the third opted to move from her management position to a staff nurse role. Ms. Cynthia Ayres, R.N., Administrative Director, responsible for the psychiatric and cardio-vascular services, was assigned to implement the LDRP transition until nursing management could be replaced.

One of the issues involved in the transition was clarification of the charge structure. Previously each unit charged separately for services and supplies. Now that the care was provided in a single central area, the old charge structure was unnecessarily complex. Duplication of charges was occurring and some charges were being missed because no one was assuming responsibility.

Ayres decided to use the CQI process to develop a new charge process and to evaluate the costs and resource consumption of the service. Ayres had not been a strong supporter of the CQI process when it was first introduced into the organization. She had felt that the process was too slow and rigid, and that data collection was difficult and cumbersome. Several teams were organized and assigned to look at specific areas of the LDRIP process.

To reach a simplified charge process, as well as a competitive price, all aspects of the process had to be analyzed. Meetings were held with the nursing and medical staff. Management of the OB patient and physician preferences in terms of supplies and practices were analyzed. A number of consensus conferences were held to discuss observed variations. Each of the six obstetricians, for example, specified a different analgesic for pain control. Each drug appeared effective for pain control, but their cost per dose ranged from $10 to $75. The physicians agreed that the $10 product was acceptable, because the outcome was the same.

Another standard practice was sending placentas to the pathology laboratory for analysis after every normal delivery. This involved labor time, lab charges, and a pathologist's fee for review. The total procedure cost $196. When questioned about the practice, the current medical staff did not feel it was necessary medically nor the current practice nationally, but that they were just following the rules. Upon investigation, the team found that an incident involving a placenta had occurred 15 years ago that led the service chief (since retired) to order all placentas sent to the lab. The obstetricians developed criteria for when it was medically necessary for the lab review of a placenta. This new rule decreased the number of reviews by 95%, resulting in cost savings to the hospital and to patients.

The charges team reviewed all OB charges for a 1-year period. They found that in 80% of normal deliveries, 14 items were consistently used. The other items were due to variations in physician preferences. The teams and the physicians met and agreed which items were the basic requirements for a normal delivery. These items became the basic charges for package pricing.

The charges team met weekly for at least 1 hour for over a year. Some meetings went as long as 5 hours. Initially, there was a great deal of resistance and defensiveness. Everyone wanted to focus on issues that did not affect themselves. The physicians objected that they were being forced to practice "cookbook medicine" and that the real problem was "the hospital's big markup." Hospital staff continued to provide data on actual hospital charges, resource consumption, and practice patterns. The hospital personnel continued to emphasize repeatedly that the physicians were responsible for determining care. The hospital's concern was to be consistent and decrease variation.

Another CQI team, the documentation team, was responsible for reviewing forms utilized previously by the three separate units. The total number of forms used had been 30. The nursing staff were documenting vital signs an average of five times each time care was provided. Through review of policies, standards, documentation, and care standards, the number of forms was reduced to 20. Nurses were now required to enter each care item only once. The amount of time spent by nurses on documentation was reduced 50%, as was the cost of forms. Data entry errors were also reduced.

The excess costs that were removed were not all physician-related. Many had to do with administrative and nursing policies. Many were due to old, comfortable, traditional ways of doing things. When asked why a practice was followed, the typical response was, "I don't know; that's just the way we've always done it." The OB staff are now comfortable with the use of CQI. They recognize that although it requires time and effort, it does produce measurable results. The OB staff are continuing to review their practices and operations to identify opportunities to streamline services and decrease variation.

Pharmacy and Therapeutics Team

In late 1987, a CQI team was formed jointly between the hospital's pharmacy and therapeutics (P&T) committee and the pharmacy leadership. Their first topic of concern was the rapidly rising costs of inpatient drugs, especially antibiotics, which were costing the hospital about $1.3 million per year. They decided to study the process by which antibiotics were selected and began by asking physicians how they selected antibiotics for treatment. They reported that most of the time they order a culture of the organism causing the infection from the microbiology lab. A microbiology lab report would come back identifying the organism and the antibiotics to which it is sensitive and those to which it was resistant. Some physicians reported that they would look down the list until they came to an antibiotic to which the organism was sensitive and order that. That list was in alphabetical order. A study of antibiotic utilization showed a high correlation between use and alphabetical position, confirming the anecdotal reports. Therefore, the team recommended to the P&T committee that the form be changed to list the antibiotics in order of increasing cost per average daily dose. The doses used would be based on current local prescribing patterns rather than recommended dosages. The P&T committee, which included attending physicians, approved the change and reported it in their annual report to the medical staff. Exhibit 9 shows what happened to the utilization of "expensive" antibiotics (more than $10 per dose) from 1988 to 1991. These costs were not adjusted at all for inflation in drug prices during this period. The estimated annual saving was $200,000.

Given this success, the team went on in 1989 to deal with the problem of the length of treatment with antibiotics. Inpatients did not get a prescription for a 10-day supply. Their IM and IV antibiotics were continued until the physician stopped the order. If a physician went away for the weekend and the patient improved, colleagues were very reluctant to alter the medication until he or she returned. The team wrestled with how to encourage the appropriate ending of the course of treatment without hassling the physicians or risking undue legal liability. They settled on a sticker that went into the chart at the end of 3 days stating the treatment had gone on for 3 days and that an ending date should be specified, if possible. The hospital newsletter and the P&T Committee annual report noted that the physician could avoid this notice by specifying a termination date at the time of prescribing. This program seemed to be effective. Antibiotic costs again dropped, and there were no apparent quality problems introduced as measured by length of stay or by adverse events associated with these system changes.

In 1990, the team began an aggressive drug usage evaluation (DUE) program, hiring an Assistant Director, Pharmacy Clinical Services, to administer it. The position had to be rigorously cost justified. DUE involved a review of cases to determine whether the selection and scheduling of powerful drugs matched the clinical picture presented. If the physician prescribed one of three types of antibiotics known to represent a risk of kidney damage in 3%–5% of cases, for example, the DUE administrator ordered lab tests to study serum creatinine levels and warn the physician if they rose, indicating kidney involvement. There was a sharp decline in the adverse effects caused by the use of these drugs. This program was expanded further to looking at other critical lab values and relating them to pharmacy activities beyond antibiotics, the use of IV solutions

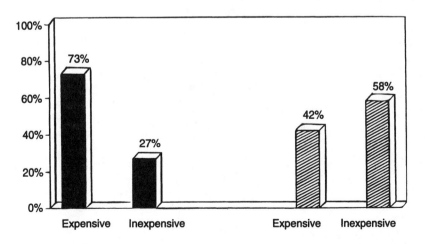

Exhibit 9. Utilization of "expensive" antibiotics (more than $10 per dose) from 1988 to 1991.

and potassium levels, for example. By 1991, the unadjusted antibiotic costs for roughly the same number of admissions had dropped to less than $900,000.

LOOKING AHEAD

One of the things that had concerned Kausch during 1991 had been the fact that implementation had varied from department to department. Although he had written in his annual CQI report that the variation had certainly been within the range of acceptability, he was still concerned about how much variation in implementation was appropriate. If maintaining enthusiasm was a concern, forcing people to conform too tightly might become a demotivator for some staff. This issue and the four mentioned in the introductory paragraph should all be addressed in the coming year.

APPENDIX A: PLANNING CHRONOLOGY FOR CQI

Initiation Plan: 3–6 Months, Starting May 25

May 25:	Develop initial working definition of quality for WFRMC.
May 25:	Define the purpose of the quality improvement council and set schedule for 2 P.M.–4 P.M. every Tuesday and Thursday.
May 25:	Integrate HQT into continuous improvement cycle and hold initial review.
June 2:	Start several multifunctional teams with their core from those completing the leadership workshop, with topics selected by the quality improvement council using surveys, experience, and group techniques.
June 2:	Department Heads complete "CEO assessment" to identify customers and expectations, determine training needs, and identify department opportunities. To be discussed with assistant administrators on June 15.
June 16:	Present to QIC the task force report on elements and recommendations on organizational elements to guide and monitor QIP.
June 20:	Division meetings to gain consensus on department plans and set priorities. QIC reviews and consolidates on June 21. Final assignments to department heads on June 22.
June 27:	Draft initial statement of purpose for WFRMC and present to QIC.
June 29–July 1:	Conduct first facilitators' training workshop for 16.

July 1:	Task force reports on additional QIP education and training requirements for:
	    Team training and team-members handbook
	    Head nurses
	    Employee orientation (new and current)
	    Integration of community resources (colleges and industry)
	    Use of HCA network resources for medical staff and board of trustees

July 19:	Task force report on communications program to support awareness, education, and feedback from employees, vendors, medical staff, local business, colleges and universities, and HCA.

August 1:   Complete the organization of the Quality Improvement Council.

Implementation Plan: 9 Months

Fall: Pilot and evaluate "patient comment card system"

Oct. 21:   QIC input to draft policies/guidelines regarding: forming teams, quality responsibility, and guidelines for multifunctional teams. Brainstorm at October 27 meeting, have revisions for November 10 meeting, and distribute to employees by November 15.

Oct. 27:   Review proposals for communicating QIP to employees to heighten awareness and understanding, communicate on HCA and WFRMC commitments; key definitions, policies, guidelines; HQT; QIP; teams and improvements to date; responsibility and opportunities for individual employees; initiate ASAP.

Nov. 15:   Prepare statements on "On further consideration of HCA's Quality Guideline"; discuss with department heads, hospital staff; employee orientation; use to identify barriers to QI and opportunities for QL Develop specific action plan and discuss with QIC.

Dec. 1:   Identify and evaluate community sources for Q1 assistance—statistical and operational—including colleges, companies, and the Navy. Make recommendations.

Early Dec.:   Conduct Quality 102 course for remaining department heads. Conduct Quality 101 course for head nurses and several new department heads.

Jan. 1, 1989:   Develop and implement a suggestion program consistent with our HCA quality guidelines, providing quick and easy way to become involved in making suggestions/identifying situations needing improvement; providing quick feedback and recognition; and interfacing with identifying opportunities for QIP.

Implementation Plan: Next 9 Months

Aug. 1:   Survey department heads to identify priorities for additional education and training.

Sept. 14–15:   Conduct a management workshop to sharpen and practice QI methods; to include practice methods;

to increase management/staff confidence, comfort; to develop a model for departmental implementation; to develop process assessment/QIP implementation tool; to start quality team review.

September: Develop a standardized team orientation program to cover QI tools and group process rules.

Fall: Expand use of HQTs and integrate into HQIP—improve communication of results and integration of quality improvement action plans. Psychiatric pavilion to evaluate and implement HQT recommendations from "patient comment card system"—evaluate and pilot.

October: Incorporate QIP implementation into existing management/communication structure. Establish division "steering committee functions" to guide and facilitate departmental implementation. Identify QI project for each department head/assistant administrator. Establish regular quality reviews in department manager meetings.

December: Evaluate effectiveness of existing policies, guidelines, and practices for sanctioning, supporting, and guiding QI teams. Include opportunity form/cross functional team sanctioning; team leader and facilitator responsibilities; team progress monitoring/guiding; standardized team presentation format (storyboard). Demonstrate measurable improvement through Baxter QI team.

Monthly: Monitor and improve the suggestion program.

January: Pilot the clinical process improvement methodology.

All Year: In all communications, written and verbal, maintain constant message regarding WFRMC commitment to HQIP; report successes of teams and suggestions; and continue to educate about principles and practices of HQIP strategy.

January: Successfully demonstrate measurable improvement from focused QIP in one department (medical records).

Spring: Expand use of HQTs and integrate into HQIP. Pilot HQT in rehab center. Evaluate and implement physicians' HQT. Pilot ambulatory care HQT.

Summer: Expand use of HQTs and integrate into HQIP. Human resources—Pilot HQT Payers—Pilot HQT

APPENDIX B

Universal Charting Team Focus-PDCA Outline

F   Opportunity statement:
At present, six departments are utilizing nine full-time equivalents 92 hours per week for charting separate ancillary reports. Rework is created in the form of re-pulling in-house patient records, creating an ever-increasing demand for chart accessibility. All parties affected by this process are frustrated because the current process increases the opportunity for lost documentation, chart unavailability, increased traffic on units creating congestion, and prolonged charting times, and provides for untimely availability of clinical reports for patient care. Therefore, an opportunity exists to improve the current charting practice for all departments involved to allow for the efficiency, timeliness, and accuracy of charting loose reports.

O   Team members include:
Debbie Wroten, Medical Records Director—Leader
Bernie Grappe, Marketing Director—Facilitator
Joan Simmons, Laboratory Director
Mary Gunter, Laboratory Patient Services Coordinator
Al Clarke, Pulmonary Services Director
Carol Riley, Pulmonary Services Assistant Director
Marlene Rodrigues, EKG Supervisor
Patti Travis, EKG
Debra Wright, Medical Records Transcription Supervisor
Mike West, Radiology Director
Lori Mikesell, Radiology Transcription Supervisor
Debbie Fernandez, Head Nurse

C   Assessed and flow charted current charting practices of departments.

Clarified and defined key quality characteristics of the charting process:
   Charting timeliness—number of charting times per day, consistency of charting, and reports not charted per charting round.
   Report availability—indicated by the number of telephone calls per department asking for reports not yet charted.
   Chart availability—chart is accessible at the nurses' station for charter without interruption.
   Resource utilization—staff hours and number of hours per day of charting.

U   Gathered data on departments' charting volumes and time spent charting.

S   Data gained through the pilot indicated that significant gains were available through the effort to justify proceeding with the development of a universal charting team.

P   The team developed a flow chart of the charting process using a universal charting team rather than previous arrangement. In order to pilot the improvement, the group decided to set up a UCT using current charters from the three major charting departments—medical records, laboratory, and radiology. The team also developed written instructions for both the charters and participating departments. A subgroup of the team actually conducted a 1-day pilot before beginning extensive education to ensure that the UCT would work as planned and to be sure that the charters from each of the large departments were well versed on possible situations that might occur during the pilot.

D   Piloted proposed universal charting team using current charting personnel from radiology, laboratory, and medical records to chart for all departments.

C   Pilot results were positive and indicated the UCT concept offered significant advantages over the previous charting arrangements.

Results were:
> Timeliness/chart availability—Pilot reduced daily charting to four scheduled charting times daily for all departments. Smaller departments did not chart daily prior to pilot. The charting team also reduced the number of occasions that charters from different departments were on the nursing unit needing the same chart.
> Report availability—Telephone calls were reduced and nursing staff, physicians, and participating departments specifically asked for UCT following the pilot.
> Resource utilization—Number of staff hours spent charting and preparing to chart was reduced from 92 hours weekly to less than 45 hours. The improvement also allowed the use of less expensive staff for charting.

A   The group reached consensus that the easiest configuration for the UCT would be to set up a separate UCT that would serve the needs of the entire hospital.

This was to be proposed to administration by the team as the conclusion of their efforts. However, an unanticipated hospital census decline made impractical the possibility of requesting additional staffing, and so forth. Consequently, the group reevaluated the possibility of continuing the arrangement developed for the pilot using the charting hours to the smaller departments on a volume basis. It was discovered that this had the effect of freeing the professional staff in the smaller departments from charting responsibilities for a very minimal allocation of hours floated to the larger departments, and it increased the availability of charters in the larger departments for other activities. The payroll department was then involved in order to develop the proper mechanism and procedure for floating hours.

This modification of the previous pilot was piloted for a month with continued good results. Streamlining of the hours floating process may be necessary to place less burden on the payroll department.

Because no major changes were required following the pilot, the group has elected to adopt the piloted LJTC format. Allocation of charting hours is based on a monthly review of charting volumes for each department. In the event that one or more departments experience a significant increase/decrease in charting needs, the group will reconvene and the hourly allocation will be adjusted.

Lessons Learned

Because of the size and the makeup of the team, which included a number of department heads, it was found helpful to set up a smaller team of three supervisors who actually knew and owned the charting efforts in the major departments. This group designed and assessed the initial pilot and actually piloted the pilot before bringing departmental charters into the process. As a result, overall team meetings were primarily used to brief department heads and gain their feedback and consensus.

PART IV

Human Resource Management and Organizational Dynamics

22

A New "Brand" for Senior Health Plus

Rosalie Wachsmuth

Aging and Disability Services Administration, State of Washington

Robert C. Myrtle

University of Southern California, Los Angeles, California

THE HEART-WARMING COMMERCIAL

It was the end of the day, and Jamie Richards was exhausted by the time she reached home. She turned the television on to catch the end of the evening news but when she saw the commercial for Senior Health Plus (SHP), a not-for-profit Medicare HMO, she let out a big groan. It wasn't that she hated the ad; she definitely thought that it was catchy and appealed to seniors. Nowhere during the 30-second spot was there any mention of managed care or HMOs. Instead, Wilma, an attractive and vibrant member of SHP's Medicare HMO plan, explained to viewers how SHP had changed her life. After Wilma's hip replacement, SHP had provided her with extensive in-home and personal care services that not only sped up her recovery but also helped her to remain independent at home and in control of her life. The commercial ended with heart-warming shots of Wilma riding a bicycle alongside her grandchildren.

Although Jamie had seen the ad many times before, she couldn't help but feel proud. Her company, SHP, had touched that woman's life, and she knew everything that Wilma had said was true. But when Jamie imagined being back at SHP's corporate offices, she grimaced. Thoughts of the inflammatory complaints she received each day, the sarcastic whispers across cubicles, the unhappy faces in the halls, and the demise of employee morale bombarded her all at once. She thought it was ironic that SHP had become so successful at projecting a positive and appealing external image. If the public knew what it was like to work at SHP, they would certainly have a different opinion of the organization. She shook her head as she wondered about what had gone wrong at SHP.

A GOLDEN OPPORTUNITY

Ten months ago, Jamie joined SHP as the Vice President of Human Resources. She had left her long-time position as Director of Human Resources at Mature Health, a rival senior health plan, for many reasons. Her previous job had been a challenge mainly due to the difficulties of boosting employee morale in the fast-paced, ever-changing managed care environment. She had found that most employees were negatively affected by the stigma of working for an HMO. In Jamie's opinion, HMOs had developed a bad reputation and were one of the most universally hated organizations.

At Mature Health, Jamie had learned a lot about managing the culture of an HMO, but she wanted to apply her skill set to a different organizational setting. When the opportunity to work as the VP of Human Resources at SHP appeared, Jamie jumped at the opportunity. She heard that SHP was a different type of Medicare HMO. For the majority of its 20-year history, it had been known as a grassroots organization focused on preserving the independence of seniors. She was impressed by the CEO's track record of pioneering creative approaches to overcome medical and social challenges. He had guided the organization from a small senior services organization to its current state as an impressive health care system for elderly people.

Jamie was enticed by the idea of joining an organization that had a history of pioneering new ways of serving the elderly. She believed that an organization like SHP, with a strong grassroots foundation, had the power to not only change the way that managed care was delivered to seniors but also remove the stigma of HMOs. In addition, she was attracted to SHP because she felt that the employees there would have more passion for their work when compared with employees at other HMOs.

SHP'S EXPONENTIAL GROWTH

Jamie had come on board during an exciting time at SHP. The organization had been experiencing phenomenal growth both in its Medicare HMO membership and employee workforce. Membership over the past several years had skyrocketed from 10,000 to a whopping 20,000. When Jamie joined SHP, membership was soaring near the 35,000 mark and the number of employees had nearly tripled to more than 400. These numbers were small when compared to the size of rival HMOs, but they were still astounding statistics considering SHP's massive growth rate over the past 3 years.

For these reasons SHP's executive management team saw a need for creating the VP of Human Resources position. SHP's culture was undergoing drastic change to accommodate the huge growth in its workforce. In addition, the executive team planned on adding another 80 positions by the end of 1999 to alleviate the heavy workloads.

SHP was also expanding geographically to meet the needs of its customers. Shortly before Jamie's arrival, SHP had relocated its administrative offices and most of its departments from a modest grassroots base located in the heart of Santa Ana to a posh corporate building in Newport Beach.

They had also created three additional area offices within the past year. This brought the total number of area offices scattered across Southern California to seven. The executive team was concerned about maintaining organizational continuity across the sites and wanted the corporate offices in Newport Beach to be the flagship. That is, the corporate offices would set the standards, and the area offices would be expected to follow suit. The executive team thought that a VP of Human Resources was not only necessary to manage the needs of the growing workforce but also to maintain uniformity across the sites.

Jamie was excited about the challenge of molding SHP's workforce. She knew that her actions would have critical effects. She was in the position to change the culture to meet the needs of the growing organization. She was excited to mold a workforce that was embedded in the grassroots beliefs of SHP. Jamie believed that the employees would be eager to develop a new culture that retained the pioneering spirit of SHP.

She was strongly attracted to SHP's vision of maintaining the independence of seniors. The company had developed four core corporate values: passion, integrity, respect, and responsibility. SHP believed that its employees should be driven by the needs of its customers. Thus, they are expected to seek "innovative solutions on issues affecting their health, independence, and lifestyle choices." In addition, the employees' behaviors should be motivated by the desire to "do the right thing." Also, not only does SHP expect employees to protect and enhance the well-being of its customers but also to value and respect each other as fellow workers. Jamie felt these values set SHP apart from other HMOs and it made her even more eager to mold the workforce.

THE BEGINNING AND END OF A HONEYMOON

Jamie had always been told that the first 90 days of a new job were the honeymoon phase. Everything at SHP seemed too good to be true, at first. She was surprised at how quickly she had been welcomed onto the executive team considering her position was so new. The members reassured her that she would be playing a crucial role at SHP and that they respected her track record. Many of the other executives had also worked at rival HMOs. In fact, it seemed like everyone had jumped ship to join SHP.

During the second day of work, she learned that one of SHP's long-time employees had suddenly died. It was the first time in SHP's history that a current employee had passed away. Understandably, the staff was in shock. Jamie knew that her reaction to the situation would be critically evaluated by the entire organization. She quickly interviewed staff members who were close to the employee and distributed a company-wide memo informing SHP's employees of the death. Jamie also arranged for a company-wide memorial service for the employee and declared a special moment of silence in remembrance of her.

Jamie's delicate handling of the situation impressed the executive team, her human resources staff and employees throughout SHP. They commended her, and she gained immediate respect from the Human Resources staff. Jamie felt that she had proven herself to the executive team and her department and validated the need for her position. After the first 2 weeks on the job, however, it seemed like the honeymoon phase had come to an abrupt end. It was then that she realized that there was a lot about SHP that she didn't know and would soon uncover.

THE BRANDING CAMPAIGN

The CEO had suggested that Jamie meet with Rita Lansing, the VP of Marketing as soon as possible. He raved about Rita's performance and declared that she was single-handedly positioning SHP for the new millennium. Her marketing department was currently immersed in an intense branding campaign. They were conducting focus groups with older adults from the community to find out everything they thought about the colors, shape, and even the symbolism behind the new brand.

The CEO felt very strongly about developing a brand for his company. He wanted to differentiate SHP from other Medicare HMOs by creating a symbol. He explained to Jamie:

> I have always dreamed about creating a brand for SHP. This brand would help consumers identify the unique services that come from our company. A brand name would not only provide an added value to our company, but also give a name for consumers to associate our services with. Seniors tend to be loyal to brand names that symbolize high quality. Just as Windows 2000 is purely Microsoft and Kleenex is the essence of Kimberly-Clark, my vision is to have the public recognize SHP by our logo and know that we deliver high-quality senior services that set us apart from other Medicare HMOs.

Upon hearing this, it clicked in Jamie's head exactly how crucial her role was in this branding process. Creating a brand wasn't just a physical action; it required a change of thought within the company. She would have to encourage the development of a more corporate, professional culture that was consistent with the brand. This branding campaign was an essential part of shaping the organization's culture. It was the basis for many changes.

This task, however, seemed rather overwhelming to Jamie. How could she develop and establish a uniform corporate culture across all eight SHP sites? The atmosphere was drastically different at each separate office. The satellite sites were professional but did not project the same image as the corporate offices. If the culture of the corporate offices represented SHP's new image, then it was crucial for the other sites to replicate it. This was significant because SHP's clients often visited the satellite sites and rarely interfaced with the corporate offices. Thus, it would be important to uphold the SHP image at the satellite sites.

The first thing that Jamie wanted to do was arrange an appointment with Rita. Jamie was eager to meet Rita and find out how she could help carry out the CEO's vision. The brand development sounded exciting, but Jamie was surprised by the amount of time and resources that were being devoted to the creation of the brand. She was, however, extremely interested at finding out exactly what this branding campaign was and to have her questions answered by Rita. Also, Jamie was very concerned about having the employees in on the development of the brand. She felt their involvement was crucial because they would be representing the brand.

STARTING OFF ON THE WRONG FOOT

When Jamie arranged to meet with Rita, she was surprised by her abruptness. Rita said that she was very busy but was willing to spare a few minutes to fill Jamie in on the brand development. Jamie was puzzled by Rita's chilly treatment especially when she compared it to the friendliness of the other executive members.

At their meeting, Jamie was further taken aback by Rita's take-charge manner. The 15-minute meeting did not go as Jamie had envisioned. Not only had Jamie wanted a longer, more in-depth meeting, but she also had hoped that the two of them could discuss where their roles fell into the organization and how they could work together to make the branding campaign a success. Jamie knew that the employees would need a stake in the campaign in order for them to buy into it. She hoped that by including them on the brand development process, this would slowly initiate an organizational culture change and foster employee buy-in.

Jamie was astonished when Rita promptly told her that the marketing department was going to execute the brand development without any help from the rest of SHP. Rita argued that the brand research was confidential and she didn't see the need for employee involvement. She wanted to perfect the brand to meet the CEO's vision not the employees' and therefore did not want employee input. Rita believed that employee buy-in would be the easiest part. If she were successful at creating a distinct, high-quality brand, no employee would argue against its implementation. In fact, Rita argued they would feel privileged to represent SHP's new brand and automatically be motivated to reinforce the brand's high quality.

Jamie was astounded by Rita's logic. She tried to reason with Rita and explained to her that in order for the branding campaign to be successful at reinventing the company's image, Rita would need SHP employee buy-in. Many of the employees had been with the organization when it was a small, grassroots oriented senior services organization. If they did not get involved with these changes, they would surely resist the change.

Rita would not budge. She said her past experiences with brand development had taught her that the process should exclude employee involvement. Rita pointed out that she would fully involve the employees during the unveiling of the new brand. She explained that her department was already planning an unveiling ceremony where all of the employees would be introduced to the new brand.

WORKING INDEPENDENTLY

After that encounter, Jamie felt that her hands were tied. How could she manage the changing organization if Rita wasn't even going to include her in the brand development? Jamie viewed her participation in the branding campaign as a critical part of being the VP of Human Resources. She approached the CEO for guidance but backed down when he told her that Rita was highly experienced and knew what she was doing. Again, Jamie saw how important the brand was to him. He seemed so impressed by Rita's progress that he couldn't see past anything else.

Jamie set off to reorganize her department and the company structure so that it would be in alignment with what she perceived to be the new emerging corporate culture. Her department was very supportive of her. They jointly decided to create a way to open the communication lines between the employees and administration. Jamie viewed communication as one of SHP's current major weaknesses. Thus, she implemented a new medium for communication called the CEO's MessageBoard, created a policy that encouraged employees to eat lunch in the lunchroom instead of at their desks, and revamped the dress code to fit SHP's new corporate image. Her department also worked in conjunction with the executive team to revamp SHP's organizational structure. She thought that these changes should have been implemented long ago.

The CEO's MessageBoard was a hit with the employees. They loved the fact that they could anonymously submit messages to the CEO and have them answered on the company's on-line server. They felt comfortable voicing their concerns and the CEO gave his own input and answers to the questions. It was also available for the rest of the organization to view on-line. Jamie thought that the MessageBoard had helped to create a firm sense of partnership between management and staff while enhancing opportunities for employee growth and development.

The lunchroom policy did not receive rave reviews. Employees felt as if the HR department was telling them how to use their lunch time and felt that it was infringing on employee individualism. Yet, Jamie did not alter the policy. She felt that it was important to encourage employees to interact with each other away from their desks.

Jamie also felt that the organizational structure changes were greatly needed because of the high levels of duplication and geographic problems. Now that SHP had taken residence in their Newport Beach building, Jamie began working with the facilities director to reorganize the employees' workstations. She had wanted to arrange them all in appropriate work units. The employees, however, resented the cubicle changes and thought that HR was imposing a major inconvenience on them. Furthermore, 3 months after the cubicle swapping, the CEO announced that SHP would be relocating to a larger building with more space the following year. This added to the employees' annoyances with Jamie's department.

INTERDEPARTMENTAL CONFLICTS

Problems with marketing and interdepartmental organization made Jamie's job even more difficult. As Jamie and her department set out to make further changes, such as revamping the company newsletter and creating a newsletter for the consumers, she noticed that Rita was stepping into her territory.

During one pivotal executive meeting, Jamie unveiled the newsletters that she and her staff had spent weeks developing. Right there in front of the CEO, Rita expressed her disapproval and pointed out that they would not fit in with the consistency of the brand. Rita explained to the CEO and the executive team that in the future, any internal and external communication documents should be evaluated and approved by her department first. This was because the documents could wear away the brand integrity. Rita said, "Unfortunately good brand management does not always allow for individual creativity. We need to present a consistent image not just externally but internally as well."

Jamie left the meeting fuming. She could not believe what had just happened. Not only had Rita made her look foolish in front of the entire executive team, but she also implied that Jamie didn't know how to do her job correctly. She approached the CEO afterward with her concerns about Rita's infringement on her departmental duties. But Jamie knew he would be no help when she saw the look on his face as she mentioned the brand. He asked her if she had seen the final draft of the brand. She shook her head. His eyes lit up as he described how phenomenal it was. Rita had produced exactly what he had envisioned over the last 20 years. He said he was astounded and could not believe how excited he was. When Jamie voiced her concerns, he reiterated what Rita said regarding the importance of maintaining the brand integrity. He also mentioned that they were preparing to copyright certain terms that would be used to refer to their case managers as "Healthy Care Managers" and the senior services department as "Living with Independence." This would prevent other Medicare HMOs from stealing or copying the services that were unique to SHP.

Jamie was speechless. It was obvious that she could no longer depend on the CEO for support. Rita had him wrapped around her finger.

UNVEILING THE NEW BRAND

Two months later, the marketing department was set to release its new brand for SHP. They had organized a huge unveiling ceremony for the brand and asked Jamie's department for help. Jamie, although still upset from her encounters with Rita, decided that it would be in her best interest to cooperate with marketing. She had hoped that there would still be an opportunity for them to establish good interdepartmental relations.

She had agreed to lend her staff and HR would be in charge of spreading the word about the unveiling ceremony. Jamie began to feel more positive about the ceremony, especially since it now would appear to the employees that HR had played a big part in the brand development. Everyone was given the morning off to attend the ceremony at corporate headquarters.

The only glitch was that marketing had ordered polo shirts, caps, and lunch boxes with the new brand for employees. Because of the budget limits, however, they didn't have enough items to distribute to all of SHP's employees. Thus, Rita made the decision to only distribute items to permanent employees who had been with SHP for over a year.

Jamie objected to that proposal and pointed out that it could create animosity among the employees and temporary workers. Yet, Rita argued that it was too late to do anything about it and that it made sense to only offer long-standing employees the branded items. Jamie backed down and gave in. She had enough to worry about with the planning of the ceremony. She was scheduled to speak after the CEO and wanted to project the right image. The recent changes that she had made at SHP hadn't gone as smoothly as she had wanted, and Jamie knew that the ceremony was the perfect opportunity to redeem herself.

As Jamie had predicted, however, the employees were not only upset about the inequitable distribution of shirts, caps, and lunch boxes, but they were also resentful toward the new brand. Although they enjoyed having the morning off to attend the ceremony, they didn't understand exactly why SHP was revamping its external image. Many commented that SHP had sold out its grassroots heritage for a more corporate, snobby image. To make matters worse, they directed their anger toward the HR department. The employees had assumed that because HR had publicized the event, they were the major movers behind the brand development.

SIX MONTHS LATER

Six months after the unveiling ceremony, the situation between the HR department and SHP's staff had only worsened. While the marketing department had developed a whole new set of rules and regulations that accompanied the use of the new brand and the trademarked terms (Healthy Care Manager and Living with Independence), the executive team had given Jamie the job of enforcing the standards.

At first, Jamie had welcomed the chance to be in control of this area. She had thought that it would provide her with more control to mold SHP's employees and regain their trust. The employees, however, viewed the brand rules as a huge nuisance and resented the fact that they had to follow them. They felt that Jamie and her department were forcing SHP's staff to adjust to a new corporate image. They accused the HR department of eliminating the pioneering spirit of SHP by implementing a barrage of rules that accompanied the brand and the new culture.

Jamie was appalled by the situation. The employees were misinterpreting her actions. She, more than anyone else, wanted to maintain SHP's grassroots, pioneering spirit. It seemed that the only people who did not oppose her changes, however, were members of the executive team. They appeared to adjust well to the new emerging corporate culture. She finally realized that they were beginning to feel comfortable at SHP, because it was now so similar to the other HMOs they had left.

The executive team was troubled by the reactions of their employees. They did not understand why they were so against the changes. To make matters worse, the popular MessageBoard had evolved into a company therapy board. Departments used it as a medium to promote name-calling while others griped about the morale at SHP, whined about parking fees, and complained about dress codes. Even more disturbing to Jamie was that all of SHP's dirty laundry was being aired throughout the company. Instead of promoting good communication, the MessageBoard had turned into a disaster. Yet she was afraid of eliminating the MessageBoard because so many employees felt it was the only venue they could use to communicate their concerns.

LOOKING AHEAD

As Jamie turned off the television, she realized that the situation at SHP had reached a critical state. Already, she had droves of employees quitting their jobs, others were interviewing with SHP's competitors, and low employee morale was beginning to affect the quality of customer service. While the marketing department's branding campaign had been so successful at projecting a positive public image, the employees who upheld SHP's reputation were not supporting it. The way the cards had stacked up against her, Jamie knew that the executive team would blame her for the situation. Thus, Jamie would have to choose her next move very carefully. The only problem was that she didn't know which way to turn.

23

Autumn Park

Cara Thomason
Terrace Senior Living, Rancho Santa Margarita, California

Robert C. Myrtle
University of Southern California, Los Angeles

Brad Douglas, the Executive Director of Autumn Park, was so tired and frustrated as he once again looked over the resident file of Mildred Puce. Brad was preparing for the afternoon meeting with Mildred and Hannah Meeks, a registered nurse, and Director of Assisted Living of Autumn Park. Brad firmly believed in the company's principles, values, and beliefs (PVBs) on how to deal with resident issues and problems, yet everything he is doing with Mildred is going against those PVBs (see Exhibit 1).

THE HISTORY OF AUTUMN PARK

Autumn Park is one of the thirteen properties owned and managed by Abbot Retirement Communities (ARC), which owns and manages high-quality, full-service rental retirement communities nationwide, offering independent, assisted, and dementia care. ARC is passionate about enhancing the lives of seniors and is committed to delivering exemplary service with integrity, dignity, and compassion.

Statement of Principles, Values, and Beliefs

We are committed to exemplary service delivered with integrity, dignity, and compassion. Our communities for seniors are distinguished by warm, secure, and friendly environments.

We will enhance each resident's lifestyle by:
• Responding immediately to resident's needs and concerns.
• Offering high quality, creatively designed programs.
• Encouraging independence.
• Promoting a sense of community and friendship.

We the staff are committed to:
• Teamwork
• Being professional
• Open communication
• Fostering a learning environment
• Continuous improvement
• Profitability

We live by a standard of conduct that encompasses honesty, accountability, personal development, and a passion for excellence.

Exhibit 1.   These principles, values, and beliefs are referred to whenever important decisions are made at Autumn Park.

ARC is a family-owned company that was founded in 1990. The President and CEO of ARC, Anthony Abbot, was given a retirement property by his family as an investment. The original plan was to manage the property and improve its appearance and services, and then resell it for a profit. Abbot became so interested in managing the property that he decided to keep it and expand the business.

Abbot had a vision to grow ARC as a unique and enduring company dedicated to meeting the changing needs of the residents and their families. He wanted to create working environments where associates were appreciated and inspired to develop as individuals and where strengths and abilities were nurtured and rewarded. He wanted to own a company of high-quality retirement communities and services delivered with a warm and friendly feeling. He was committed to responsible growth, operational excellence, and superior financial results. He did not want the largest company in the industry; he just wanted the best.

In 1996, Abbot and his executive team wanted to develop a property from the ground up. Abbot wanted to build a high-end retirement community. The properties he had acquired previously were all middle- to upper-end properties, in appearance and price. Abbot was able to meet with the County Development Planning Department for a new city in Southern California. They found a center location for the property and bought the land. Also during this time, ARC moved their corporate office from North Carolina to Southern California.

ARC broke ground for Autumn Park in 1999, with an anticipated opening in March of 2000. Autumn Park was a community for independent and assisted living residents, with an additional neighborhood for dementia care. The goal for Autumn Park was to have no more than 40% of its residents on assisted living.

BACKGROUND OF MILDRED PUCE

In September of 1999, Mildred Puce visited the trailer that was advertising for Autumn Park while it was being built. After several visits with the marketing team about what Autumn Park could provide her, she gave her deposit in November of that year. Mildred already lived at another continuing care retirement community (CCRC), yet she was attracted to Autumn Park's centralized location; it was near shops, restaurants, churches, and grocery stores. Autumn Park offered what she had before, plus more services.

Autumn Park's marketing team was looking to fill up their new property as soon as possible. They were taking deposits and applications from anyone who was interested and seemed appropriate; but Mildred was different. Although she was already living in another CCRC, Mildred was in a motorized wheelchair, younger than 60, had multiple sclerosis, and the use of only her head and left arm. Autumn Park accepted her deposit based on the criteria that they had to have an exception letter from the state because she was under the age requirement to live in a CCRC, had special needs, and required a Vera body lift.

Due to unforeseen circumstances, Autumn Park's opening was postponed till July of 2000. In March, Autumn Park received doctor's orders that Mildred needed a Vera lift to get in and out of bed and to the toilet. The orders also indicated that she was able to operate the lift with little assistance. She also needed a motorized chair due to her disability and therefore needed a handicapped-access apartment. The Life Enrichment Assistant Coordinator of the CCRC in which she lived also wrote a letter to Autumn Park saying how wonderful a resident Mildred was and how sorry they are that she is leaving them.

In May of 2000, Autumn Park received another order from Mildred's doctor that stated Mildred could self-administer her own beta injections. The marketing department collected all of her information but did not share the information with the clinical staff to assess at that time. The physician disclosed all of her disabilities for the clinical staff to examine and consider in their assessment.

The assessment is done prior to the resident's moving in, and if the clinical staff does not feel that Autumn Park can take care of the needs of that person then the move-in is denied. The assessment is based on observation and conversation with the resident, along with a physician assessment of the resident's medications, diagnoses, disabilities, and abilities (see Exhibit 2). ARC policy states that after the initial assessment, the resident must be reassessed 30 days after the move-in date.

If the assessment indicates that the resident needs to be on assisted living, the resident is charged an additional $400 a month to go into assisted living, Level I, and another $300 for each additional level of assisted living care.

The original assessment given to Mildred, prior to her moving in, put her at a Level I for assisted living. Mildred was assessed at 10 minutes for bathing and showering, 15 minutes for grooming, and 15 minutes for assistance in transfers. Mildred also indicated in her assessment that she is fully capable of taking care of her two cats.

Autumn Park opened its doors July 1, 2000. During the first month of operation, the Executive Director resigned and the Director of Assisted Living was let go. In the interim of hiring replacements, the corporate staff brought in regional directors to fill in. By the end of August, Brad Douglas was hired as the new Executive Director of Autumn Park and Hannah Meeks was Autumn Park's new Director of Assisted Living.

Meeks reassessed Mildred at the end of August, 2 months after her move-in date, at a Level III. Mildred was taking 45 minutes of the caregivers' time for her showers, which were given three times per week. Mildred was also having the caregivers spend 20 minutes each day helping her with her oral care. It was also discovered that the caregivers were spending an extra 15–30 minutes with Mildred each time she had to use the restroom. Much of that time was spent helping her in and out of her Vera lift. It also took caregivers 20 minutes to transfer Mildred in and out of her bed, which they did once in the morning to get her out of bed and once at night to get her back into bed.

Each apartment at Autumn Park has two emergency call cords (e-cords), one in the bedroom and one in the bathroom. The e-cords are to be pulled only in case of emergencies. Once the e-cord is pulled, it shows up on a computer at the front desk, where the receptionist radios a caregiver to go to that specific room. If a resident wants a caregiver's help that is not an emergency the resident calls the front desk. After the receptionist receives that call, he or she radios a caregiver to go to that room for assistance. Since the e-calls are considered emergencies, they are put in top priority over the phone calls. It was discovered that Mildred was pulling her e-cord every 30 minutes to get the caregivers to help her with minor things, such as taking out the trash, turning on her lights, or feeding her cats.

Instructions for Level of Care Assessment

Bathing/Showering:
- 20 minutes—Resident requires daily bathing/showering due to incontinence
- 10 minutes—Requires total assistance, substantial assistance, or standby assistance during bathing/showering including help in and out, supervision/assistance with washing, shampooing, toweling, dressing, and so forth; bath/shower 3X/week; assist with dressing daily
- 5 minutes—Resident requires verbal reminders, clothes laid out, bathing items prepared, some assistance with buttons, zipper, and so forth
- 2 minutes—Resident requires minimal assistance, including reminders and follow-up
  Staff member does not need to be present during bathing and dressing
- 0 minutes—Independent

Oral Care:
- 10 minutes—Total assistance or standby assistance with and/or reminders for oral care including care of dentures, partials, and so forth
- 5 minutes—Reminder and setup only
- 2 minutes—Reminders only and follow-up check daily
- 0 minutes—Independent

Grooming: (includes hair care, shaving, and make-up application)
- 15 minutes—Total assistance or standby assistance daily
- 7 minutes—Reminders, setup, and follow-up only
- 0 minutes—Independent

Toileting/Incontinence:
- 50 minutes—Assistance and/or reminders to resident to use the bathroom every 2–3 hours; assistance with protective undergarments, assistance with removing and/or re-applying clothing; changing bed as needed
- 25 minutes—Reminders and directing only and/or frequent accidents (more than 1X/week)
- 10 minutes—Assist with cleanup of occasional accidents
- 0 minutes—Independent

Medication Management:
- 20 minutes—Total medication administration (4 plus X a day/dosing or more than 6 medications a day)
- 15 minutes—Supervision of medication administration (3X a day/dosing or 3–6 different medications a day)
- 10 minutes—Supervision of medication administration (2X a day/dosing or less than 3 medications per day)
- 5 minutes—Weekly medications set up only, or supervision of medication administration for P.R.N.s only
- 0 minutes—Independent

Mental Status/Behaviors:
- 60 minutes—Disoriented, requires 24-hour supervision and monitoring; occasional redirection

(continued)

Exhibit 2. Level of care assessment criteria at Autumn Park.

(continued)

- 30 minutes—Disoriented, frequent reminders needed, but some direction or redirection required or depression requiring constant encouragement and frequent individual socialization
- 20 minutes—Mild disorientation, occasional behavior problems, needs reminders daily or depression requiring daily encouragement
- 10 minutes—Mild disorientation, no behavior problems, follows routines or some depression requiring occasional encouragement
- 0 minutes—Independent

Transfers/Ambulation:
- 10 minutes—Always assist with transfers; pushing wheelchair to meals, activities, or standby assistance for ambulation with walker
- 5 minutes—Occasional assistance for wheelchair transport to meals, activities, or standby assistance for ambulation with walker
- 0 minutes—Independent

Other Treatments:
- Other treatments, including follow-up of therapies, dressing changes, customary care, Una boots, whirlpool treatments, application of ointments, blood sugar, frequent vital signs, or treatment. Record estimated/actual time per day to perform treatment. This includes weights or vital signs, more than once a month, daily bed change due to incontinence, and so forth.

Legend:

0–45   Minutes of care per day is   Level I

46–90   Minutes of care per day is   Level II

91–135   Minutes of care per day is   Level III

Greater than 130 minutes per day might require Alzheimer's care or nursing care. Each additional 40 minutes will be billed as an additional level.

Douglas, Autumn Park's new executive director, and Meeks also noted that Mildred was abusing her privileges with Autumn Park's scheduled transportation. Autumn Park owns a bus that is wheelchair accessible, and has a capacity for 20 people. The bus is normally used for scheduled outings and activities for the residents. Autumn Park also owns a Town Car that is used for doctor's visits and unscheduled errands. One hundred and forty residents must share these two vehicles. Although Mildred was aware of her restrictions on transportation since she could only use the bus, she still demanded that the bus take her to her doctor's visits on her schedule. She was not concerned that the bus was being used for another scheduled activity.

Mildred was constantly complaining that the caregivers don't understand her lift and don't understand English. She was continually pulling the e-cord. Once her present rent increased due to the time spent on her, she came back to Autumn Park with her attorney claiming discrimination under the Americans with Disabilities Act saying that Autumn Park only raised her rate, and no other resident's rate.

Every time Autumn Park showed her the minutes, she insisted that they were not right. She then dictated to Meeks which caregivers she wanted to care for her. Such a request was considered private duty in Autumn Park, which constituted a rate increase. Mildred once again claimed that Autumn Park was discriminating against her and threatened to sue.

In November of 2000, Meeks discovered that Autumn Park did not have any of the exception letters on Mildred's conditions to the state— injections, age, lift, and disability. Douglas and Meeks hoped that after they filed the exception letters, the state would not longer allow Mildred to live at Autumn Park. Yet, the exception letters came back approved by the state.

Also in November, Autumn Park gave Mildred a 30-day period to evaluate the minutes spent on her care. She was to keep a record and the caregivers were to keep a separate record of the minutes they spent with her. Yet, it was soon discovered that she manipulated the caregivers when to document the minutes and when to stop. Mildred denied any accusations that she manipulated the caregivers in their documentation of her care. Due to the dispute on how to record and how the minutes reflected the care, Mildred and Autumn Park redid the evaluation in January 2001.

Also, in January, a letter was sent to all residents at Autumn Park that there was a change in the price structure of assisted living. Instead of $400 for Level I, and $300 for Levels II and III. It will now be $500 for each level of care.

In March of 2001, a second evaluation of the minutes of care for Mildred was conducted. Mildred still didn't feel that the minutes documented a true reflection of the care she was given. Once again it was discovered that Mildred was manipulating the caregivers, because many came forward to talk about it with Meeks. Also, several of the caregivers wanted to quit because they no longer wanted to care for Mildred. They claimed she was verbally abusive and yelled at them. Mildred denied that she ever raised her voice to a caregiver or spoke to them in a derogatory way. She said that the caregivers must have interpreted her orders incorrectly. Also, in the span of 5 months, three caregivers were receiving workers compensation because they hurt their backs trying to care for her. Mildred still demanded only certain caregivers to care for her, and now she wanted no male caregivers giving her showers.

By this time, Douglas and Meeks were very frustrated with Mildred. They wanted her out of the property but didn't know how to dismiss her without getting sued or causing negative publicity. Douglas decided to visit the Executive Director of the CCRC Mildred lived in prior to Autumn

Park. The Executive Director agreed with Douglas about how difficult and manipulative Mildred was. She also told Brad that, "once we got her 30 day move-out notice we were jumping up and down in the halls. We wrote glowing letters about her just to make certain that Autumn Park would take her." Douglas was completely at a loss on what to do about Mildred Puce.

In May of 2001, Autumn Park talked to the ombudsman about the difficulties they were having with caring for Mildred. The demands she was putting on Autumn Park and the caregivers were causing a great deal of stress. The ombudsman agreed with Autumn Park that Mildred Puce had been a difficult resident.

In June, Mildred complained to the same ombudsman that her personal rights were being violated since Autumn Park was still allowing a male caregiver to give her a shower. The ombudsman then called state licensing agent on Autumn Park. The State Licensing Agent came out to Autumn Park and talked to Douglas and Meeks about the difficulty they had in caring for Mildred. Autumn Park provided the agent with all the information they had on Mildred including documentation of what skill level they provide for her in care and how Mildred needed more.

By this time, Mildred had developed severe edema in her legs due to poor circulation. This swelling in her legs has caused them to weigh around 50 pounds each. This increased the risk of caregivers injuring themselves when they lift one of her legs to reposition them in her wheelchair or her lift. If this edema persisted, her skin would break down, causing open, weeping wounds. If this happened, she would be immediately sent to the hospital.

Under the California state regulations, Title 22, a residential care facility for the elderly is obligated to give a resident a 30-day notice to move out if the facility feels that they can no longer provide the care a resident needs. Yet, if Autumn Park gives Mildred a 30-day notice, she will sue Autumn Park on the basis of the Americans with Disabilities Act. Mildred also threatened that she will call the local media about Autumn Park's treatment of a handicapped resident. Therefore, Douglas had made certain that he told the state licensing agent that Autumn Park can care for Mildred but not to her specifications.

Also, under these state regulations, a facility can refuse to permit a resident to return to the facility after a resident has been hospitalized, if the facility believes that they can no longer care for the resident. The regulations state that a resident in such a facility must have skilled health professionals take care of any open wound, skin tears, and/or pressure ulcers. In such cases, hospitalization may be necessary to receive such care or the facility will have an approved exception from the state that a home health nurse will care for the resident until their wound has healed.

As Douglas looked over Mildred's file, he felt that his hands were tied. Mildred needed custodial care not skilled nursing care. Yet, Mildred was a victim of her own circumstances since she could not afford the one-to-one care due to her insurance. Community Care licensing agents had even evaluated Mildred, and they all agreed that Mildred Puce was not appropriate for a CCRC and needed a different level of care.

Douglas also thought about what the ARC corporate staff told him. They stated that anything is better than negative public press about Autumn Park or ARC. "Do what it takes to provide her care; avoid a lawsuit and negative publicity at all costs."

At the meeting with Mildred, Brad will offer Mildred with three legal options: 1) to get care from another agency that meets licensing requirements, 2) to move to another facility with more skilled care, or 3) to offer 12 hours of one-to-one care that will cost Mildred $7,000 a month.

24

Hammond General Hospital

The New Contract Food Service

Raymond L. Hilgert
Washington University in St. Louis, St. Louis, Missouri

Cyril C. Ling
Illinois Wesleyan University, Bloomington, Illinois

Edwin C. Leonard, Jr.
Indiana University—Purdue University, Fort Wayne, Indiana

Hammond General Hospital is a 334-bed general hospital located in a small southwest town of approximately 45,000 people; it serves a county-wide population of approximately 140,000. The area is heavily dependent on manufacturing and supports several industries; however, there is considerable unemployment and good jobs are not readily available.

Hammond General is one of the largest employers in the city. The administrative team was fairly young and aggressive, but administration also felt a genuine obligation to provide a safe, pleasant, and positive work environment for hospital employees.

From *Cases, Incidents and Experiential Exercises in Human Resource Management, 3rd edition* by Hilgert/Ling/Leonard. © 2000. Reprinted with permission of Custom Publishing, a division of Thomson Learning: www.thomsonrights.com, Fax 800 730-2215.

THE CONTRACT FOOD SERVICE DEPARTMENT

Dave Smith came to Hammond General Hospital in October to become director of food service. Smith was an employee of Universal Hosts Company, a large, national food service corporation that had just been awarded the management contract for the department. The previous director of food service had been employed by the hospital in the same capacity for the last 28 years and had been a registered dietitian (R.D.). Prior to Smith's arrival, the hospital had always operated its own food service.

At the time, approximately 15% of all hospital food service departments in the country were contracted. Universal Hosts Company had approximately 50 such contracts, making it the fourth largest in the industry. The general procedure was for the contractor (Universal Hosts) to supply a director and an assistant director, as well as to provide support systems such as recipes, production systems, and accounting procedures. The company charged the hospital for the salaries and benefits for the management team and a negotiated fee for all other services. The director would report to the hospital's assistant administrator (John Block) as well as to the company's district manager.

When Universal Hosts Company assumed management responsibility for Hammond's food service department, the department had 58 full-time equivalent employees (FTEs). This consisted of 40 full-time employees and 25 part-time employees (see Exhibit 1 for an organization chart and Exhibit 2 for selected managerial profiles). Dave Smith and Doris Horn were the two managers employed by Universal Hosts. All others were hospital employees.

The clinical staff was headed by Chief Dietitian Cynthia Thomas, R.D. and consisted of three clinical dietitians and four diet clerks. Operations were to be headed by Universal Hosts' new assistant director, Doris Horn, R.D. Her responsibilities included food production, sanitation, patient tray lines, and the employee cafeteria. Three supervisors reported to her, one each for mornings and afternoons and one as a relief supervisor. Pat Stone, R.D., was placed in charge of all catering events and was made responsible for coordinating new projects and changes that would come with the change in management.

RESISTANCE TO THE NEW DEPARTMENT MANAGEMENT

Dave Smith described his reception at Hammond General Hospital as follows:

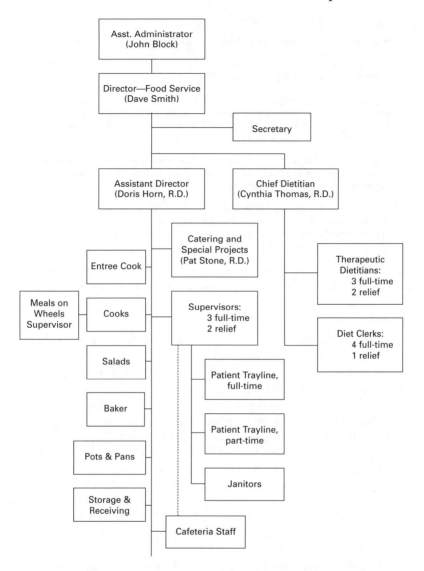

Exhibit 1. Organizational chart for Hammond General Hospital's food service department.

Prior to assuming official control of the department, I spent a week there getting to know the people and learning the current system. I immediately met resistance from the acting director, Pat Stone. Stone felt she should have been promoted and that an outside food service was not needed. She had been acting director for 6 months and prior to that had been the assistant director for 10 years. Further resistance was quickly

Dave Smith: Thirty-two years old. Held a bachelor's degree in business administration (BSBA) from an eastern state university; had been with Universal Hosts Company for almost seven years, five as an assistant director of food service at two other hospitals.

Doris Horn, R.D.: Twenty-five years old. Held a bachelor's degree in nutrition from a state university in Illinois; had been with the Universal Hosts Company for only one month but had been an administrative dietitian in another hospital for two years.

Cynthia Thomas, R.D.: Twenty-six years old. Held a bachelor's degree from a state university in Michigan; had been a clinical dietitian at Hammond for three years before becoming chief dietitian.

Pat Stone, R.D.: Fifty years old. Held a bachelor's degree from a private institution in the East; had been assistant director of food service at Hammond General for ten years; prior to that, had been an administrative dietitian in the military service.

Exhibit 2.   Managerial profiles for Hammond General Hospital's food service department.

made obvious by the entire dietitian staff, who all felt that the director should be a registered dietitian (R.D.). There was also concern among the nursing staff at the hospital that a man had taken a position that traditionally had been held by a woman.

After encountering nothing but resistance wherever I went, I made an appointment to see the assistant administrator to whom I reported at the hospital. His name is John Block, and he had been at Hammond General for only 1 month himself. In fact, his first assignment was to hire an outside contract company and then approve me as the director.

Upon hearing my problems, John smiled and said, "That's nothing; I understand the entire city is upset that a big company has taken over the food service department. The hospital's board of directors is having second thoughts, and the president of the hospital, Dan Schultz, is not comfortable with my selection of you as director."

But John Block then explained to me the reasons for contracting with Universal Hosts to run the department:

- The department was considered to be overstaffed by 10 FTEs.

- The food and supply costs were excessive in comparison with industry standards.

- Department morale was at an all-time low; the department had supported a recent unsuccessful attempt by the Teamsters to unionize all hourly employees in the hospital.

- The medical staff was unhappy with the quality of the cafeteria food.

- Overtime pay in the department was the highest in the entire hospital.

- Performance evaluations had not been taken seriously for several years.

- Ordering of food lacked systematic procedures and was not well related to dietary planning or cost estimates.

Block summed it all by saying that the department was run last year the same way it was 28 years ago. There have been no new systems, improvements, or changes in management philosophy for more than a quarter of a century.

A few days after this conversation, John Block was admitted to Hammond for emergency surgery, and he would be out for 2 months. Dave Smith was now virtually alone to succeed or fail.

INTERVIEWS WITH SUPERVISORS AND EMPLOYEES

Following his talk with Block, Dave Smith conducted a series of interviews with selected supervisors and employees. The following comments were made in these interviews.

Sally Manley, A.M. supervisor: We are supervisors in name only. We make no decisions, take no disciplinary actions, are not involved in performance appraisals, and are not involved in interviewing new hires. If we do discipline someone, it is usually overturned.

Jane Harper, P.M. supervisor: The morning shift does everything wrong. There is no procedure that we do the same as them. People that cross shifts don't know what to do. When we ask management for a decision as to what to do, they say "do whatever will work for you." Also, we have no authority to discipline, so no one pays any attention to us.

Sheila Rafferty, relief supervisor: This place is a zoo. No one knows what they're supposed to do. There is no direction and no management whatsoever. The employees do what they please, and nobody does anything about it.

Millie Park, head cook: I have been here for 20 years, and this place gets worse each year. No one in there [the office] ever comes out here. I'll bet they don't even know what's on the menu today. They order food and don't even take inventory. I'll bet there is $30,000 of outdated food in the basement. Also, no one else can cook. They pay dishwashers as much as cooks, so we have two cooks who can't even read a recipe—if we had recipes, which we don't.

Pat Baker, cook: We never have enough food to cook what is on the menu. We are always running out, and we get blamed. We can't cook what we don't have. Also, everyone else in the other departments thinks everyone in the kitchen is a stupid jerk, when they are the only stupid ones [management].

Lora Lee Butram, cafeteria cashier: We run out of food halfway through lunch. No one in the kitchen knows what is going on. Everyone in the hospital thinks everyone in this department is an idiot.

James Willson, janitor: They want us to clean the kitchen. I don't even have a good broom or a mop. Half of the time, I don't even have soap to use on the floor. How can I clean the kitchen?

Jean Allen, diet clerk: They want us to have a high school diploma plus a year of additional schooling. Yet, we don't make any more money even though we do as much as dietitians.

Ed Norton, maintenance foreman: They should close food service and have McDonald's deliver. No one in that whole department can do anything right.

Allie Crow, head nurse: The patients don't get what they ordered. The trays are late and incomplete, and the food is cold. If a patient has a problem, we can't get a dietitian to come visit them.

Noreen Watson, housekeeping supervisor: We are supposed to clean the cafeteria at night. Food service is supposed to clean it during the day. They don't. It is a mess, and no one can do anything about it.

Delphine Mason, director of human resources: I think there are a lot of good people in food service. I think they care, but they need help and a lot of it.

THE MANAGERS MEET

Several days after assuming responsibility for the food service department, Dave Smith met with his assistant director, Doris Horn. Her comments were: Let's bomb this place and go home. It's hopeless! Look what we face:

- No one wants us here.

- Our budget is unrealistic; it's based on having people that can, at least, walk and chew gum at the same time.

- Pat Stone, the previous assistant director, thinks she should be the director and hates you for taking her job.

- The chief dietitian is 100 pounds overweight (Great example, eh?), and she is afraid of her "old school" dietitians who don't want to leave their desks.

- There are no systems of any kind.

- The place is filthy.

- The whole hospital hates the department.

- The supervisors can't manage people and don't.

- Administration thinks we will have the best food service department in 1 year because our salesman said we would.

Why did I take this stupid job?

Dave Smith replied. "We will fix this department the same way you would eat an elephant, one bite at a time. Let's get'em all—managers, dietitians, and supervisors—in here and start right now."

25

Appalachian Home Health Services

Kathryn H. Dansky

Pennsylvania State University, University Park, Pennsylvania

Frances Matthews, the director of clinical services at Appalachian Home Health Services, Inc. (AHHS), was concerned. AHHS needed to hire a nurse quickly. One of the staff nurses had just handed in her resignation because her husband was being transferred out of state. The nurse who was leaving gave AHHS 2 weeks' notice, which complied with the agency policy; however, it still left the agency in a bind. Matthews knew that recruiting and interviewing home health nurses was a time-consuming process, and, even after a nurse was hired, several weeks of orientation were usually required before the nurse could perform independently. She knew that all of the regular staff nurses were working to capacity and that the loss of even one nurse would have major implications. She walked over to Kate Hennessey's office to discuss the situation. Hennessey was the director of administrative services. Matthews and Hennessey had started AHHS 4 years ago. Together, they made all final hiring decisions.

Matthews knocked on the door, saw that Hennessey was sitting at her desk, and walked in. "Sue is leaving. She sure picked a bad time to move!" She laughed halfheartedly, and said, "We need to replace her quickly. Do you have any brilliant ideas?"

From Dansky, K.H. (1991). Appalachian Home Health Services. In G.E. Stevens (Ed.), *Cases and exercises in human resource management* (5th ed., pp. 246–251). Homewood, IL: Richard D. Irwin, Inc.; used by permission of the author.

Hennessey sighed, and responded, more in the form of a statement than a question, "We don't have any decent applications on file, do we?"

"Nope."

"Great. Well, let's get our ad into the paper today, maybe something will turn up."

BACKGROUND

AHHS is a private, not-for-profit home health agency, located in a rural area of a midwestern state. The stated purpose of AHHS is to provide health care services at home to elderly individuals, persons with disabilities, and persons with short-term, specific health care needs that could be handled at home.

AHHS is a "fee-for-service" health care organization; it provides in-home services, then bills for the services, either to a public or private insurance carrier (e.g., Medicare, Medicaid, Blue Cross/Blue Shield), or to the patient directly. AHHS receives all (100%) of its revenue from billed services. As a private organization, it does not receive government subsidies or tax support.

Competition in the home health field is intense, particularly in rural areas, where the need for services fluctuates. Because services are expensive to provide, it is critical for agencies to generate a volume of visits sufficient to cover fixed expenses plus make a small profit. Competition for AHHS comes primarily from Care One, Inc., a multicounty operation that has been established in the area for well over 10 years. AHHS surpassed Care One in total number of visits after its second year of operation and has been steadily growing. Many of the physicians in the area, however, continue to use Care One, and Care One receives more referrals from nonlocal hospitals than does AHHS.

AHHS currently has 32 employees, including 15 registered nurses (full time and part time), 8 nursing aides, 1 physical therapist, 1 speech-language therapist, and 7 administrative staff. All but two employees at AHHS are female.

REFERRALS FOR SERVICE

Most of the business generated for AHHS is in the form of referrals. Hospitals (social workers, discharge planners) account for more than 70% of patient referrals; of this total, approximately 85% are from the two local hospitals and 15% are from out-of-town hospitals. The second most frequent source of referrals is the general public; former patients, potential patients, family members, clergy, and the like may request services directly. Approximately 20% of referrals come from this source. A small number of referrals come directly from physicians. Although this source is less than 10% of the total, it is important to the AHHS, because of the power and status that physicians have in the community.

PATIENTS WHO RECEIVE HOME HEALTH SERVICES

Most of the individuals who receive in-home care are elderly. They usually have a chronic illness that requires monitoring or have a need for rehabilitation therapy following an acute episode, such as a stroke or hip fracture. Some patients have disabilities and require ongoing therapy at home. Some are convalescing from a hospital stay, and need short-term care (e.g., dressing changes). Others have a special type of medical need that does not require hospitalization, such as intravenous antibiotics or chemotherapy.

Most of the patients cared for by AHHS are indigenous to the area, live in rural areas, and are religious. Although not all patients fit this description, it is fairly safe to say that the patient population is elderly, traditional, and conservative.

THE ROLE OF THE HOME HEALTH NURSE

The registered nurse is the central caregiver in the home health field. The nurse must be able to function independently and comfortably in the patient's home, and must be capable of performing a wide variety of clinical procedures (e.g., giving injections, inserting catheters, obtaining specimens). Furthermore, the R.N. is considered both a "case manager" and a "gatekeeper" in coordinating medical, health, and social services (see Table 1). This position requires high-level skills in nursing and communications. Nurses with a bachelor of science in nursing (B.S.N.) and experience in home health or community nursing are usually sought for these positions.

ANSWERS TO THE AHHS ADVERTISEMENT

After Matthews left, Hennessey asked the office manager to run off a copy of their standard classified ad for a home health nurse (see Exhibit 1) and take it to the local newspaper's office. The next day, the newspaper carried the ad in the classified section. The ad ran for 3 consecutive days.

Table 1. Job description for home health agency registered nurse

Definition

The registered nurse administers skilled nursing services to a patient in accordance with a written plan of treatment established by the patient's physician. The incumbent is directly responsible to the Nursing Supervisor and ultimately to the Director of Patient Services.

Qualifications

1.   Graduate of an approved school of professional nursing

2.   Current license to practice as a registered nurse in this state

Responsibilities

1.   Conduct initial patient assessment and evaluation

2.   Evaluate the ongoing needs of patients on a regular basis

3.   Initiate the patient's plan of treatment and any necessary revisions

4.   Provide those services that require substantial specialized nursing skills

5.   Initiate appropriate preventive and rehabilitative nursing procedures

6.   Prepare and maintain clinical notes

7.   Coordinate care with allied health professionals

8.   Inform the physician and other personnel of changes in the patient's condition

9.   Counsel the patient and family in meeting nursing and related health needs

10.   Participate in in-service and continuing education programs

11.   Supervise and teach other nursing personnel

Applicants were requested to call the office, or to send a résumé to the director of clinical services.

AHHS received two responses to the ad. One was a résumé from a student at a nearby technical college. The college had a 2-year (associate degree) registered nurse program, and the applicant was in the last quarter of her second year. Matthews read over the résumé. She knew, from past experience, that R.N.s from 2-year programs lacked many of the skills for this type of work. She decided not to interview this applicant.

The other applicant, Margaret Jenkins, called to express interest in this position; the conversation was pleasant and informal because the women knew each other. Jenkins had lived in the area all of her life, had family there, and was well known for her community activities.

Jenkins is a registered nurse, with a B.S.N. from the local university. She had most recently worked for 8 years for Dr. Edward Smith, a general practitioner in town. Prior to that time, she had worked at the state mental health center. References from both employers indicated that she was

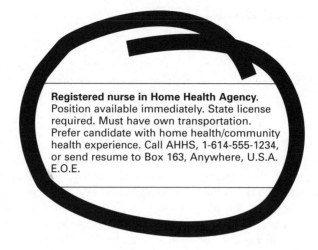

Registered nurse in Home Health Agency.
Position available immediately. State license required. Must have own transportation. Prefer candidate with home health/community health experience. Call AHHS, 1-614-555-1234, or send resume to Box 163, Anywhere, U.S.A. E.O.E.

Exhibit 1.   Sample classified ad for a home health nursing position.

hard working, responsible, and professional and got along well with patients, staff, and physicians.

Eighteen months ago, Jenkins was involved in a domestic violence situation in her home. During an argument with her husband, according to the press, Jenkins was physically attacked and the argument ended in the death of her husband. Jenkins was charged with murder. During the course of the trial, most of the details were made public. Episodes of violence had occurred previously, resulting in a separation of Jenkins and her husband, with a restraining order against the husband. Jenkins testified that on the night of the fatal argument, she was home with her two children when he appeared and threatened all three of them. While her husband was beating her, she managed to pick up a kitchen knife and kill him. The court convicted her of involuntary manslaughter and sentenced her to 10 years in prison. While she was in prison, her attorney petitioned for early release, based on her standing in the community and the fact that she was the sole support of two young children. Also during this time, several concerned friends led a successful campaign to have her nursing license reinstated. (The state board of nursing had revoked her license to practice nursing, a standard practice for convicted felons.)

Jenkins' immediate concern was finding employment. Dr. Smith, her former employer, was semi-retired and not able to rehire her. When she saw the AHHS ad in the paper, she thought it was her answer. Now that she had her license back, she could begin working immediately.

THE INTERVIEWS

Because of Jenkins' good work record and because no other suitable applicants were available, Matthews asked Jenkins to come in for an interview, and set up an appointment for that afternoon. The procedure at AHHS was for all R.N. applicants to be interviewed first by the nursing supervisor, then by the two directors, Matthews and Hennessey.

Jenkins walked in to the AHHS offices and greeted everyone warmly. A Caucasian woman of average height and weight, she appeared to be in her mid-thirties. She was on time, was dressed appropriately, and looked a little nervous. Barbara Jones, the nursing supervisor, introduced herself and led Jenkins into the conference room. A half-hour later, Jones brought Jenkins to Hennessey's office, where the second interview would take place. Jones went in first and briefly summarized her interview. Although she had a positive overall impression, she was concerned about Jenkins' lack of experience with home health procedures, particularly interviewing and assessment skills. Because this part of the job was so important to the overall plan of care, it was essential that R.N.s have experience in this area. She then left the office and Jenkins went in.

Jenkins sat down with Hennessey and Matthews. The three women discussed AHHS policies and general personnel issues, including benefits. It was clear that Jenkins had the abilities and skills needed, she knew the geographical area well, and could communicate effectively with area physicians. Her only weakness was that she did not have home health experience. Her personal life was not discussed, but she did remark at one point, "You know, I really need this job." At the end of the interview, Matthews thanked her for coming, and said, "You do meet many of the qualifications, but I'm not sure if you're the right person for this job." Jenkins smiled grimly and said, "I wouldn't blame you if you don't want to hire me." With that, she picked up her things and walked quietly from the office.

Matthews and Hennessey looked at each other. "I don't know," Hennessey said. "I don't know either!" responded Matthews. They usually based their hiring decisions on qualifications plus "intuition," and usually agreed on an applicant's suitability. This case was different, however, and neither was sure whether they should hire Margaret Jenkins.

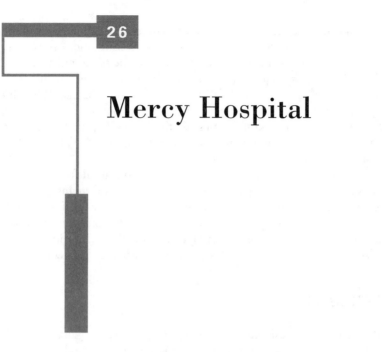

26

Mercy Hospital

Mercy Hospital is a general hospital with 300 beds. There are two larger general hospitals in the city, one of which is owned by a for-profit chain, and one smaller hospital. The investor-owned national hospital chain that operates Mercy is highly regarded in the industry for its innovative approach to hospital management. It recently undertook an advertising program highlighting the quality of its professional staff and extolling the virtues of its patient-care programs to the Bay Village community.

Two years ago, Mercy began an affiliation with the medical school of the local university. It was thought by both boards of trustees that there would be a mutual advantage from such an affiliation. For Mercy, there was prestige to be gained from a university affiliation, and some cost advantages as well. For the university, there were medical resources and a training site.

Because the residency programs are fairly new, they are still being developed and are subject to a certain amount of experimentation. Besides the residency programs, several fellows are pursuing further specialization and doing research. Most of the hospital facilities are at their disposal, and,

Adapted by permission of the publisher from WHAT MANAGERS DO, 4th edition, by William R. Allen and Harold L. Gilmore, pp. 211–228, © 1993 by the American Management Association (1-800-262-9699). All rights reserved.

in their clinical research, they are permitted to involve the patients in the hospital. Laboratory animals are also on site for various kinds of research.

The chiefs of medicine and surgery as well as the pathologist-in-chief and the radiologist have joint appointments in the hospital and the medical school. They are therefore full-time, salaried physicians. The joint appointments mean that the medical school pays part of their salaries, and, in addition to clinical responsibilities for the hospital patients, they also carry teaching responsibilities in the residency programs. The chief of medicine is also the director of medical education.

An active and varied program of in-service education for nurses has been developed during the past year and a half. Several members of the medical staff, particularly the chief of medicine and an attending cardiologist, have contributed significantly to designing and executing the program. Parts of the program use videotaped lecture–demonstrations, which have also been used for nursing education in the other hospitals in the city.

THE PROBLEM

David Chadwick, president of Mercy Hospital since January 1993, returned to his office after his summer vacation in 2002, to find on his desk a letter from Helene Swenson announcing her resignation as vice president of nursing services.

He was dismayed by the news, for he had not suspected that problems in the hospital could have caused her resignation. He had hired Swenson just over a year before, and she was only beginning to be able to deal effectively with the serious problems that had plagued nursing. In fact, he had expected that definitive and positive changes would become evident by the end of the coming year. He was sure that, at that time, nursing service would take its proper place in the total health care program.

Chadwick had known for some time that the administration of the hospital had problems that needed careful attention and probably some reorganization. It was with that in mind that he had hired a management consultant earlier that summer. As he returned to work, he was looking forward to the consultant's help, and he planned to work regularly with the consultant during the coming year.

This resignation by the vice president of nursing had an immediate effect on his priorities, and he quickly set out to deal with the crisis. Chadwick believed that he had to do everything possible to change Swenson's mind. She was too valuable an executive to lose, especially because she had already analyzed the urgent deficiencies in the nursing service. Besides, Chadwick knew that the problems must be serious if they prompted so conscientious a person as Swenson to take this drastic step.

Chadwick telephoned Swenson and asked her to come to his office, adding that he was very distressed by her resignation. He suggested an immediate conference, because he was anxious to hear why she was resigning. As Chadwick listened to Swenson's comments and complaints, he learned more about the nature of problems in the hospital. He realized that his problems were shared by the other executives and especially by his immediate subordinates. He considered most of the people to be experienced and competent; but because the work of each depended heavily on others, he thought a possible source of some of the confusion and ineffectiveness lay somewhere in the relations among the executives.

Chadwick asked Swenson to withdraw her resignation and to wait until the situation could be analyzed more carefully. He promised that in the meantime he would investigate the specific issues she had raised, discussing with the people immediately involved those issues that had led to her resignation. She made it very clear that these problems impeded her work to the point where she alone could no longer deal with them. Chadwick decided he had to mediate between Swenson and several other members of the administrative group to find workable solutions.

On a more general level, Chadwick decided to undertake, with the consultant's help, a thorough analysis of hospital organization, including various individual responsibilities. The consultant agreed with Chadwick that the understanding that might result would be very helpful in reaching a long-term solution.

Actually, this work had begun early that summer when Chadwick had hired the consultant to examine the hospital organization, including nursing services but excluding the medical staff organization. He had spent considerable time with the consultant in clarifying his own role as president. They had begun by examining his relations with the board of trustees, specifically his relations and work with the various committees of the board. Then they had examined his working relations with other executives in administration and physicians who headed the primary clinical departments.

Chadwick felt confident that he had the support of the board of directors in his efforts to modernize and upgrade the quality of care at Mercy Hospital. The board had worked closely with him in arranging the affiliation with the university. He had received superb performance evaluations and expected another at the end of the year—provided he could find a solution to the problems in the administration that seemed to be indicated by Swenson's sudden resignation.

As a result of the news of Swenson's resignation, Chadwick wanted to shift the consultant's emphasis to a close examination of the work of his subordinates and their relations with each other. As a first step in that direction, he suggested to Swenson that she and the consultant should spend as much time as necessary to pinpoint the problems she had to get the analysis under way.

THE "LEPER COLONY"

Chadwick had hired Swenson as vice president of nursing services after firing the incumbent he had inherited from his predecessor. Swenson had held a similar job in another hospital, having begun her career in nursing administration first as manager of operating rooms and later as associate vice president of nursing at a large teaching hospital in a neighboring city.

On assuming her position at Mercy Hospital, Swenson discovered that the situation in nursing service was worse than she had been led to believe. Not only was there a serious shortage of nurses, but also only a handful were competent. Worse still, she found it was nearly impossible to recruit more staff, because the hospital had the reputation of being an undesirable place to work. She had once remarked, "From the way people react to my recruiting overtures, you would have thought we were running a leper colony!"

Nursing standards were among the lowest she had ever seen. "I would be very reluctant to advise any sick person to come here as a patient, and you can appreciate what it means to me to have to say that. Except for one or two nurses and two of the managers, professional discipline and responsibility barely existed. Nurses simply disappeared off the floor for varying periods and the patients were left unattended."

There were no educational activities, so there were no attempts to introduce innovations in nursing practice and no way to inform nurses about developments in clinical nursing. There was a running feud between most of the nurses and attending physicians, and mutual hostility and mistrust with members of the house staff. In short, Swenson had found precious little that would attract new nurses to the hospital.

Daily routine included an overwhelming amount of paperwork. There were forms to be filled out for every administrative department of the hospital, from human resources to accounting. Yet, despite the time invested in filling out and submitting forms, Swenson had difficulty gaining access to even the minimal information to plan the work load and use her scarce nursing staff's time effectively. Work schedules for day, evening, and night shifts never seemed to match the demands.

Although a new system for payment had been implemented at the time she joined the hospital, Swenson had never seen it work satisfactorily. Every week there were discrepancies between the payment people received and what they thought it had been agreed they would receive.

She had, after more than a year of effort, reached a point at which she believed that some headway had been made in her own area. Still, she was far from satisfied with the help she got from her colleagues. Several serious clashes with the vice president of human resources finally precipitated her decision to resign.

In view of Chadwick's promise to try actively to solve the problems that she thought needed immediate attention, Swenson was persuaded to stay. But she cautioned, "I cannot go on doing the work that I think needs to be done around here unless something changes. I must know what I have the right to expect from Frank Samuels [the vice president of human resources] and Michael Ryan [the associate vice president], and I must have some assurance that it will be done.

"I must also know and understand what they want me to do and what they have the right to ask me to do. After all, if we all know what our jobs are and how our jobs coordinate, we all can concentrate on our own work and stop devoting our energies to working against one another and constantly having to call on Mr. Chadwick to mediate our differences."

A SERIES OF COMPLAINTS

Swenson discussed the situation in several sessions with the consultant and now and then with Chadwick. Referring to the organization chart (see Exhibit 1) she said, "I have studied it for hours trying to figure out what it means in terms of my relationship with some of these people. But it tells me very little, except that I am responsible for a certain number of units in the hospital and that Mike [Ryan] is to run such sections as admitting, central supply, and the pharmacy. We don't actually have an assistant vice president yet, although a new person is supposed to join us in a couple of weeks.

"Each time we have any problems with these activities, I can complain my head off to Michael. But as often as not, he continues to do what he wants and disregards what I tell him. Or he tells me that things are going wrong because somebody in my area is inefficient. In the end, because he clearly ignores some of the things that I tell him, I must complain to the boss. I wish I didn't have to, but I do."

Swenson admitted that if Ryan were to suggest that she alter some part of her department and she disagreed with him, she would also refuse to follow his suggestions. The only way in which the work in nursing and the work in the pharmacy, for instance, could be coordinated was for her and Michael and the chief pharmacist to go together to Chadwick. They always seemed to be able to iron things out that way.

Just recently, a disagreement had arisen about some changes in managing the pharmacy. The manner in which orders for medications were passed from hand to hand and transcribed had caused several serious errors. While physicians waited for medications to be given to a

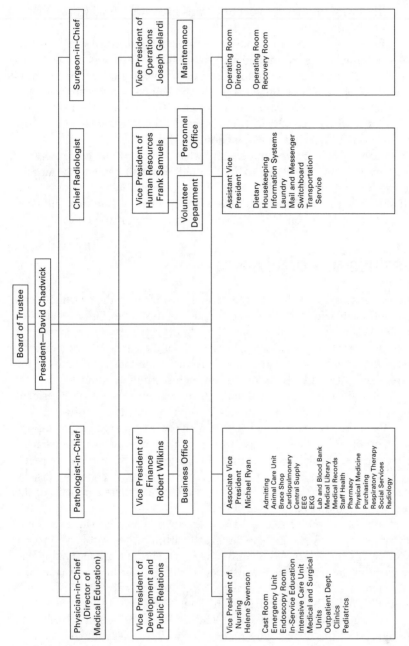

Exhibit 1. Organization chart for Mercy Hospital.

Board of Trustee

President—David Chadwick

Physician-in-Chief
(Director of
Medical Education)

Pathologist-in-Chief

Chief Radiologist

Surgeon-in-Chief

Vice President of
Development and
Public Relations

Vice President of
Finance
Robert Wilkins

Vice President of
Human Resources
Frank Samuels

Vice President of
Operations
Joseph Gelardi

Business Office

Volunteer
Department

Personnel
Office

Maintenance

Vice President of
Nursing
Helene Swenson

Cast Room
Emergency Unit
Endoscopy Room
In-Service Education
Intensive Care Unit
Medical and Surgical
Units
Outpatient Dept.
Clinics
Pediatrics

Associate Vice
President
Michael Ryan

Admitting
Animal Care Unit
Brace Shop
Cardiopulmonary
Central Supply
EEG
EKG
Lab and Blood Bank
Medical Library
Medical Records
Staff Health
Pharmacy
Physical Medicine
Purchasing
Respiratory Therapy
Social Services
Radiology

Assistant Vice
President

Dietary
Housekeeping
Information Systems
Laundry
Mail and Messenger
Switchboard
Transportation
Service

Operating Room
Director

Operating Room
Recovery Room

patient, nurses transcribed the orders onto a requisition to the pharmacy. After filling the orders, the pharmacist posted them on a daily tally sheet to produce a list showing all of the medications that had been dispensed to hospital patients. This sheet then went to the business office to be charged to the patient's bill. Besides creating errors in transcription, the method required time in nursing, pharmacy, and the business office.

Swenson and the chief pharmacist had met and worked out a simple system to avoid all this. The new method was obviously an improvement, and neither she nor the chief pharmacist could understand Ryan's objections. The doctor would henceforth write the order on a form with several copies. One copy would go to the pharmacy as a requisition, another would go directly to the business office, and the other copies would be used in the nursing station for the patients' records and as nursing instructions so that the nurses could administer the medication when it arrived from the pharmacy.

For some reason, Ryan objected. Only when Swenson and the chief pharmacist presented the plan to Chadwick and he endorsed it enthusiastically did Ryan agree to the change. "And it works beautifully!" Swenson told the consultant.

In Ryan's favor, however, she said she had gladly accepted his advice on budget procedures. Because he was well versed in how to set up departmental budgets, she had done exactly as he had told her. Ryan had to coordinate many of the day-to-day operations, including many medical aspects such as the various laboratories, radiology, the emergency unit, and the outpatient department. His suggestions for coordinating work among these medical and paramedical units and nursing were accepted by almost everyone, including the physician-in-chief and Swenson. He seemed to have a comprehensive view of the way these activities meshed. Also, because none of the individuals, such as the chief pathologist, the physician-in-chief in medicine, and Swenson, knew the details of the operations outside their own departments, it was Ryan who moved from one to the other and suggested ways of getting more efficient interaction toward the outcome, namely patient care.

"You know," said Swenson, "I don't understand the situation with Mike. When he is making suggestions to all of us, such as when the patient-care committee was trying to coordinate the work of the chemistry laboratory, the outpatient department, and my nursing people, he is straightforward and decisive. But the moment I try to work with him on some coordination problem that involves one of his departments, like admitting, pharmacy, or dietary, he seems hesitant and evasive. Even when he promises to straighten things out, like the tie-ups in getting materials out of central supply, he never seems to take the promised action."

Swenson recalled one issue that had lingered unresolved for several months. It involved the dietary department, the admitting office, and nursing. The problem was that many hours passed after a new patient was admitted before dietary supplied a meal. The nurses on the unit were upset at this delay because it prevented them from offering some small gesture of welcome and hospitality to the new patient. First the nurses complained to the dietitians, but the dietitians passed the blame to the admitting office, and the admitting office offered the explanation that the attending physicians often neglected to specify diets for their patients. Without any instructions from a physician, there was no request to dietary to supply a meal.

For weeks Swenson asked Ryan to take some action to coordinate the work of the doctors, admitting, and dietary so that these delays could be eliminated. Despite his assurances and promises, however, more time passed with nothing done. In her view, Ryan should have specified some policy to admitting and dietary that would guide them if a physician's order was not immediately available. "Certainly tea and a piece of toast couldn't hurt anyone who is not going to be anesthesized shortly. And it would be a way of saying to patients that they were being cared for and welcomed." Swenson said that most of the time the nurses themselves decided to order something from the kitchen and give it to the patients, but the head of dietary was against this kind of action, claiming that it brought risk to the hospital. She had to have doctors' orders before any food was provided to a patient. The nurses, however, had developed relationships with some of the dietary servers, who understood the problems the nurses were having and who were usually willing to allow the nurses to order something.

Regarding the outpatient department, Swenson was frankly at a loss about her responsibilities there. The manager of the department was a nurse subordinate of Swenson's, but Chadwick had said that, although Swenson was accountable for the nursing service in the outpatient department, Ryan was responsible for "everything else." Swenson's attempts to get Chadwick to clarify this statement had been unsuccessful. She had the impression that responsibility for the outpatient department moved back and forth between her and Ryan. Although it was clear that Ryan had to coordinate the role of the physicians with nursing and paramedical services, and that this involved difficult problems of scheduling, Chadwick had not made it clear to her in what way the outpatient department was different from inpatient nursing units, for which she was totally responsible.

Swenson told the consultant that, apart from these particular problems she had cited, she was really much more concerned with trying to understand what her attitude toward Ryan should be. She recognized Chadwick as her boss. It was he who decided with her what her main objectives were, and he provided the resources she needed to do her job. Furthermore, because of the importance of nursing, she knew that reestablishing efficient and effective nursing services was a primary consideration for the hospital. Therefore, within reason, she could get almost anything she wanted from Chadwick. True, the two of them sometimes differed about the priorities of means and ways of accomplishing main objectives. Sometimes he would get his way, other times she would get hers.

When it came to Ryan, however, she thought that on certain matters his advice seemed to lack authority. She accepted his ideas and believed they were generally helpful to her and to others when the issue was clearly within an area of his expertise or when it concerned the coordination of work across the various hospital departments, but she was less inclined to accept his views when one of his own departments was involved. And why did he back off and become indecisive when just the two of them tried to iron out their common difficulties? Swenson said that, when they both went to Chadwick to iron out their differences, "Mike often 'chickens out' on me when the problem involves his departments. In the presence of the boss, he just fails to state his views openly and leaves me to stick my own neck out. I guess that's his way of looking good."

THE MAKING OF THE CRISIS

As the discussion between Swenson and the consultant proceeded over several weeks, she described her relationship with the vice president of human resources, Frank Samuels, and how problems in that relationship had led to her resignation.

Samuels had joined the hospital several months after she did. At the time, she had looked forward to working closely with him. Because one of the most critical problems in nursing was human resources, or rather the lack of them, she had hoped to receive much-needed help from Samuels. "But it was my expectation that I would call the shots. I felt that I was entitled to ask for help from Frank. I didn't expect that his help would be thrust on me in accordance with his judgments of what I needed."

Very few months had passed before Samuels realized, from discussions with Swenson, that recruiting nurses was a top priority. He decided that one of his most important tasks should be a recruiting trip through the southeastern states. Samuels recommended the project to Chadwick and succeeded in convincing him that one of the senior nurse managers should accompany him on that trip.

Swenson had opposed the idea, but because she had not had time to plan her own recruiting strategy and had no alternatives to offer, Samuels was authorized to take the trip. "I felt it was absolutely wrong, but I didn't know exactly why. I wish I could have been more convincing in opposing the project, because I *knew* it would not work."

This expensive trip produced only one recruit, who turned out to be unsuitable after Swenson interviewed her and checked her references. If this had been only her opinion, she would have admitted that she might have been all too ready to turn down this find because of her opposition to the whole recruitment approach. Because she needed nurses very urgently, however, she asked one of her colleagues at a neighboring hospital to do some reference checking for her. What Swenson learned confirmed her own judgment and information.

She began to understand better the underlying reasons for her disapproval of Samuels's trip after she began getting feedback from people in her profession at the colleges and hospitals that Samuels and the manager had visited. There are certain rules to be observed when nurses are recruited. Educators in nursing and nurses themselves want to talk to members of their own profession. Samuels did not know enough about nursing services at Mercy, he did not know where the current staff had been trained, and he did not know enough about the subtleties of nurse–doctor relations in the hospital to discuss these matters. Also, the fact that he was a male recruiter in a predominantly female profession was not in his favor.

"Frank just had no idea how to deal with nurses. He also had no way of knowing what were the peculiar requirements of nursing service in this hospital. And he did not realize how bad our reputation was because he could not read between the lines of the many refusals he got. Frank could not offer any nurses the kind of inducements that might have brought them here as a challenge, because he doesn't know what might challenge today's bright young nurse. And taking an older manager along did not do our image any good. She didn't represent our group."

For a while this trip and its failures greatly annoyed Swenson, especially because her own reputation suffered from it. It took some time until the word got around why she had not done the recruiting. After his failed trip, Chadwick excluded Samuels from recruiting nurses.

Swenson told Samuels that she would welcome his contribution to devising and implementing a payment plan that would provide fair remuneration and make possible simple and easy calculations of pay for both nurses and nonnursing staff. She had hoped this would eliminate the cumbersome and error-ridden situation she had inherited.

Also, she desperately needed a way to maintain up-to-date information on nurse staffing patterns and schedules. She asked Samuels to look into her particular needs in nursing service and advise her on a scheduling system she might adopt.

At about the same time, Chadwick asked Samuels to compile an employee handbook that would describe clearly and attractively the whole range of working conditions, pay, and benefits applicable to all employees.

Swenson expected that Samuels would complete this handbook as quickly as possible, because it was essential in her recruiting program, but the deadlines passed several times. So she decided to develop a handbook for exclusive use in nursing. When it was done, however, Chadwick reprimanded her. Although he was also exasperated by Samuels's procrastination, he considered it essential that Samuels be the one who put the handbook together. After all, it would be a policy document for the whole hospital, committing the entire institution to an internally consistent and equitable system. It could not be oriented to any particular segment of the hospital's employees.

Swenson reacted with anger and frustration. She was frustrated because she had expected Samuels to meet her time targets, although she had never spelled them out. She was angry because her independent but necessary action had brought Chadwick's disapproval. So, although in the early months of working side by side in the hospital she had often sought Samuels's advice, her disappointment with his ineffectiveness in meeting her needs turned into hostility and mistrust. Increasingly, the two avoided each other.

Besides the expectation Swenson had regarding the handbook, Samuels's advice on staffing control, and a clear scheme for payment, she had other expectations of cooperation and help from Samuels that had not materialized. For instance, she asked that one of his subordinates recruit and preselect clerks, secretaries, and nurses' aides. When these tasks were not done, Samuels responded to her queries by claiming that his people had no time for them. Also, he turned down her many requisitions for staff with the explanation that they were not included in her budget.

Her feelings were aggravated by Samuels's instructions to her and to her staff. These instructions interfered with what she believed were her decisions. She cited his interference, for example, in the decisions on selection and termination made by her and several other people in the administrative group. Samuels had made a big issue out of her decision to hire a secretary whom he had fired from his department. Although she finally gave in, she did not understand his stubbornness in opposing her on this matter.

Some months before the incident with the secretary, she had decided to add to her administrative staff a personnel assistant who had worked for Samuels and whom he had fired. Swenson hoped that, with the help of a person experienced in the personnel policies and procedures of the hospital, she could overcome some of the problems of the excessive workload. Particularly when the help she wanted had not been forthcoming from Samuels, as she hoped, she decided to have her own "personnel resource person." Assuming that the dismissal by Samuels had derived largely from a personality clash, she expected that a change in bosses would have a positive effect on the young woman. Samuels raised no objection. She therefore assumed that he would not oppose her subsequent decision to hire his ex-secretary.

"I wish Frank would stop his continuous interference in our personnel procedures. On a few occasions, Frank came after us when we revised a few job descriptions of nonnursing positions and rerated these positions. After all, it is my decision to change the work of a secretary, clerk, or assistant in our nursing education program. I do so because I see the need for such a change. Once or twice the change may be the result of a recommendation one of the nursing managers or I made. What Frank fails to see is that jobs aren't a sacrosanct, fixed, unchanging series of tasks. New things have to be done all the time! And when I decide that we are going to do other things, new things, and I want them done the best way possible, I am going to assign them to the best person I have in my organization. Naturally, when I do this, that person is going to have more responsibilities. And when I see after a while that person is getting these things done well, I want to rerate the job. It simply isn't the same job. By what right does Frank tell me this job is worth $2,000 a month when I think it's worth $2,200 a month? All I did was move it up one grade. I am not violating the whole grading system that he set up. I am only using my judgment. And my judgment tells me that the way I have changed the job content means it is a higher level job!"

Samuels was continually sending back pay raises for nursing personnel that Swenson had approved. Each time the statement that the raise exceeded what was authorized by the salary schedule accompanied these rejections. If she decided on a raise of a certain size, she was not going to be told by him that it was not authorized. After all, contended Swenson, she alone was going to answer to Chadwick for the way she used resources he had put at her disposal.

The final straw came as she was in the midst of the busiest period of the interviewing season. Her staff had spent time that they did not have putting the handbook together in anticipation of applications from newly graduated nurses following an intensive recruiting campaign. The backlog of work all around was compounded by an inability to straighten out the continuous errors in the calculation of pay rates as they were returned from the human resources office. These discrepancies convinced Swenson that the procedures for payment were unclear and conflicting and that the calculations were too time consuming and subject to error.

She had to do something about this. The exasperation of her administrative staff affected her as well, and she went to Samuels and asked him once and for all to untangle this mess. His response was that no other department had difficulties with the pay rates and the calculation of individual salaries. He did not know whether there was any point in repeating his explanation for the umpteenth time. That response, along with his persistent imposition on the time of her administrative staff and managers by his demands for information about the nursing complement and other statistical information, triggered her letter of resignation.

SWENSON'S OTHER COLLEAGUES

Even taking their different personalities into account, Swenson still wondered why she had more trouble with Samuels and Ryan than with the vice president of finance, Robert Wilkins, and the vice president of operations, Joseph Gelardi. Both had always been extremely helpful.

As she increasingly avoided contact with Samuels, Swenson turned to other colleagues, particularly Wilkins. She solicited Wilkins's help for clarification of the payment system, thinking that because he issued the payroll checks, he would understand the system. Yet discrepancies persisted.

On several occasions she turned to Ryan for advice on matters that were clearly in Samuels's domain. He did not turn her down, but in trying to please her, he came into direct conflict with Samuels. Just recently, when Chadwick learned that Ryan had advised her one way while Samuels had advised her another, Chadwick severely reprimanded Ryan for making a decision that was not his to make.

Although Gelardi did not exactly perform miracles when Swenson asked him to make some complicated alterations in a nursing station, at least he completed the work within a reasonable time. Some of his suggestions were so helpful that the occasional delays in getting the big jobs done were forgiven by the nurses at the station and by Swenson herself. She expressed relief that Gelardi was at least one of two people she could rely on to get things done.

As for Wilkins, he had been very cooperative in accepting the changes in the system for requisitioning and issuing medications that she and the chief pharmacist had worked on. Wilkins also needed information from nursing service to produce the monthly reports to the administrative groups and to the board of trustees. Once he had established the frequency and format of the information he wanted from Swenson and her staff, however, the reporting became routine, and Swenson did not feel that Wilkins's demand for periodic information from nursing was an imposition. This situation, she thought, was in considerable contrast to the degree and extent to which Samuels imposed on her and her staff. She was, however, at a loss to explain the difference, except that she had the impression that the sheer quantity of information that Samuels demanded was greater. Perhaps, she conceded, it was also harder to gather because the system was unclear.

Swenson hoped that Chadwick's reassurances would bring the resolution of problems she had been battling unsuccessfully. She had reason to rely on his promise to clear up the relationship with Frank Samuels in particular. She doubted that the two of them could start from scratch, but at least they could eliminate this continuous friction. She expected that, if the irritations and obstacles in her relations with some of her colleagues could be mitigated through the concentrated communication and analysis afforded by the consultant, and if Chadwick could see himself and the organization with greater clarity, there would be clearer sailing over the next 8–10 months. By that time, she was sure, the results of her efforts to develop better services would demonstrate that her decisions had produced satisfactory results, or, as Swenson herself put it, "Mr. Chadwick can have my head."

ASSIGNMENT

After reading the case, review the situation of the various executives and managers at Mercy Hospital as they attempt to identify reasons for dissatisfaction with their relationships and performance. Place yourself in the role of an external consultant to the president, and prepare a report in the form of a memorandum to the top management of Mercy Hospital. Clearly indicate what you believe are planning problems, assess present organization and staffing decisions, analyze the leadership styles demonstrated, assess the existing control systems, and suggest areas that need improvement.

27

Watergate Nursing Home

Donna Lind Infeld
The George Washington University, Washington, D.C.

Dorothy J. Moon

BACKGROUND

Watergate Nursing Home is a 178-bed private, not-for-profit nursing facility (NF), located in Washington, D.C. Watergate is owned by a not-for-profit corporation, which is headquartered in New York City. It owns and operates 10 other units throughout the northeastern United States, but Watergate is the only one in Washington, a large minority market. It is the second largest facility owned by the system and the only one with more than 50% (51%) public pay residents. The company purchased Watergate 5 years ago, and the operation has been running smoothly since. Recent information, however, suggests there may be trouble.

Watergate has historically had very low employee turnover. This is especially true for the management staff. All but two department heads started when the company took over more than 5 years ago. The administrator, Mr. Merrian, is well liked and personally oversees every detail of the operation. The corporate regional supervisor, who had been Mr. Jones until Ms. North replaced him 2 months ago, visits the facility monthly. Merrian and his staff quietly wish for the old days. North has a reputation

---

as being very modern in her management ideas, whereas things have typically been traditional at Watergate. North has notified the management staff that she will be visiting them for 2 weeks beginning next Tuesday. The idea does not please the staff. Even though they have heard that North is nice, anybody from corporate staff is an outsider, a bother, and someone who gets in the way.

North arrived on schedule. In the weekly department head meeting, North reassured the staff that her visit is her usual way of getting to know the facilities she supervises. She also informed them that she does not want to interrupt their day-to-day activities. She asked each to set aside at least 2 hours at their convenience to meet with her. She asked that they send their department manuals to the conference room, which will be her temporary office. She promised to provide constructive feedback and to have a closing meeting to discuss her findings. During the 2 weeks North used document review, interviews, and observation to collect data. Some of her findings are described in the following sections.

THE ADMINISTRATOR

Merrian started with the corporation more than 5 years ago when Watergate was purchased. He is 48 years old, has a bachelor's degree in business administration, and is very active in the American College of Health Care Administrators. Previously he had been the director of personnel for another NF. He completed an administrator-in-training program at that facility and received his license to practice nursing home administration. He had worked as an assistant administrator for 2 years prior to starting at Watergate. Everyone likes Merrian. He has a good sense of humor; he is very personable with the staff, residents, and family members; and he seems to believe in providing good quality care. His one weakness is his difficulty with confrontation. He does not want to hurt anyone's feelings and, therefore, avoids situations that might have this effect.

While reviewing the organization chart in the administrative manual, North noticed that it had a position designated for an assistant administrator (see Exhibit 1). She did not, however, remember such a position in the budget. Neither had there been any mention of needing or recruiting for such a position. The way the organization currently functions, all department heads report to Merrian in a hierarchical arrangement. Perhaps this explains why Merrian is so rushed. He is clearly a hard worker and is at Watergate from early morning until late evening. He maintained an open-door policy to residents and their families, so they frequently dropped in during the early evening.

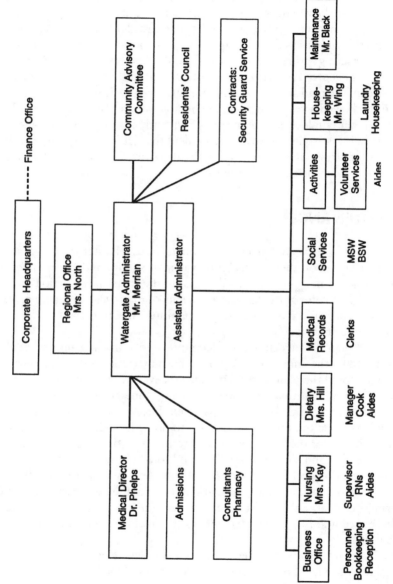

Exhibit 1. Organization chart for Watergate Nursing Home.

DIETARY

Ms. Hill, the dietary supervisor, reported no problems in her department. Nonetheless, her budget showed a sudden rise in raw food cost. The department had been over budget for the past 2 months. When questioned, she said it was due to frequently running out of food. She claimed she is ordering proper amounts and could not explain the shortages. Shortages occurred primarily on weekends, but Hill denied there was any change in weekend staffing or other unusual events. Employee attendance records showed a recent increase in absenteeism and lateness. North also noticed that employees were meeting frequently in small groups when no supervisor was around. Merrian is confident that Hill will handle the problem. After all, she had been running the department well for 5 years. She had always had the answer in the past.

MAINTENANCE

North visited the maintenance department next. Maintenance was cited for deficiencies on the last health department survey, and she wanted to know how the new procedures submitted in the "plan of correction" were working. Problems at the last survey included no preventive maintenance schedule, staff failure to attend safety committee meetings, and an out-of-date maintenance manual.

The plan of correction included a preventive maintenance schedule developed by the engineer at corporate headquarters. The health department accepted the plan, and Watergate was expecting a follow-up survey. North determined that work was not being done according to the new schedule. When Mr. Black, the department head, was questioned, he said he did not have the time or manpower to do it. He felt no ownership or responsibility for the schedule. He was committed to taking care of emergency repairs and the daily small "fix-it" jobs. He had to supervise the employees, do special skilled jobs, and complete the paperwork. He did the paperwork last, if at all. North also noticed that he was very impatient during her visit, and that yesterday he had missed another safety committee meeting. Black was interrupted with an electrical problem early in the visit.

In the middle of their meeting, Black was called away to lead the fire brigade. A fire had broken out on the third floor! North hoped it was not serious, but she welcomed the opportunity to see the fire plan in operation. She joined Black as he responded. The third floor staff had already begun executing the fire plan when Black, Merrian, North, and the rest of the fire brigade arrived. When the fire department arrived, things were progressing according to the plan. The fire department took control and extinguished the fire, which was contained in one patient room.

There were no injuries and little damage to the area. Residents and staff remained calm. The fire chief commended everyone involved for their quick and appropriate responses. Investigation showed that a resident discarding a lighted match in the trash basket in his room caused the fire. This was hard to explain because policy requires close supervision of all smoking. North made a mental note to see how Merrian reviewed this incident.

NURSING

The nursing department appeared to be running smoothly. Survey reports had been good, staff morale was high, and care was of high quality. When asked how she would improve the department, Ms. Kay answered, "Better relations are needed between doctors and nurses." Because doctors are required by regulation to visit patients only every 60 days, it is difficult to maintain their commitment. The nurses had become very discouraged because many doctors were not actively interested in their patients' care. The last time Dr. Cutler came to visit Ms. Jacobson, for example, the nurses on duty were in a meeting. He did not bother to look for them to explain why he was changing her treatment regimen. Kay has met with Dr. Phelps, the medical director, several times about this problem, but it persists. As medical director, Phelps was responsible for the quality of the facility's medical care, and he was the personal physician for those residents who do not have their own doctor. He can try to encourage other physicians to be more active in the home, but coming to visit is a big demand on a physician who may have only one patient in Watergate. Nurses were becoming frustrated and Kay worried it would cause burnout. In preparing for the last survey, nurses did a great deal of extra work bringing physicians' orders up to date. Some traveled to doctors' offices to get their signatures. Merrian was aware of the problem, and he, too, had met with Phelps. Kay had complete confidence that Merrian was dealing with the problem.

HOUSEKEEPING

North moved on to the housekeeping department, where the director, Mr. Wing, welcomed her. He is very proud of his department and wanted North to know there were no problems. When asked why absenteeism was so low but turnover was the highest of all departments, Mr. Wing was quick to answer proudly, "When they are sick and cannot come to work I

don't tolerate it. I don't take any of those doctors' notes for an excuse."
When asked what Merrian thought about this, Wing replied that he had
never discussed it with him.

"Mr. Merrian is so busy, I do not bother him with little things like
this. After all, he is the best boss I have ever had. He does not bother me,
as long as things are clean around here and I don't spend more than my
budget. That is all he asks. I understand him and he understands me. I
don't like anybody looking over my shoulder. You know what I mean? Mr.
Merrian hires good department heads, and he lets us do our job. We love
him around here. That is why this facility is so good."

As North talked to employees in the department, she sensed a great
deal of tension and dissatisfaction; they were doing their jobs only because
they felt threatened. One worker described working for Wing as being like
slavery. They said they had tried to talk to Merrian, but he would not talk
to employees without their department head present.

RESIDENTS

The daughter of a long-time resident interrupted one of the meetings
between Merrian and North. She demanded to know what had happened
to the television set missing from her mother's room. Merrian had no explanation, but he was sure that Ms. Green, charge nurse on the floor, could
straighten it out. Green was called and reported that, when she returned
from her weekend off, she noticed the television was not there, but she
thought a family member had taken it. It did not occur to her that it had
been stolen, and she did not make a report. Merrian promised the daughter there would be a full investigation. He reminded her that residents and
families brought property in at their own risk, but he was confident the set
would be found. After all, there had been no mention of any unusual occurrences in the weekend security report. Just to double check, Merrian
planned to call the guard service to make sure its report was complete.

In the most recent "level of care report," North noticed that several
residents were being considered for reclassification to a lower level of care.
This would result in their discharge because Watergate is not licensed to
provide housing for independently functioning older persons. It would be
desirable and very effective if the facility could provide living units for
older people who did not need nursing services. The facility could provide
residents of independent living units with primary health care on a fee-for-
service basis. This would provide continuity of care as well as additional
revenue.

As North went through the facility, she sensed a happy feeling among
the residents. The environment was pleasant, there were many activities to

keep them busy, and there were few complaints. The facility had a good reputation in the community. There has been a long waiting list in the past, but it began shrinking last year.

The volunteer coordinator has had no trouble recruiting community volunteers, and there were active, sincere volunteers at almost all resident events. Just this morning North overheard one of the residents, Ms. Hass, telling a volunteer about a large amount of money missing from her room. The volunteer was very sympathetic because she knew Ms. Hass before she moved to Watergate. They both belong to the large Lutheran church two blocks away. Many of the volunteers also belong to that church. Hass was quite forgetful, and sometimes confused, but until now she had managed her own funds. She received a large monthly retirement check and could have had the amount of money she claimed. North thought it best to have the social worker follow up on the conversation.

PLANNING

Several months ago, Merrian was asked to submit a 5-year strategic plan that was to include expanding existing services. Corporate headquarters has not yet received it. North was responsible for discussing this matter with Merrian. North noticed an apartment building for sale two blocks from Watergate. This might be the opportunity the company was looking for because it could meet the needs for independent residents. She wondered if Merrian had begun his strategic plan or knew anything about the building. This would be the topic of their next meeting.

Other department visits were uneventful; the departments were running well. North met with all department heads and reported the results of her survey. She spent several hours privately with Merrian. As a result of this meeting Merrian developed short-, medium-, and long-range plans. Finally, North prepared a report for the corporation.

CONCLUSION

North knew that her work was cut out for her in bringing Watergate up to corporate standards. Because Medicare and Medicaid have initiated a survey process that pays primary attention to patient care issues, dining areas and eating assistance, and medication distribution (drug passes), she was particularly concerned about Watergate's adequacy in these areas. She knew that, as a new corporate regional supervisor, she must build a good relationship with all managers and produce smoothly operating facilities with minimal deficiencies. She believed she must show progress within 6 months.

Despite her specific concerns, North noted that the home maintained good relationships with family members and had relatively happy residents. This could be a result of the personalities involved, and she wanted to be sure that the changes resulting from her recommendations did not disrupt this essential quality of the Watergate Nursing Home.

28

Suburban Health Center

Bruce D. Evans
University of Dallas, Irving, Texas

George S. Cooley
Long Green Associates, Inc., Long Green, Maryland

The situation gave Helen Lawson good reason to pause. She had been supervisor of Metro City Health Department's Suburban Health Center for only 2 months and reflected that things had been going well. Yet, Lawson had one problem that, unfortunately, threatened to overshadow all of the good things, and she was not sure how to avoid trouble.

Dr. Morgan had just left her office, and he had merely added fuel to the fire. He was the staff doctor for a state-funded health project. He had come to plead that Dorothy Wilson be fired. Wilson, it seems, was the problem. As one of Lawson's staff nurses and one of only three in the office with a bachelor's degree in nursing, Wilson had been with the Suburban Center for 3 years. When Lawson was first hired, she had planned to rely heavily on Wilson, but so far she had not been able to do so.

Lawson knew, of course, that she did not have the authority to dismiss Wilson, because they were all municipal employees. She had had trouble convincing Morgan of this. He had been adamant. He had tried previously to have Wilson discharged because his people were unable to work with her. His staff had said her attitude conveyed that they were intruding in her domain and that she resented them. Wilson's actions did appear to reflect this attitude.

Morgan had related several incidents indicating that Wilson was a very weak communicator and that both her resentment and inability to communicate resulted in almost no coordination. Because coordination in community health services is very important, Morgan believed it was essential to replace Wilson with someone more mature who could work effectively with the state agency. Lawson had listened. Although reiterating the limitations of her authority, she promised to look into it further.

Appointments and lunch gave Lawson a brief respite from Morgan's comments. On her return, however, she felt compelled to carry through on her promise quickly. The first step was to review Wilson's personnel file carefully. To do so, Lawson called for her clerk to bring in the file. In passing she said, "Billie, why don't you go to lunch now. Ms. Wilson will be here to cover the phones." Billie replied excitedly, "Oh no, Ms. Lawson! I'll just wait for the others to get back. Wilson can't handle them. I can never make out messages that she leaves after answering."

With the exchange ended, Lawson turned to the file. She had glanced casually at all the personnel files previously, but she had not looked thoroughly to see what they might reveal. Wilson's job application reflected that she had held eight assorted jobs in the 6 years preceding her application for this job. Lawson wondered what caused these job changes.

Pertaining to her education, Wilson's file reflected that her degree had been earned only after course work from five colleges and universities. Also, her excessive tardiness had delayed her attaining full employment status. Finally, her most recent performance report had been downgraded to "satisfactory" from her previous "excellent" ratings.

Armed with this, Lawson decided to meet with Lila Moran, the previous supervisor who had left to take a part-time position closer to her home. At her office, Moran added further information. "I confess I wasn't able to handle Wilson," she said. "I was afraid of her and did not want to confront her. After all, she is really a big woman and can be intimidating. Certainly her ratings were inflated, but I only did so to avoid trouble. Ms. Wilson's work—especially her reports—was often substandard. She often refused to do things, but the others covered for her in the office, so I let it go."

WILSON'S BEHAVIOR

The past 2 days' input weighed heavily on Lawson. Throughout all her subsequent findings, she recognized that Wilson's performance was continually unsatisfactory. As a result, Lawson felt compelled to begin and maintain a file on Wilson's performance. Despite incidents that had been related to her, Lawson found no specific deviations committed to writing. The depth of the problem was highlighted by the fact that it took less than 2 weeks to accumulate several memos in Lawson's file. Wilson's less-than-satisfactory performance, it seems, was hardly a rare occurrence.

One thing Lawson noted again and again was that Wilson consistently failed to leave word with anyone when she left the office. Not only did she fail to sign out, but also she failed to even mention where she was going or when she would return. This happened even at peak workload times when the entire staff was needed. Wilson seemed oblivious to these needs and went about tasks that could as easily have been scheduled for slower periods.

Lawson also noticed that Wilson always took 2 hours for lunch on Fridays. The staff jokingly seemed to know what she was doing and had covered for her often. Although Lawson did not object to occasional long lunch hours, the regularity and seeming secrecy bothered her.

In one specific incident, Wilson was gone for more than an hour one afternoon. When she returned, Lawson asked where she had been. "I went to get gas," she said. "I only use this one brand, and there is no station on my way home." Lawson asked her why she could not go out of her way after work. Rather than answering, Wilson appeared hurt and just stared away. Reacting to an awkward situation, she went off to sulk and was moody for the rest of the day.

Lawson next reviewed Wilson's time sheets and written reports. All employees were required to account for how their time was spent and report on the families for whom they were responsible. These reports resulted from periodic visits to the families' homes. Lawson noted that Wilson's sheet reflected consistently longer transportation and visit times than did those of the other staff nurses. Furthermore, Wilson's reports were poorly organized and provided scant information to justify the time spent. The reports did not reflect why she made the visit, what problems if any were noted, and what actions she planned to take to correct them. Rather, she gave a hazy narrative paragraph to show the visit was made.

When Lawson asked her about this, Wilson again seemed hurt, but she also indicated in a rather hostile manner that many of these problems were not her fault. "My district is the most spread out. I also find many families not at home. That's why my transportation time is higher. I can't help that." She also laid much blame on the coordinating agencies. "It's often the agencies' fault. They don't coordinate properly. I can't do it all myself." She said further that she often failed to get proper and adequate information because someone else slipped up.

LAWSON'S PROBLEM

Lawson considered this information for a few days and decided to discuss the situation with Betsy Graham—her immediate superior at the health department—in the hope that she could provide some useful guidance. Graham began by saying, "Yes, I was aware that Moran was having a personnel problem at Suburban, but it never officially got up to me, so I took no action. My main contact with Wilson came when Moran decided to leave. Wilson was senior there, and could have taken over your supervisory position, but she expressed no interest in it. She apparently had no desire to move up or accept more responsibility. The job remained essentially vacant until you arrived. Everyone pretty much looked after themselves."

Graham was unable to give Lawson any more first-hand information, nor did she seem to have any concrete advice for Lawson. Lawson puzzled over the facts as she drove back to the office. She realized there was sufficient information before her to solve the problem, but what she had not been able to do was put it together properly to come to the right conclusion. As she reached the office, she tried to sort out the issues, identify the causes of the problem, and decide what to do.